The Eco Anti-Diet

Plus Confessions

by

The Barbi Twins

Bloomington, IN  Milton Keynes, UK

authorHOUSE™

AuthorHouse™
1663 Liberty Drive, Suite 200
Bloomington, IN 47403
www.authorhouse.com
Phone: 1-800-839-8640

AuthorHouse™ UK Ltd.
500 Avebury Boulevard
Central Milton Keynes, MK9 2BE
www.authorhouse.co.uk
Phone: 08001974150

First published by AuthorHouse 4/24/2006

ISBN: 1-4259-2722-X (sc)

Library of Congress Control Number: 2006903470

Printed in the United States of America
Bloomington, Indiana

This book is printed on acid-free paper.

Photo Image Consultant: Daniel DiCriscio

DEDICATION

To Cozy the cat, a Katrina victim, who won the lotto by going to Best Friends.

CONTENTS

INTRODUCTION:
WE LOST MORE THAN MOST PEOPLE
WEIGH!

How did we lose our weight and keep it off?
How did we recover from bulimia?

Hi, I'm Sia, I'm a recovering DIETER. My twin sister, Shane, is also a DIET survivor. Formally known as *the Barbi Twins*, we had our seven and a half minutes each of fame. Some claim we brought in the "cheap" look. We couldn't care less, as long as we looked THIN! Between my sister and me, we lost 100 pounds, over and over, no joke! Who better to talk about doing every diet known to mankind (and a few that were meant for pets), than my sister and me? We were known as the "Calorically Challenged Clones." We were so out of control, grocery clerks had to weigh us going in and out of the stores. Our photo shoots went from our being *model-thin* to "Oh my God . . . you're fired!" It took us awhile, but we finally figured out that DIETS DON'T WORK! Some of the titles in this book are a parody of other diet books, because diets don't work! There are many diet books being marketed, but obesity and body obsession are two of the fastest-growing epidemics. We learned that most books sell gimmicks and shortcuts in a "one-size-fits-all" package, which always backfires. Because of this, we are getting fatter as a nation. Diets are about deprivation, always excluding a certain food group. We are not meant to starve, nor eat the same things day after day. Continual diet failures lead to our depression and low self-worth, defining ourselves by our weight-loss struggle. This eventually creates obsessive behavior, which has leaked into every part of our life. Sound familiar?

My sister and I, like many people, have experienced every type of diet dilemma. We were always asked *"How did you lose weight?"* or *"How did you recover from bulimia?"* This led us to seek a simple way to share our *keys to success and clues for our recovery* with others. We participated in all the research pertaining to every type of diet, statistic, information, and weight-loss program mentioned in this book. We accumulated all our research and made a formula to help find a solution for weight and diet issues:

Research = Formula = Solution

In order for us to accomplish any goals, we needed "tools." Tools are *instruments* which help us achieve our goal. My formula is divided into two separate categories, Physical Tools and Mental Tools. The Physical Tools are *tools* which help us achieve our physical goals — health = weight loss, fitness, etc. The Mental Tools help us achieve our mental goals; learning to commit, confront, and making our life manageable = freedom from obsession.

Physical Tools:

      21 Questions (which help determine your health and future)
+   Lifestyle Quiz *(and supplement guide)*
+   Body Type Quiz *(and exercise guide)*
=   *Food plan* (specially designed for each individual per situation)

Mental Tools: Find out "what's eating you" or "what you are eating over"

      7 simple motivational techniques which help you learn …
+   How to learn to commit, confront and replace "triggers" (food and situations)
=   **FREEDOM** from the obsession over food and body image

I named my food plans "The Eco Anti-Diets." Eco Anti-Diet food plans are ecologically friendly (mostly raw, live food without animal meat). They are also different from other diets because they are specially designed for each individual, taking into account their circumstances. This means, unlike a diet (a one-size-fits-all), the Eco Anti-Diet food plan can change daily, according to your situation and preference. Eco Anti-Diets are not rigid, but act more like guidelines. I include guiltless allowed/disallowed treats, so no one feels deprived. This helps lift any food addiction. It also allows people to "wean" themselves off of sugar and heavy meat. The Eco Anti-Diet strategy prevents sabotaging your food plan. Eco Anti-Diets are also an anti-aging formula. I used my twin for diet, health, and fitness experiments. We concluded from our research that everybody responds differently. This book also *combines* the *Physical* and *Mental Tools,* because it's NOT about the weight and diet. That is "symptom chasing." If symptom chasing were that simple, you wouldn't continually buy into diets which are proven to fail. We know this firsthand.

We've come a long way. At one time, our goal was to own a donut shop. We graduated to searching for a "cure" for FAT. We came to a point of surrendering all diets and the obsession that went with them. We would like to confess our downfalls and reach out to our fellow sufferers. Our recovery is based on sharing our simple methods to help others with their diet dilemmas. I wrote this book without a ghost writer, using my sister as my "guinea pig" and my muse. (She finishes all my sentences.) <u>Anyone</u> can achieve their goal with the simple formula we created. Our motto is "What builds a cell, builds health." We stress that **HEALTH** should be the goal, then fitness and beauty (or weight loss) will be the by-product! That's how we did it!

Please understand that this book is basically an "interview" with my twin. The information, surveys, polls, and statistics included in this book are clinical studies gathered from my observation of my twin (deja vu) and our friends. Other information and research came from the compilation of books, articles, and lectures that we have collectively learned throughout our years, and from the trials and errors that we have actually lived. Scientific experiments are normally tested on twins, so we had that advantage. We are not doctors and we do not pretend to be. We present information in a "fellowship format" by sharing our experience, strength, and hope, and it is in no way is meant to replace or supersede actual doctor's advice. We insist on you consulting your physician or health care provider with anything pertaining to diet, fitness, or medical issues.

In view of the complex, individual, and specific nature of health and fitness problems, this book, is not intended to substitute for professional medical advice. We, the authors, and publishers, expressly disclaim any responsibility for any liability, loss, or risk, personal or otherwise, which is incurred as a consequence, directly or indirectly, of the use and application of any of the contents of this book.

CHAPTER 1:
<u>DANGER</u>: WIDE LOAD AHEAD!

"Bait and Switch" fads used for the FAT EPIDEMIC hitting America!

My sister's idea of diet "research" was reading fortune cookies and astrology charts. What a bimbo.

Wow, we live in such a dichotomy! First, we foolishly believe that there is ONE diet or diet-aid, which will be the "magic bullet" for all of us, all of the time. Obviously, one size does not fit all, believe me. (I've tried to "squeeze" into all of them!) We are a nation that buys into the "billion-dollar diet business" (usually recycled and renamed diets), over and over, while most Americans are gaining weight. It's as if the diet conglomerates pulled a bait and switch on us. Think about this contradiction: We pay billions of dollars to maintain a diet-image nation, while we keep getting fatter! These two growing epidemics, *diet–image obsession* and *obesity* (let alone other diet-related diseases), are growing at such an alarming rate that by the time you read these statistics here, they will have reached shockingly new heights. I have observed:

- ☞ There are at least 1 billion adults worldwide who are considered overweight.
- ☞ There are 300 million of this 1 billion who are considered clinically obese.
- ☞ 70% of Americans are overweight and over 40% are obese.
- ☞ Most Americans are gaining about a pound or two per year, the equivalent of a mere 10 or 20 calories per day.
- ☞ While the average American is gaining 1-2 pounds per year, the obese American is gaining 3 or more pounds per year.
- ☞ Over half of our nation's population is heading towards obesity, and it's not slowing down.
- ☞ More than a quarter of the population is obese.
- ☞ Approximately 59 million people are classified as obese.
- ☞ Medicare reported that the average person costs approximately $6,700 a year, while the obese person costs approximately $13,000 a year.

☞ 22 million worldwide children under the age of five are overweight or obese.

☞ Our children's obesity has tripled since 1980.

☞ Obesity is rising as the #1 health problem with American children

☞ Our children are appearing with many adult diseases related to poor diet, never seen before this time or in other countries.

☞ Type II diabetes, brought on by obesity, was once an "adult" disease, but now kids as young as 10 suffer from diabetes.

☞ It is now predicted that, unlike any other time in history, many children will not outlive their parents because of weight-related diseases.

☞ The number of overweight children ages 6-11 doubled from 1980 to 2000, and tripled with children ages 12-17.

☞ Most children diagnosed as ADHD (hyperactive) or ADD (attention deficit disorder) are unnecessarily medicated, rather than changing their diet. When raw fruits and vegetables replaced the sugar in their diets, most of these kids no longer showed signs of hyperactivity or ADD.

☞ Eating disorders affect at least 10 million women and 1 million men in the U.S.

☞ Eating disorders with men are rising, but at a lower estimated rate because they are more embarrassed to "come out."

☞ More than 3/4 of teenage girls are on some diet or are worried about their weight.

☞ Preteens are starting to worry about their weight and diet.

☞ Children as young as 5 years old have been a patient of an eating disorder clinic.

☞ Victims of eating disorders are at higher risk of death than any other mental illness.

☞ 15% of eating disorder victims die as a result of their disorder.

☞ Women in their forties and fifties are now showing signs of bulimia and anorexia.

☞ Binge eating is now affecting women in their forties.

☞ 70% of Americans 55-74 years old are overweight or obese.

☞ At least 1/3 of women who are in some weight-loss clinic or program are unknowingly binge eaters. * 89% of women have been on some sort of diet during their lives.

☞ More than 3/4 of female athletes show signs of an eating or body disorder.

☞ Osteoporosis is a growing disease, not because of the lack of calcium, but the excess of dieting and exercising of most American women.

☞ The U.S. has more fat-free diet snacks, low-carb diets, other fad diets, gyms, and fancy fat farms, etc. than any other country, and yet we are have the highest disease rate related to weight.

☞ Our food is rejected by other countries because it's loaded with addictive additives, which enhances weight problems.

☞ Other countries, such as France, have about a quarter of America's obesity problem.

☞ Most of the causes of death are related to weight or diet problems.

☞ 1 out of 2 women die from weight- or diet-related problems in the U.S.

☞ 95% of most number-one selling books, shows, fashion tabloids, magazines, etc. are related to diets or how someone looks.

☞ The average height and weight for a supermodel is 5'10", 110 pounds.

☞ The average height and weight for a normal American female is 5'4", 164 pounds.

☞ Yet most women compare themselves to this image that only represents about 2% of Americans.

☞ Most women either torture their minds, thinking they should be this thin, or they torture their bodies, trying to get that thin.

☞ We are spending over a billion dollars a year to buy into the diet rage, while we are getting fatter.

☞ When televisions were introduced to other remote areas or countries, eating disorders rose as well.

☞ It's obvious that we are getting fatter as a nation when airlines are reported to raise their fees because customers, as a whole, are getting fatter, which uses more fuel!

What does this tell us? That we are a nation ready and willing to buy any gimmick, at any cost, and yet it's obvious that diets don't work! In fact, we are getting worse. We live in a paradox; our restaurants serve oversized meals, the media constantly advertises fast foods, and our schools sell junk food, while diets are constantly being promoted. It's true the media and oversized servings can perpetuate the problem; however, we shouldn't blame them when it's all about supply and demand. We are the ones (customer/audience) who do the requesting and buying. Nonetheless, our constant focus (obsession) is on diets and thin celebrities. We just keep gaining more weight, no matter how many diets we buy into.

I've observed that we all repeat the same fixes, gimmicks, fads, etc., over and over, and yet we expect different results. Ever hear the saying, "Insanity is repeating the same action over and over, and expecting a different result"? This is the exact pattern that we all seem to use with weight and health issues! Billions of dollars are invested in promoting different ways of making you think that there is one certain diet or one shortcut. This was glaringly apparent during our recent university lectures. The audiences were totally uninterested in the diet research and warnings.

They just wanted to hear about the "magic bullet" for losing weight. How did we lose weight? What did we use? We could have made a mint by selling any gimmick diet. But it was more important to share our recovery from diet obsession, at no cost. Diets simply made us fat and then "fat efficient" (effortlessly saving fat). We binged after each diet fad we endured (a.k.a. "Calorically Challenged Clones"). So, it wasn't surprising that our bodies became so fat-efficient that it didn't take long for us to be right back where we started. This made us move our food and diet obsession into bulimia. Just like diets, bulimia stopped working.

Finally, we found the "magic bullet" — *educating* ourselves and collecting that information to make formulas targeting our weight problems and diet issues. As soon as that made sense, we made **health the goal** (making the body work for us rather than *working* for our body), and let **the way we looked (our weight) be the by-product**! Ironically, it wasn't a battle anymore. Unfortunately, most people want a quick remedy without research. They buy the popular short cut fix, thinking it's "an easier, softer way," when it's all been done previously and *failed*. That is why it is so important to do research. My sister and I made it easy for the reader to help determine their own food plan and motivational and recovery exercises by the personal questionnaire and quizzes. This easy format is divided in such a way that any body type can use one of the given choices. We want to bust the myths and excuses for weight problems and inspire the hopeless. Our excuses were bad affirmations which told us why we didn't want to be healthy. But we can tell you from our experience that for every excuse, there is a reason why you CAN achieve your top health and fitness goal. And we will help you. Excuses are like farts; we all smell them, but no one admits to them.

Genetics or metabolism are the usual excuses for diet and fitness issues. Genes are also very controversial when discussing health and weight. As twins, it was easier for us to see how genetics play a major role in health, fitness, or diets. We believe genetics only become a dominating factor when health is not a priority. Let's take a look at two different people. Let's say one individual has excellent genetic characteristics, and other has poor genetic characteristics. Moreover, the person with good genes also has an excellent metabolism, excellent health, good insulin response, and is not prone to any diseases. On the other hand, the person with poor genes fights family diseases and hereditary traits that the other doesn't. If they both share the same health habits, which they are in control of, then the one with excellent genes will prevail with superior health and fitness. However, if the one with poor genes chooses a radically extreme health and recovery regimen over the one with good genes (who applies regular health habits), the one with poor genes will prevail with better health and fitness, nine times out of ten. *You are what you eat if you eat correctly, but if you eat poorly, you become your genes.* I know this from being a twin and experimenting with each other. Metabolism and poor genes (or other medical problems) have always been the *scapegoat* for most weight and health problems. On the contrary, I believe TRADITION is the dominating culprit. Tradition is used as a euphemism for your habits that you learned growing up and incorporated into your adult lifestyle. What you apply to your health is more powerful than what you were given. Don't make the mistake of thinking your habits and traditions dictate your life. Believe it or not, we only use less than 10 percent of our brain consciously (discipline), while the other 90 percent awaits our *habits*. I have seen people with cancer or other debilitating diseases rise above the rest because of their extreme discipline and health choices.

A lot of successful athletes have had to overcome some form of handicap or misfortune before they could even be up to par. Eventually, their extreme discipline, focus, and right health choices put them ahead of the normal athlete. Lance Armstrong is a good example, along with some other super-athletes.

Poor diet and weight problems CAUSE almost all medical conditions, rather than the other way around. Some complain that their breathing problems, cramping, back problems, thyroid problems, urinary infections, and so forth, prevent them from exercising or eating right. They never seem to connect their poor health habits to their declining health problems. Furthermore, all their excess medications cause edema, hunger, and insomnia. People addicted to over-the-counter remedies or prescription drugs are the ones who want to buy a quick fix, without learning about their body or why they have these problems. It is almost impossible to help someone with medical problems if they continue to symptom chase. Some instances might be justifiable, but what I have learned is that we are a nation addicted to "medicating" ourselves for every ailment. We use this same mentality (symptom chasing) for our weight problems.

I have discovered individuals who have cured chronic and fatal diseases by diet alone. If you participate in research, as I did, you can find methods other than overmedicating yourself. These other alternative methods for recovery prove to be extremely successful. I'm in no way suggesting you forsake your doctor's advice; you should always consult with your doctor or find one who will work with you.

For Shane and me, our research went beyond what doctors normally study. Doctors study pathology (the behavior of a disease), not health. Shane and I studied at health institutions that had patients who had given up on doctors, or vice versa. This is where they believe doctors cure disease A by creating disease B. They also believe that *you become your genes if you don't incorporate good health habits*. It's true we initially wanted to find the "cure" for FAT, but rather we learned the truth about health. These patients at the institutions were given a grim prognosis by doctors but found recovery in alternative health and radical diet regimens. By sharing these experiences, we want to give people hope that there are other *options* to thoroughly research. We have also observed a lot of chronically ill patients who did away with their drugs (carefully monitored by some doctor or supervisor), and targeted their health problems with radical and extreme diet alternatives.

For every medical excuse I've heard (why they gain weight or can't exercise), I've heard the same number of success stories. These success stories broke all the conventional medical rules by simply applying extreme health and diet alternatives without drugs or surgery. It's as if doctors give out "form letter" advice, always prescribing drugs and/or surgery for every problem, regardless. My sister's and my entire health problems were due to our diet abuse. So why symptom chase? We knew we could correct poor health by reversing our health habits. If a diet can make you sick, then it can also help you get well.

Most people "set themselves up" by placing themselves around people, places, and things that invite or encourage their poor eating habits. There is a saying that "environment is stronger than willpower." Your health and well-being should be a priority. You shouldn't make yourself fit into your environment. You should consciously surround yourself with a health-friendly ambience. Create one, if you can. Too many times, mothers shamelessly use the excuse of keeping junk food snacks around for their kids. Why would any mother want to teach her kids to eat poorly? Eating habits are learned behavior. Of course, fast food is convenient for the person on the go. But so are "nature's snacks," fruit, nuts, seeds, etc. It's a matter of priority, and health should be first. Then there is the "holiday excuse." Perhaps someone is "forced" to eat their family's pasta because it's a family tradition. Your family's tradition may also result in the same health and weight problems for you. Ironic how we conveniently become modern, rather than traditional, when it comes to dating, goals, careers, and styles. But we can't insult our family by refraining from fattening family buffets. Yes, there are excuses if you want them. Nevertheless, there are alternative solutions for each of them, too, if you want to explore or experiment with them.

Genetics, medical conditions, traditions, and environmental influences can all be major factors with weight and diet issues, if you ALLOW them to rule your life. The mind is a powerful tool that can rule your life or be ruled by your life. We simply must know that it's possible to reverse the myth that we are dictated by genes, medical conditions, traditions, and environmental influences. After all, if people have used such destructive behaviors as their "survival mechanisms," then it's not impossible to *disassemble* the destructive patterns by replacing them with healthy methods of recovery. You can begin your lifestyle change with this book.

In order to accomplish any goal, you need *tools*. Tools are instruments which help you achieve your goals. My sister and I want to share our self-help plan (formula) to give a solution for others who also have weight issues and eating disorders. This self-help plan (formula) is divided into two categories, Physical Tools & Mental Tools.

Physical Tools:

    21 Questions (which help determine your health and future)

+   Lifestyle Quiz (and supplement guide)

    <u>Body Type Quiz (and exercise guide)</u>

=   *Food Plan* (specially designed for each individual per situation)

Mental Tools:

    (find out what you are eating over)

+   7 motivational techniques which help you learn....

+   How to learn to commit, confront, and replace "triggers" <u>(food/situations)</u>

=   Freedom from the obsession over your food and body image

People would always ask my sister and me, *"How did you lose weight?"* or *"How did you recover from bulimia?"* This book is sharing our simple <u>keys to success and clues to our recovery</u>. Keep in mind that your goal should be *HEALTH,* not weight loss. The by-product of *health* **IS** beauty and fitness (weight loss). Physical and Mental Tools need to work synergistically, in order to work. These tools can change according to you and your circumstances. For instance, I would not have the same tools as my sister, Shane, nor would I keep the same tools that I had in the beginning of my recovery. That is why one diet for everyone doesn't work. One size does not fit all! My food plans are different than diets (which deprive and symptom chase), because your daily diet should vary according to your body type, activity, health, and preference. No one should share the same diet with someone else, nor eat the same thing every day.

Remember, the food addict is in the habit of using food emotionally, as an escape or to medicate themselves. This book teaches how to reach those feelings without food, but also how to use the correct foods to chemically balance the body, without deprivation. I will also show which trigger foods to avoid. They can be replaced with something just as fulfilling, but won't cause compulsive overeating. In addition, I will show how other foods can actually help our hormonal balance and metabolism, giving us fulfillment, energy, sanity, and motivation.

Diets don't work, period! If they did, our nation wouldn't be getting fatter and diet books/aids wouldn't be bestsellers. We are not meant to be deprived or overweight. Something is wrong if we feel deprived while constantly battling weight. Chapter 5, Mental Tools, helps you deal with your feelings and commit to your food plan. Incidentally, you are a *food addict* if you've had a constant or long-term struggle with weight, food, or body image. I would no more try to help an alcoholic (when intoxicated) deal with their issues than try to aid a food addict with theirs, if they still insist on "practicing" their destructive eating habits. Thus, if you have reached this far into this book, you have realized that a continuous problem with weight or obsession with food/body is not about being thin or needing to be "in control." (Weight/body obsession is just the symptom of the real problem.) It's about making a life-changing experience, so your life (weight, sanity, etc) becomes manageable. My sister and I *finally* got it…. so can you!

CHAPTER 2:
POPULAR DIETS – "ONE BLONDE'S MEAT IS ANOTHER BLONDE'S POISON"

Want to know my no-fail diet trick? I would put perfume on my food, so I wouldn't retrieve it out of the trash. Brilliant!

The term "diet" is defined as: "foods eaten sparingly; following a regimen or a pattern of eating usually used for weight loss or medical reasons." Diets come in all shapes and forms. So do we. There should never be one diet for everyone. One size does not fit all! It's unfortunate that the word *diet* sells without any merit or research. Today, the term *diet* is a euphemism for quick- fix or gimmick. While I was researching the most popular diets, all the librarians and bookstore clerks had the same remark, "None of them work, or they wouldn't keep coming back." Protein diets are on their way out, as they have been numerous other times in diet history. The same diets have been around for years. They are just renamed and repackaged to look like a new rage. Simply put, they are *recycled failures in the disguise of a current event*. With so many brilliant people in the world, wouldn't you think a solution for weight loss would have been found by now? People don't like the simple truth. Ironically, people would rather BUY a simple fix.

Most popular diets use some type of medical theory or generalization, which doesn't work. For example, I may have the same blood type as my twin sister, but we reacted differently to the same diet. That was the great thing about being a twin.... "twin experiments!" My body reacted differently, at different times to the same diet, according to my health and circumstances. Diets that are dictated by blood types, for instance, don't work or hold true all the time. Another example of this would be when I suffered adrenal exhaustion from over-exercising, and my body had a surplus of insulin with a high set point. A *set point* is where your weight maintains at a certain level, no matter what your diet or exercise routine is. I was too tired to starve or eat meat-protein meals. There wasn't ANY diet that would work for me. When I suffered from pernicious anemia, my body could only digest plant energy and natural nutrients, which was contrary to what doctors often advised (meat and iron supplements).

Diet is another term for deprivation, depletion, and depression. Diets exclude certain food groups or types of foods, which deprive your body and deplete needed nutrients. Eventually, as I have found, this leads to depression as well. Foods work synergistically with our hormones and brain chemicals. Serotonin (neurotransmitter — calms), epinephrine (adrenaline), and endorphins (hormone — pain/emotions) are all compromised when you diet, which takes a toll on our bodies mentally and physically. Omitting necessary nutrients causes the body to overcompensate for their absence. Subsequently, the imbalance or absence of hormones and brain chemicals leaves you tired, weak, depressed, and many times, sick. The body becomes enervated (drained nerves). No wonder people despise dieting or end up sabotaging them! Popular diets are always compared to good old-fashioned balanced eating. The popular diets usually result in quick and temporary weight loss, while normal healthy eating habits give a better long-term effect. It's a known fact that every time you diet, you train your body to lower its metabolism and become "fat efficient" (effortlessly clinging to fat). When you diet, you starve yourself physically and mentally. Whether you have a weight problem or not, when you finish or "blow" your diet, you will gain back all the lost weight and at <u>least five pounds more</u>. Does everyone think they are the exception to this rule? Obviously....YES!

In this book, I place all diets in these five basic categories. I will go over the pros and cons of each type of diet in each category. Below the various diet definitions, I also listed today's popular diets, which may be included in each specific category.

The five diet categories are:
1. Protein or low-carbohydrate diets
2. High-carbohydrate diets
3. Calorie or fat gram count diets
   (including Glycemic Index)
4. Gimmick diets (including *all-you-can-eat* diets)
5. Deprivation diets (including fasting, food replacements, and cleansing diets)

<u>PROTEIN or LOW-CARB DIETS</u>

Protein diets, as I've mentioned, are on their way out. Why? Because they are a "temporary gimmick" which won't last, and sometimes doesn't work at all, as with my sister Shane. Many celebrities endorse them, and restaurants and grocery stores are catering to the low-carb craze. Protein is one of the four basic nutrients. Protein is essential for growth and development. It provides energy and is important in the manufacturing of hormones, antibodies, enzymes, and tissues. Complete proteins contain all the essential amino acids (the building blocks of all proteins). This doesn't mean that we can't receive proper or complete protein without animal protein. Soy products, beans, and grains contain protein, and are a "complete protein." (For example, combinations of grains with legumes.) Although fifty to sixty grams of protein is usually recommended, our nation eats far too much. I have found that most of us can survive very well with a mere twenty grams of protein every other day.

Protein diet gurus claim too much insulin is the cause of weight gain. Insulin is the hormone produced in the pancreas, which regulates glucose levels in the blood, and the lack of which causes diabetes. The appeal of protein diets is the "all-you-can-eat" feature of this particular food plan. The large amount of fat calories makes you feel full and satiated. Protein diets advise the dieter to omit or limit carbohydrates (the fuel). This forces the body to break down fat for fuel. This fat breakdown continues no matter how many calories you consume (theoretically), as long as it's not carbohydrates. Protein diet gurus also claim that carbohydrates, unlike protein, cause insulin spills which stop the fat-burning/muscle-building process. More recently, revised protein diets (which included low-carbohydrate content), claim the protein and fat block the insulin spill caused by carbs. They would exclude certain carbs (or extra carbs), that caused higher insulin spills. *Low-carbohydrate* is the term frequently used for anything with seven grams or less of carbohydrate per serving or twenty-one grams or less per day.

Apparently, high-protein diets are based on the premise that if you eat a big carbohydrate-packed meal and do not use those future glucose calories as fuel, the pancreas secretes an excess of insulin. This drives the glucose too quickly into the cells. When those glucose stores are filled to capacity, the liver breaks down the extra energy molecules and handily stores them as fat. The fat cells can store unlimited amounts of fat. However, I have found the body stores ALL incoming excess calories as fat. This includes extra calories from protein and dietary fat. So why avoid carbs in moderate, digestible portions? Most people lose weight, at first, with protein diets because when they start their diet, it's usually after a binge. The excess weight loss is usually water weight as well. Initial dieters usually eat considerably less, protein or not, than they did before their protein diet. Protein diets leave the pancreas *dormant,* causing an insulin overflow when the protein dieter returns to any normal amount of carbs, causing a bloated, lethargic feeling and ongoing hunger.

Protein diet gurus also claim you can accumulate enough energy from protein without needing carbohydrates for fuel. Carbohydrates, unlike protein, need insulin to break down into fuel. The protein diet gives you a false sense of weight loss (water weight) because it has a diuretic effect. A baby is made up of 75 percent water. A man is made up of 50-70 percent water. Water helps the skin's elasticity, but we lose it as we age. You can imagine what the protein diet does to the skin and the aging process. It also gives you a false stimulant effect, which makes you think you have energy immediately preceding a meal. Nitrogen-based proteins (animal protein, particularly meat) do not have any (or very little) carbohydrate content. This forces the body into an unnatural state of ketosis (the act of burning fat, rapidly, without burning glucose), thus creating fatigue, coated tongue (halitosis—bad breath) and severe water loss. Drinking water is vital with protein diets, but add lemon for the natural sodium. This will prevent you from losing your electrolytes (helps dehydration).

During protein diets, the kidneys are overworking because of the diuretic effect it creates, which later may cause severe kidney damage. Protein diets also have been known to create headaches, nausea, constipation, and muscle cramping, due to the loss of electrolytes. Liquid protein diets have been proven unsuccessful, both with weight and health issues. Dieters who've endured long liquid protein diets have been reported to have severe kidney damage, sluggish metabolisms, and always regain their weight, plus more.

High-protein diets also result in high intake of cholesterol, since they are usually high in animal fat. When your liver and digestive system are working overtime, it enhances the dizzy or lightheaded feeling you receive while dieting. Body builders consume high quantities of protein to help their muscles grow. This is a fallacy because protein cannot be stored. Incidentally, exercise, not egg whites, makes you grow. Bigger does NOT mean stronger or being a better athlete. On the contrary, mega-protein consumption results in bulk, which actually creates a sluggish athlete. Lean muscle creates a more efficient athlete. When I'm scouting for the best horse, I don't look for a bigger horse. I look for good conformation, a horse with long and lean muscle tissue, which permits the horse to perform better. An athlete should never consume more protein (in grams) than half of his body weight in pounds.

Normally, this is how the body works: If the blood delivers more glucose (the body's main source of fuel from breaking down the foods we eat) than the body needs, the hormone insulin signals the liver and muscles to take up the surplus. Then it is stored as future fuel or is converted into fat. Exercise can also utilize the surplus. You don't have to sacrifice carbs, you just need to limit the amount, watch for the quality, and exercise.

The popular protein or low-carb diets are including healthier tips and then renaming them. Some include "magical" nuts, such as the macadamia nut, and emphasize Mediterranean fats, such as olive oil and Omega 3. The essential fatty acid (Omega 3) can be found in salmon, flax, and nuts such as walnuts. These are good hints, but you don't need to eat a protein diet in order to include these healthy choices. These recent protein/low-carb diets usually constrict carbohydrates to 30 to 40 grams a days.

When I suffered pernicious anemia, the doctor gave me the usual instructions: eat meat and take iron. Anemia can be a symptom of a vitamin C deficiency, not just iron, folic acid, and B12. As I said, plant proteins and chlorophyll were the only foods my exhausted body could absorb. When my adrenal glands were exhausted from too much exercise, protein diets made my body acidic. This complicated the health problems I already endured. Protein diets never worked for me because my body recognized saturated fats as sugar, causing an insulin over-secretion. The body is sophisticated enough to learn every trick and then compensate for it.

Most people eat a diet made for carnivores, which we are not. Our bodies have a harder time digesting meat protein. The hydrochloric acid used for digesting meat is unnatural for the body. This digestive aid has to eventually be manufactured by our body. Our intestines are longer than carnivores. Meat meals can take up to ten hours of digestion, while other plant proteins only take a few hours. This leaves the body open for diseases while the meat ferments in the intestines (acidosis), struggling to digest. This accumulation of toxins promotes parasite infestation and chronic diseases. Furthermore, our cattle and poultry are raised with the use of antibiotics and other chemicals. Animal protein, particularly red meat, contains phosphates (as in sodas), which leeches calcium. Calcium deficiency is the root of all diseases. Meat is connected to most health problems.

Fish is poorly regulated and inspected. Our polluted waters are contaminating our fish supply. There has also been recent concern over high mercury levels in such commonly eaten fish as herring, swordfish, tuna, and mackerel. "Chunk light" tuna has the lowest mercury levels of the bunch. You should avoid these fish when pregnant. Salmon is highly rated because it is known as an anti-inflammatory food which contains large amounts of Omega 3, the essential fatty acid. "Farm-raised" salmon (and other fish) is rated poorly, because of the pollutants or antibiotics. The best fish to buy is wild fish. People don't realize most fish is dyed, like farm-raised salmon. It's recommended that you eat no more than nine to twelve ounces of fish per week (two to three servings). Shellfish are filter feeders and considered fairly dirty. Food poisoning is common with shellfish, particularly poorly cooked or undercooked. Fish oils should be taken in careful amounts because they are usually loaded with concentrated amounts of toxins. Fish oils go rancid easily, as well, causing free radicals.

Protein diets, as a whole, overwork your kidneys, liver, and other organs, further escalating the aging process. Heavy-protein meals leave the body's pH very acidic, which creates the body's environment, inviting diseases to smolder. Acidosis makes the body more susceptible to diseases and causes leeching from your reserves and bones, which can cause arthritis. Meat is high in phosphates, which leeches essential calcium but can cause unnatural growth. Women who overload on meat and dairy protein are more prone to having a Caesarian-section childbirth. Dairy is a known contributor to congestion, arthritis, asthma, candidiasis, allergies, and odor problems. The saturated fat from animal products interrupts or increases the estrogen balance in women, which continues female problems, edema, and weight difficulties.

From a positive standpoint, it is better to choose a protein food, rather than a sugar/junk food. That doesn't necessarily mean meat. There are healthier choices. Incidentally, all protein is not the same. Liver may have more vitamins and minerals than other foods, but it is also the filter for the animal's body, which contain all the toxins, hormones, and chemicals they were exposed to. Your body struggles to excrete those toxins, which in turn depletes your own nutrients. Protein powders are overrated when it comes to delivering the amount of protein needed. Regardless of their content, protein powders do not give the same effect as non-fragmented protein itself. Whey is the best choice of all the protein powders. The bottom line is, if high-protein diets worked, why have they gone in and out of style continuously throughout diet history, while we have been getting fatter? You decide.

Popular protein or low-carb diets may include: *Hampton Diet, Eat to Win, South Beach Diet, Dr. Atkins Diet, The Zone, Scarsdale Diet* and *Stillman Diet.*

HIGH-CARBOHYDRATE DIETS

Carbohydrates, like proteins, are one of the four basic nutrients (water, protein, carbohydrates and fat). They are found in almost every plant food, such as fruits, vegetables, grains, and legumes. Some dairy products (e.g. milk) contain a considerable amount of carbohydrates. There are two groups of carbohydrates: simple and complex.

Simple carbohydrates (simple sugars) include fructose (fruit sugar), sucrose (table sugar) and lactose (milk sugar), etc. Complex carbohydrates are also made of sugar, however, the molecular structures contain complex chains that are longer. These carbohydrates include fiber and starches such as vegetables, whole grains, legumes, etc. The main purpose of carbohydrates is to fuel both the body's cells and the brain. Though fiber cannot be digested, the carbs convert into glucose. This glucose (fuel) is either used for energy or stored in the liver (reserves). Consuming too many carbs will result in storing fat as reserves. The fiber and sugar content has the most effect on our blood sugar. Fiber actually slows down the secretion of insulin. Therefore, the more fiber, the better the glucose delivery. Animal protein doesn't contain any carbohydrate content, except some dairy. On the other hand, many carbohydrate foods contain some protein, such as avocados, nuts, seeds, and beans. Some sea greens contain all food groups without including any harmful chemicals. This is why, in my opinion, carbohydrates are a better food choice than meat and other animal proteins.

Carbohydrate diets are unfairly compared to protein diets. Most people consume sugars and refined carbohydrates rather than whole grains, fresh vegetables, and fruits. Refined carbohydrates in excess act like sugar because they are almost completely starch. Theses refined carbs enter the bloodstream rapidly, causing an excess of insulin to balance the rise in blood sugar. In turn, the excess insulin causes the blood sugar to drop, creating an unending hunger and the same cravings—namely for sweets. Unlike refined carbs, whole grains contain bran (the outer layer) and germ (the internal embryo), antioxidants, fiber, and photochemicals. These all help fight disease, particularly diabetes II and cancer. The fiber in whole grains helps slow down insulin secretion. Whole grains contain 10-15 percent protein. The FDA claims that "diets rich in whole-grain foods and other plant foods low in total fat, saturated fat and cholesterol, may help reduce the risk of heart disease and certain cancers." People who eat live fruit and vegetables with whole grains are healthier and live longer. Whole grains are usually considered low-glycemic. (There is a slow rise in blood sugar and insulin release.) Whole oats and barley are a good choice, especially because they create a slower insulin response. Other healthy whole grains that are usually overlooked are millet, spelt, sorghum, grano, amaranth, and farro.

The best-rated diets for health are the high-carbohydrate diets. High-carbohydrate diets are the opposite of protein diets. They tend to be lower in fat and protein. Frequently recommended by nutritionists, they are often moderate and well-balanced, incorporating all the food groups. These highly rated carb diets are high in whole grains, fresh fruits and vegetables, legumes, EFA oils or fats that promote HDL (good fats). They are also very low in protein and usually eliminate animal protein such as meat. These diets are proven to fight cancer, high cholesterol, aging, diabetes, arthritis, memory loss, and high blood pressure. When high-carbohydrate diets are compared to protein diets for weight loss, high carbohydrate diets sustain better long-term weight loss.

Carbohydrates, however, hold nine times more water than protein or fat grams. Although this is healthier for the skin and bodily function, it can also give the impression that the water-weight is fat. Eventually, the body adjusts to the appropriate water balance and weight. Incidentally, when muscle replaces fat, one might experience temporary water retention. That is why I never recommend weighing yourself while your body is trying to adjust.

Simply put, eating too much of anything causes weight gain and fat storage. Just because dieters may choose a no-fat diet does not mean it is free of calories. On the contrary, fat makes you feel full. Subsequently, dieters consume more calories on a no-fat diet than they would eating a moderate amount of good fat. Fat can also be used to block insulin the way protein does. Good fats (monounsaturated fats or essentially fatty acids) can actually speed up the thermogenesis (body-heat metabolism) of the body.

The classic Food Guide Pyramid is usually the gold-standard curriculum in nutritional schools and uses a high-carb food program. It recommends that most of your daily calories should come from complex carbohydrates (grains, legumes, and cereals) rather than from proteins (dairy, poultry, meat) and even less should come from fats (oils, butter, sweets). The recent chart emphasizes good fats (Omega 3), fresh fruit, and vegetables with whole grains. Obviously this is much healthier than its previous recommendation, but too many breads and grains cause an acidic reaction in the body. This may lead to joint pain or arthritis. Certain breads, cereals, and fat-free snacks may be low in fat and calories, but they are not low in their glycemic index content (the relative potency of carbohydrates and their propensity to raise and stabilize blood sugar). That means such foods as rice cakes or carrots can be low in calories and fat, but their glycemic index ranking is extremely high, causing an over-secretion of insulin. I believe most of your complex carbohydrates should be obtained through *live* foods, such as fruits, vegetables, nuts, and avocados. Live/raw-food dieters don't have to worry about calories, fat grams, or glycemic index rating because the foods are clean, pure, easily assimilated, and easily digestible. This leaves your system more energetic and clean in order to heal, detox, and burn fat. Although I prefer a high-carb diet to a low-carb diet, it is the quality and quantity of the carbs that dictates how efficiently the diet works.

Popular high-carbohydrate diets may include: *The Mediterranean Diet, Macrobiotics, The THE FOOD GUIDE PYRAMID, The Pritikin Diet, Durhan Diet, and Longevity Diet.*

CALORIE OR FAT-GRAM-COUNTING DIETS (and GLYCEMIC INDEX)

It seems every diet, including most protein diets, count calories. I considered myself a "calorie connoisseur." I would simply scan any food item like a grocery store register and be able to guess the exact calorie amount. The average person consumes about 1,800 to 3,000 calories a day. The average weight loss diet recommends about 1,000 to 1,200 calories per day. The average calorie count to maintain your weight is about 1,800 to 2,000 per day. It is usually recommended for men to average no more than 2,600 calories per day and women should have no more than 2,000 calories per day. The quality of the calorie (where it comes from), is more important than the quantity. Calorie intake should vary and depend on your body type, activities, health, and circumstances. A calorie is not a calorie. A laboratory calorie is not the same as a digested calorie. Different foods stimulate certain hormones. Hormones, not calories, dictate your body's health and weight. An empty calorie food may trigger your insulin or estrogen, causing hypoglycemia or edema. This makes weight loss more difficult. A calorie is defined as a unit of energy equal to the energy needed to raise the temperature of one kilogram of water one degree Celsius. This is a fine definition for a Petri dish, but not for your body. Because your body is dictated by hormones, you can experience a different reaction to the same food at different times. Here's another example: take a one-hundred-calorie apple and compare it to a one-hundred-calorie chocolate candy. They have the same calorie content, but they will react differently because of the different qualities of the calories. The chocolate candy triggers your endorphins, which act like a drug (hormone pain relief and "high"). The unnatural sugar in the candy can also cause an insulin and estrogen overflow. The lack of fiber makes the candy a high-glycemic food as well. Nature put a natural insulin filter in the fiber of the apple. Apple is a better choice although it may be the same calorie content.

Too many calories cause weight gain. It's best to compare calories relatively. You have to consider not only the quality of the calorie but your own circumstances as well. If you were eating over 3,000 calories a day, it would be ridiculous to initiate a diet of 1,200 calories to lose weight. This can cause a shock to your body. It's best to gradually lower calories. You can achieve the same amount of weight loss by eliminating just a few hundred calories per day. Some athletes do well with a lot of calories. Sedentary individuals complain they gain weight eating 1,200 calories or less. Calorie counting can be misleading and turn into an obsession in and of itself. If you consume too few calories, you lower your metabolism and cause your body to sacrifice vital tissue because it's incapable of finding your reserves (glucose/fat). The body learns to save the fat for future "famines," creating a fat-efficient body. Eating too few calories can also enervate the body, which leaves no energy to burn calories. Too many calories causes weight gain and digestion problems, leading to further health complications. Instead of counting calories, choose better energy sources.

Any diet less than 1,200 calories per day is almost guaranteed to be unbalanced and nutrient-deficient. Anything from 300-800 calories per day is classified as a VERY-low calorie diet, which is asking for trouble. This can also cause the body to enter into *ketosis*. Ketosis is the body using fat without the help of carbohydrates. Ketones are the residue of ketosis. They are unwanted and abnormal cellular biochemicals, which are made only when the body does not have available fuel sources, namely carbohydrates. Ketosis makes dramatic and quick weight loss possible, but it is temporary, due to the lack of cellular water. This is a dangerous state for your body because ketosis causes excessive urination. This contributes to additional dehydration, a feeling of lightheadedness, halitosis, and nausea. Ketosis during pregnancy causes mental retardation in infants. Throughout the years, I've been told low-calorie diets can slow down the aging process.

With the right foods, low-calorie diets have been known to help cancer patients and those with other chronic diseases.

Counting fat grams is more ridiculous than counting calories. Fat is a nutrient that we need to survive. Fat performs many functions in our bodies. Once again, it's not the quantity but the quality of the fat you consume that is important. Trans-fatty acids and saturated fats are known as unhealthy and have little or no advantages. Monounsaturated fats and polyunsaturated fats (especially essential fatty acids) are healthy and necessary for cells to function. Certain fats are essential for thermogenesis in the body (body-heat metabolism). All fats stimulate, trigger, or manufacture our brain chemicals and hormones. Hormones dictate our bodies. These hormones are responsible for all bodily functions, including weight gain or loss. Eicosanoids (mini hormones that dictate all bodily action), are directly effected by the fats in our foods. EFAs (essential fatty acids, especially Omega 3) are the building blocks of eicosanoids. Therefore, the types of fats we eat are more important than the amount of fat grams. There are many high-fat foods that are very good for you, such as avocados, seeds, and nuts. The fats in these foods can lower or even replace your "bad" LDL fat. Obviously, if nature put fat into natural foods, then we are meant to consume it. Whether it's calories or fat grams, too much of anything causes weight gain and health problems. On a live, raw diet I am able to eat a large amount of calories and fat grams because of the nature of the food: pure and easily digested. This leaves the body full of energy and free to burn fat and calories. There are also diets that promote fat intake, basically excluding all the other food groups. These all-you-can-eat fat diets work the same way as the protein diets, by excluding carbs and depending on ketosis. These high-fat diets are obviously dangerous and depleting, and they rarely work in the long term, if at all.

A glycemic index chart (the relative potency of carbohydrates and their propensity to raise or stabilize blood sugar) would be a better chart reference to use instead of a calorie and fat-gram chart. Simply put, the glycemic response reflects how fast and how high your blood sugar rises after eating a certain food and how quickly the body responds by bringing the blood sugar level back to normal. Most people can quickly readjust without worrying about glycemic response. However, some chronic dieters and most of the obese population usually have abnormal carbohydrate metabolism (improper insulin response). That's when it's advisable to be careful or avoid some high-glycemic foods such as corn, carrots, peas, and potatoes. Unlike calorie and fat-gram counting, the glycemic index is reflected by the way certain foods react synergistically with our own hormones. The problem with this glycemic index chart is the poor comparison made between what's acceptable and unacceptable. Their charts will rate some junk foods, such as ice cream, as acceptable (low-glycemic) and yet rate carrots, for instance, as unacceptable just because they are a high-glycemic food. I think it's important to realize which foods are high-glycemic in order to carefully monitor your insulin, however, I don't think you should exclude healthy foods. Unlike ice cream, high-glycemic fruits and vegetables contain important nutrients that are valuable for brain chemicals and hormonal functions, such as good eicosanoids or serotonin (from tryptophan found in grain, legumes, and seeds). The object is to learn *how* to eat high-glycemic foods and *when* to eat them.

Basically, using any chart, counting, or point-value system creates a *body and food obsession*, causing a further urge to break the rigidity or ritual of your diet. It also creates a detrimental relationship with your foods as being "good" or "bad" rather than healthy or poor choices.

Popular calorie or fat-gram counting diets (and glycemic index diets) may include: *The Thin Commandments, Weight Watchers, Jenny Craig, Richard Simmons, and Glycemic Index Diet and Charts.*

GIMMICK DIETS (including ALL-YOU-CAN-EAT DIETS)

Just about all the diets could be included in this section. Whether it's relying on charts or the way certain foods react with your body, everyone is selling some gimmick. The unfortunate part of gimmick diets is that nine times out of ten they have no merit. Usually they are based on theories without scientific studies or claims that are poorly researched. Some gimmick diets add a "supernatural" food, substance, secret formula, or magical instrument that offers nothing but a placebo effect. Gimmick diets tend to generalize the diet and assume your body will react the same way as everyone else's does, all the time. This is ridiculous because everybody reacts differently. We also react differently to different foods at different times according to our mental state (stress), health and fitness, and outside circumstances.

The all-you-can-eat diets are the most ridiculous. Overeating causes weight gain and/or unhealthy deficiencies. It causes a deficiency somewhere by excluding one or more of your important food groups or nutrients. Overeating one food or food group creates allergies, which build up and sometimes cause a false-deficiency reaction because the body tries to compensate for the overload. Overeating any type of food can trigger an eating disorder as well.

Gimmick diets may include a spiritual guide or affirmation. This is a good idea because we direct our body's cells and hormones to react according to our attitude. Stress has been proven to be a direct cause of weight gain. For example, I have found, when I was under stress, my adrenal glands excrete excess cortisol which triggers excess insulin, causing weight gain. Constant stress can causes adrenal exhaustion, which eventually depletes the cortisol. Cortisol is the hormone that helps the carbohydrates and proteins metabolize. Too much cortisol can cause weight gain as well. This further disrupts the other hormones and chemicals such as epinephrine (adrenaline) or digestive enzymes. The body's elimination is disturbed and the body stores the undigested food as fat.

People suffering from eating disorders should separate their food plan choices from their spiritual program. I believe recovery is made more successful by incorporating some form of spirituality. But when someone with an eating disorder places magical thinking or shame onto their food or body, it creates an ongoing obsession with both the food and body. They relate to food as good or bad rather than healthy or unhealthy. Using the label "good" or "bad" creates a shame-based mentality, making you define yourself by your choices or weight. Shame-based individuals usually think they *are* the problem instead of thinking they have a problem. Saying a prayer before you eat is an honorable tradition. Food addicts should base their food decisions on healthy choices rather than "godly" choices. Nature's foods are basically raw fruits and vegetables. Eating things that are unhealthy is not a sin. It's a poor choice that we all have made or continue to make. It is far better to inform yourself rather than condemn yourself. When individuals base their diets on *feelings* rather than healthy choices (for a health goal), I notice they struggle with weight. The object of this book is to help you let go of your love affair with food and the feelings attached to it.

Other gimmick diets may include "magical foods" such as adding coconut oil or a grapefruit before each meal. One diet claims eating a small fatty snack before a starchy meal prevents overeating. The diet claims this blocks the insulin or trips the brain transmitter to create satiation). There are other gimmick diets that include eating or drinking a certain soup or one type of food and nothing else. There are diets that claim that eating fruit alone will make you thin. This is not a good choice for a compulsive overeater. Too much fruit can cause fermentation. I know true fruitarians. They do not have an eating disorder. They usually choose that specific eating habit for extreme health results or for a medical condition they were concerned about. The only "magical foods" are natural foods such as vegetables, fruits, and nuts. In moderation and balanced with variety, these are the foods that will give you what you need for good health, which automatically leads to your weight goal.

There is also a diet that excludes all sugars. Although I think sugar itself is a drug, not a food, you should not replace healthy fruits and vegetables that are high in sugar with sugar *substitutes* and saturated fats. Sugar itself causes an over-secretion of insulin and a chemical reaction in the brain and body much like that of a drug dose. Sugar also causes an over-secretion of cortisol and estrogen, making weight loss difficult. Long-term sugar use eventually causes hypoglycemia (excess insulin) that may develop into diabetes, which is insulin depletion. Sugar excess may also cause adrenal exhaustion (cortisol depletion) and perimenopause (excess estrogen), which may develop into early menopause (estrogen depletion). Sugar is linked to pain, arthritis, scar tissue, infections, and slow wound-healing. It is recommended to eliminate sugar ten days before and after any type of surgery. When you detox from the sugar, just like drugs, you can experience a withdrawal and craving period, creating an eventual crash. Sugar is purposely added to products such as fast food, cigarettes, and toothpaste because of its addictive nature. A high-sugar diet has been to blame for many children who are diagnosed as hyperactive (ADHD) or attention deficit disorder (ADD). I have noticed that children were fed a diet of mostly raw foods and no sugar, most of them were no long hyperactive or they showed fewer symptoms of ADD. Corn syrup is actually worse if you consider the extreme blood sugar response it causes. Sugars are renamed and repackaged, much like diets, to give the buyer the impression they are safe, healthy, or calorie free. I have found that sugar substitutes cause a backfire effect. For example, the alternative to butter is oil substitutes (trans-fatty acids). Fake fats and sugar substitutes interfere with insulin balance and blood sugar, making weight loss difficult. While I agree with omitting sugar (which is related to health problems such as infections and escalation of tumor growth), I don't believe you should replace it with another poison, such as fake sugar or fat.

A very popular diet is aimed at the carbohydrate addict. I think we are all basically carbohydrate addicts in some way or another. This diet is based on the fact that we all have one "freebee" insulin spill per day that can happen within forty-five minutes of eating a high-carb meal. This leaves the other two meals as a low-carb and low-calorie meals, which should preferably be eaten at night. Shane and I happily experimented with this diet, sharing it with all our other food-addict buddies. We came to a disappointing conclusion; this diet, like others, causes further or eventual weight gain. It also triggered our binge cycles. Obviously, this diet is better for people who normally indulge all day on junky carbs. This limits their bingeing to forty-five minutes a day and helps promote some self-control with delayed gratification. I do not, however, recommend it to any individual who suffers with eating disorders. It only accelerates the disease and doesn't teach you to choose food plans according to your health and circumstances. This sets off the food obsession and teaches you to live to eat, rather than eat to live.

Some diets are a one-stop-shopping gimmick. Some include an initial "kick-start" by starting out with few days of deprivation (ketosis), before the regular diet. Usually a low calorie/carb food plan kick-starts their diet.. Their "form letter" diet is usually disguised as your own specially designed food plan. It may also offer a doctor or give medication shots (such as vitamin B shots) with a support group. It's all common sense or cliché, yet these plans usually charge a fee. Why pay for something you can get without the cost? The twelve-step programs offer about the same thing plus a recovery program that supplements the food plan. You should choose your own healthcare provider or doctor who specializes in *your* health issues, not your food plan. Incidentally, if you take vitamin B shots without needing them, you can actually gain weight. It's best to get your B vitamins from food sources.

Other gimmicks may include food combinations. This theory is related to the digestion of your meals. While this works well with raw food dieters, it is contradicting, in theory, for other normal diets. If you are going to be a fanatic about digestive enzymes, then be consistent about the quality of foods and their effect on body's chemicals and hormones as well. Again, otherwise this is "magical" thinking. Even though everything works synergistically in the body, food combining alone will *not* fix your problems with weight. Try eating a variety of foods rather than overeating selective foods that digest together. Overeating causes insulin excess. Too much of one food or food group creates allergies and a blood sugar imbalance. It is far better to eat simple and pure foods rather than grouping all your indigestible or impure foods into one digestive category. Food combining gurus emphasize the fact that we digest different foods with different enzymes in different parts of the digestive system. This is true. Starch is digested in the mouth, with the help of enzymes found in saliva; meat is digested in the stomach with the help of hydrochloric acid. When we mix starches with protein or fruits with proteins, we interrupt the digestive process, leaving the enzymes disabled or destroyed. Starch is then rushed to the stomach undigested, corrupting all digestion and elimination, and hence weight gain occurs. Subsequently, the foods are fermented and unable to be used for fuel, so we store this residue as fat or toxins. This can further cause acidosis (abnormally high acidity in the blood and other body fluids), which disrupts your pH balance. Food combinations are used frequently by raw-food dieters and other popular diets. Though food combination makes a lot of sense (especially for raw dieters) and is an excellent regimen for the elderly or ill, it doesn't always work, especially for weight loss. Many times dieters have the impression they are on an all-you-can-eat diet and overeat the same food group at one meal. You can only extract so many nutrients from a meal. The rest is stored as fat, good food combination or not. Food combinations don't allow the meal's insulin flow (such as when eating fruit) to be blocked by protein or fat. The body can assimilate just about anything. It's far better to use portion sense and basic balance. Enzymes deteriorate as we age and from excess overeating or chemical use. I've found it far better and more fulfilling to eat "pure," small portions of what I need. Food combining did *nothing* for my weight struggles and triggered my compulsive overeating. I finally found that balance and variety made my body work more efficiently. Overdoing one digestive group never quenched my hunger. Digestive enzymes can supplement your diet, if need be. However, the food addict should learn balance, not tricks, which don't usually work.

Other popular diets focus on portion control or behavioral modification. Both are important, until they call it a "diet." As soon as a food plan becomes a diet, rather than a guideline, it becomes a rigid regimen that can be broken or "blown." Diets are a set-up for failure.

Usually the title of a diet book is a gimmick. It's the old switch-and-bait scam; it draws you in with the pretense that you get something for nothing. Some of these diets may work temporarily, but all of them eventually stop working, if they work at all. The reason is simply that our bodies learn or know every trick and will try to compensate for them. This in turns makes our bodies more diet savvy, making it more difficult to lose weight.

Popular gimmick diets may include: *Binge Busters, The Coconut Diet, French Women Don't Diet, The Maker's Diet, Suzanne Sommers Diet, Carbohydrate Addict's Diet, Lindora, Sugar Busters, Beverly Hills Diet, Blood Type Diets, Tops, The Cabbage Soup Diet.*

DEPRIVATION DIETS: (Including Fasting, Food Replacements and Cleansing Diets)

Deprivation diets can be diets that exclude solid food or a certain food (or juice) to attain certain weight or health goals. The name alone is a turn-off to anyone facing dieting dilemmas. I have witnessed carefully monitored starvation diets slow down tumor growth and the aging process. These are not good diet plans for weight loss. Eventually, starving prevents your mind or body from learning how to eat and can further any eating disorders that may already be present.

The definition of *fasting* is food abstinence. There are many interpretations of fasting. Some assume fasting is going without solid foods (juicing) or omitting entire food groups. True fasting is not ingesting *any* food or juice—just water. Very low-calorie diets or liquid fasts are usually considered fasting because they only include 300-800 calories. Carefully monitored low-calorie diets have been shown to boost our immune systems and invigorate the body and mind. This is because the extra energy usually used for digesting heavy meals is used for healing and other important bodily functions instead. This causes a rejuvenating effect on our cells, organs, and skin. Fasting relies on the body's ability to supply nutrients or adjust to the no- or low-calorie intake. It is important to specify the quality and quanity of the juice or food intake. When you ingest a very small amount of food, the body recognizes it as starving. When you fast on just water, your body automatically retrieves the body's reserves. Fasting should always be done under some type of supervision. Usually on about the fourth day, the body goes into the fat-burning process. Fasters should rest to avoid enervation (robbing from the nerve tissue). A technique fasters use to know when to break a fast is to wait until the coated tongue (ketosis) has cleared. Sweet breath and normal hunger (not cravings) manifests as well. A faster should never break his or her fast during a "fasting crisis.", (the worst part of the fast). This is when the body is detoxing and needs to rest. When the faster eventually breaks his fast, he should only eat one fruit (preferably citrus to counter dehydration) every two hours, six times a day, for the first few days. Extreme hunger returns when the faster eats. It takes twice as many days as the length of the fast to recover from fast. This is why fasting has received a bad reputation. It's not the fasting that is dangerous but how the fast is broken. Some fasters have nearly killed themselves by breaking their fast with junk food. It is unwise to follow a cleansing fast with a sudden overload of junk food. This can shock your body and create damage.

Water fasting can be dangerous, too, because it is the sodium in fruits and vegetables that retain your water balance. Water has a diuretic effect. This can be dangerous because of the lack of natural sodium and other minerals that are natural in fruit and vegetables. Sodium makes electrolytes when it enters the body, which prevents dehydration. Lemon is very good because it contains sodium that helps our electrolyte balance. Lemon can help edema (water retention) when you are bloated as well as dehydration. During long fasts, there is an initial weight loss that is enormous, but is always regained somewhat with food. This is why fasting should be done for health purposes only. The body learns to starve and lowers the metabolism. When someone ingests less than 800 calories or so per day, ketosis occurs; the body uses fat without the help of carbohydrates. Ketosis makes dramatic and quick weight loss possible, but the loss is temporary due to the lack of cellular water. This is a dangerous state for your body. Ketosis causes excessive urination (which contributes to dehydration), feelings of lightheadedness, halitosis, and nausea. Ketosis during pregnancy causes mental retardation in infants. The duration of a fast does not depend on the faster's weight. A thin person with good reserves can last longer than an overweight person who is detoxing from junk food and stimulants. Junk food detoxification may cause stress on the adrenals. Stimulants can leech your reserves as well. Fasting is a good spiritual tradition and health option but is not good for weight loss.

Hygienic is a term coined by fasting gurus. It basically means eating raw, live food in perfect food combinations. In a perfect world, we would just pick-and-eat our food. Some dieters claim anything cooked under 105-120 degrees is considered raw. There are several explanations or theories to justifying cooking under 108 to 120 degrees. One is the *sun theory*. The average temperature of the food sitting in the sun is 120 degrees. The other rationale is eating anything 108-120 degrees or under won't disrupt the food's nutrient value or enzymes process. Cooking or processing food causes cross-linkage, which makes the food unrecognizable to the digestive tract. A cross-linkage is cell damage due to certain food or toxin interaction. This is not true for all foods. Raw means raw. Some raw-food dieters include "raw" cheese or kefir. This does not apply to hygienics, who simply eat raw plant food, specifically low-sugar vegetables and fruits.

Hygienics want the *live* enzymes to work on their bodies. They combine foods this way: sweet fruits, melons, sub-acid fruits and citrus fruits, each eaten separately. The vegetables are eaten separately as well. Nuts, seeds, and avocado can be eaten with your vegetables, preferably toward the evening. Fruits are best in the morning hours. Some hygienics only eat vegetables, avocados, and very little fruit (green apples and grapefruit), if any at all. Some believe in eating these foods whole, while other hygienics prefer juice fasting. The object of eating foods whole is to keep the pulp, which slows down the insulin flow. To some, juice is considered oxidized (easily rancid), because it's not in its complete form, the way nature intended it to be. Oxidation may break down the enzymes and nutrient value. Juice experts believe a tired or sick body may need immediate energy (sugar) without the waste of fiber. Whatever the case may be, I have nothing but good remarks to say about any live, raw-food dieters. I've seen good results with both theories. However, it is not a good idea to eat raw simply to lose weight, especially if you have an eating disorder. It takes time to adjust to the simplicity of the diet. This diet should be gradual. It also takes time to acclimate to pure plant fuel to take the place of the familiar animal foods and years of corrupted meals. Weight loss may take time on a live raw-food diet. People who suffer from eating disorders treat a raw-food diet like a deprivation diet, thereby sabotaging their diet and eventually eating junk food. Unlike in other countries, most of our food is loaded with dangerous amounts of additives that are purposefully addictive. Other countries usually reject our food because it's so impure. This is why it's dangerous to follow a cleansing diet with the shock of junk food. Raw-food diets should be exclusively for people who want to change their whole lifestyle (not temporally) for health purposes only.

Liquid protein fasting has a very bad reputation. It has been reported to cause severe kidney damage, create fat efficiency, and always cause weight gain. Fat efficiency is when the body makes, creates or holds onto fat much more so than normal. This is the worst choice for fasting. It's unbalanced and dangerous, and it backfires.

Short-term juice fasting or adding lemon (or other natural nutrients) to water proves beneficial without severe side effects. Juice fasting has helped people detox from chemicals, parasites, and junk food. Again, it's a poor choice for weight loss, though. It is good to begin a diet with a cleansing regimen, without looking to the fast to be the answer to your long-term weight problems. Cleansing or not, your body can only starve so many times for so long. The body remembers every time it starves and then compensates. Long juice fasts can be enervating or cause fat efficiency, because your body has a hard time recognizing whole foods after a long fast. Juice fasting can also help combat food allergies, asthma, chronic fatigue, depression, some cancers, and many more illnesses. I have witnessed extremely ill individuals return to good health with a properly guided fast.

Food replacements are usually pre-packaged drinks that are used in place of a meal or two. These drinks are usually loaded with sugar and unnatural chemicals. The vitamin/mineral content that is offered is often in supplemented form as opposed to coming from natural food sources. It isn't any different than simply taking vitamins with a sugar drink. The sugar (a drug, not a food) leeches whatever vitamins or minerals that were added to the sugar-malt. It is true that, when you are in a rush, these meal replacements are handy. However, it is much healthier (and just as handy) to create your own meal replacement. If you filled a thermos full of a homemade smoothie of yogurt, fruit, and flaxseed, that would supply everything you need—a complete meal. It's also natural and without side effects. Food replacements do not teach you how to eat. If you are using food replacements to lose weight, you are training your body to starve during two meals and binge on the third. The object is to learn to choose enjoyable but healthy foods without freaking out. Meal replacements are usually used by overeaters who fear dealing with food. You don't learn anything when you abstain from choice.

There are some diets that are specially designed for health rather than weight loss. These diets include soy, fruits, vegetables, and natural supplements. Many of these diets are used for treating people with chronic diseases such as heart disease and cancer. These natural diets usually exclude any animal protein or sugar. I think these diets are superb. There is criticism of certain diets that emphasize too much soy because of the phytoestrogens, which some say cause estrogen complications. Soy is very hard to digest. (It's better to use fermented soy, like tempeh, which is easier to digest.) Others believe that the phytoestrogens actually bind with any estrogen surplus, helping to eliminate the excess. Soy is a complete protein with many benefits, *including* the phytoestrogens. Quite simply, soy, like any food, should be eaten in moderation.

Popular deprivation diets (including fasting, food replacements, and cleansing diets): *Slim Fast, The Master Cleanser, Dr. Weil's Diet, Hygienic Raw Food Diet, The Optimum Health Institute.*

*Note: Shane and I have tried all of the diets above, plus more. We concluded diets and gimmicks don't work! We did, however, incorporate some of the popular health strategies (without relying on them as a trick or quick fix into various non-diet food plans or **Eco Anti-Diets**. (Eco Anti-Diets are further discussed in Chapter Four.) I gave a complete thumbs-up to a few popular diets, while others only destroyed my metabolism and promoted my eating disorder. The diets that were <u>superb</u> were the ones that stressed HEALTH—not weight loss—and encouraged or included an exercise and recovery program as well.*

CHAPTER 3:
PHYSICAL TOOLS
Quiz I: 21 Questions (family disease quiz)
Quiz II: Lifestyle Quiz
Quiz III: Body Types Quiz

During my binge days, my tools were very simple. I'd use plastic wrap to sweat my binge off. I'd use a lock on my refrigerator and I'd use a rear-view mirror to remind myself of what my binge left behind: a bigger behind!

Tools are *instruments* that help accomplish your goals. Remember, when *health* is the goal, then it is an automatic byproduct that you will look and feel good. If you are unhealthy physically or mentally, you will continue to have problems or obsessions with weight and diets. Rather than symptom-chasing with a one-size-fits-all *diet* of deprivation, I gave each reader an easy formula according to your lifestyle, body type, and health history. You can change the food plan when needed or desired. I learned early on that one continuous diet eventually stops working because our bodies learn the diet trick or gimmick. Our bodies try to compensate, eventually making any diet backfire. Diets create food allergies and nutrient depletion because diets rarely allow variety. The Physical Tools are reinforced by the Mental Tools. This makes the journey enjoyable, without having to wait for results…they will come.

How did we lose weight? How did we recover from bulimia?

Let me share the keys to success and the clues to our recovery: Physical and Mental Tools

The **Physical Tools** are composed of three simple quizzes: the 21 Questions, the Lifestyle Quiz, and the Body Type Quiz. Your answers from these three simple quizzes will direct you to your own specially designed food plan. I refer to my food plans as "Eco Anti-Diets" (further discussed in Chapter Four). Eco Anti-Diets are used in the same way as anti-aging (fights aging), antibiotics (fights infections), anti-oxidants (fights free radicals), and anti-viruses (fights computer malfunctions). Eco Anti-Diets fight *bingeing and diets*: deprivation, depletion, depression, and diet abuse. This makes it easy to refrain from sabotaging your food plan. Because Eco Anti-Diets are healthy, they also fight aging (anti-aging). The Eco Anti-Diets are a cleaner and easier way of achieving your weight goals. The Physical Tools are the first part of our research we put together as a formula (quizzes) to give a solution (food plan), for weight and diet issues.

Research=Formula=Solution *to your weight and diet issues*

    21 Questions (which determine your health and future)
+   Lifestyle Quiz (and supplement guide)
    Body Type Quiz (and exercise guide)
=   **Food plan** (specially designed for each person per situation)

The **Mental Tools,** further discussed in chapter five, are a supplement to the Physical Tools. They reinforce a complete lifestyle change to good habits. The Mental Tools are motivational techniques that help you learn to COMMIT to your food plan, CONFRONT the issues you eat over, and REPLACE trigger foods and situations. This will help free yourself from the cycles of dieting and body/weight obsession. In other words it's about FREEDOM.

~ ~ ~ ~ ~ ~

The Physical Tools:

The Physical Tools are the following three quizzes which will determine which food plan is best suited for you. The first quiz is the 21 Questions, which helps determine your health and family disease history. The second quiz is a Lifestyle Quiz, which will help determine the best description of your lifestyle. The third quiz is a Body Type Quiz, which simply describes your body structure. Each quiz has one final question, which makes a total of 3 answers to the three quizzes. According to your answers (one answer per quiz), you will be assigned a color. When you have finished all three quizzes, you will have a total of 3 colors (one per quiz). All three colors (the combination), will direct you to your own specific food plan.

QUIZ I
21 QUESTIONS: That Help Determine Your Health and Family Disease History

Genetics are not always kind. Neither is my sister. My sister once informed me that the definition of a second-born twin is a "defective clone." I can deal with that...

21 Questions will help determine where your health status lies and where your health will take you—if you continue with the same health habits. Let's say that your health habits are similar to your parents. If so, in all likelihood you are on the same health path as your parents, meaning whatever disease they are confronting you will be facing as well. Hereditary factors seem to be more influential if you live the same way (or worse) than your parents and family lived. On the other hand, making radical health changes lessens hereditary traits. Health habit changes, when radical, can be more powerful than genes! *You become your genes when you have poor health habits.* Or...*you are what you eat when you eat well, but if you eat poorly, you will fulfill your genetic destiny.* The following questionnaire will help clear the way to the right health path in order to improve your overall health.

Your annual checkup should include the following lab work. Discuss the results with your doctor.

1. Your pH balance, which should be near 7.4, and fall between 5.0-8.0.
2. Your ketones reading should be negative, which means you are NOT diabetic.
3. Your glucose should range anywhere from 70-110.
4. Your cholesterol should range anywhere from 140-200.
5. Your HDL (good cholesterol) should range anywhere from 2.0-4.5.
6. Your LDL (bad cholesterol) should range anywhere from 70-130.
7. Your triglycerides should range anywhere from 30-150.

✋ If you don't fall within these parameters, consult with your doctor. This chapter will help you understand where you are in relation to your health.

The first quiz of the Physical Tools is 21 Questions. You simply circle **Yes** or **No** for each answer. At the end of this questionnaire, you will be asked how many times you answered **Yes** or **No**.

☞ Circle **Yes** or **No** after each question. Decide what best describes you, your health, and your family disease history.
(If you aren't sure, circle **No**.)

1. Do you or your family have a history of weight related or chronic diseases such as heart disease, diabetes, or obesity in your family?	Yes	No
2. Have you dieted more than half of your adult life?	Yes	No, just lately
3. Do you gain weight easily, particularly in the mid section or get cellulite easily?	Yes	No
4. Do you have a tendency towards sweets and snacking?	Yes	No, not really
5. Would you prefer large protein meals as opposed to sweets and snacks?	Yes	No
6. Do you eat throughout the day?	Yes	No, just at meals
7. Do you mostly eat late at night?	Yes	No
8. Are your eating habits strictly feast-or-famine?	Yes	No
9. When you diet, is your tongue unable to coat? (In ketosis, or when burning fat, the tongue creates a white coating).	Yes	No or don't know
10. When you are under stress or in a heightened state of emotion, do you practice your poor eating habits or drug of choice (compulsive overeating, binging, compulsive dieting, anorexia, over-exercising, bulimia, or BDD)?	Yes	No
11. Do you suffer from bloating, headaches, and mood swings frequently?	Yes	No
12. Do you feel hungry no matter what you have eaten?	Yes	No, never. I am full after a normal meal.
13. Do you get light-headed easily and feel a lack of energy most of the time?	Yes	No
14. Are you susceptible to colds, allergies, candidiasis, and viral infections?	Yes	No
15. Do you constantly have cold feet or cold hands?	Yes	No, never
16. Do you constipate easily or suffer from constant diarrhea?	Yes	No
17. Are you easily depressed or have you lost the desire for things you once enjoyed (sex for example)?	Yes	No
18. Did all diets stop working for you?	Yes	No
19. Do you suffer from insomnia or have trouble getting to sleep?	Yes	No
20. Do you feel worse following exercise?	Yes	No
21. Do you use any stimulants or over-the-counter drugs, including caffeine, cigarettes, or diet aids?	Yes	No

Warning: You don't have be the drama queen my sister was. She wheeled herself into the emergency room after answering "Yes" to almost all of these questions.

LET'S DETERMINE HOW MANY "YES" ANSWERS YOU HAVE...

1. *Count your total number of* **Yes** *answers you circled* _____

2. *If you answered* **Yes** *to 18-21 of the questions, your health is poor. Circle this color–RED*

3. *If you answered* **Yes** *to 14-17 of the questions, your health is fairly poor. Circle this color–PURPLE*

4. *If you answered* **Yes** *to 7-13 of the questions, your health is fair. Circle this color–WHITE*

5. *If you answered* **Yes** *to 3-6 of the questions, your health is fairly good. Circle this color–BLUE*

6. *If you answered* **Yes** *to 0-2 of the questions, your health is good. Circle this color–GREEN*

☞ Following the brief answers to the 21 Questions, there are two remaining quizzes (Lifestyle and body type). You will be assigned one more color per quiz, according to your answers. Your three colors (combined), will determine which food plan is best suited for you.

Brief Answers to the 21 Questions

1) If you come from a long line of **chronic diseases in your family history,** you will have to be more diligent than the average person when making your lifestyle choices. You may be prone to hypoglycemia and diabetes. Too much caffeine and saturated fat can be just as damaging to the insulin balance as sugar abuse. Dental problems can be the symptom of a disease or part of the cause of a disease. A compromised immune system forces the body to leech minerals from other reserves such a teeth, hair, and bones. Longtime sugar use also robs the B vitamins. Longtime meat eating creates phosphate buildup, which leeches your calcium. A lack of a few vitamins or minerals can cause disease just as much as the buildup of toxins. Throughout my years, I have experienced that certain types of diets can be more powerful than drugs or surgery, in most cases. I have seen individuals (hygienics or raw-food dieters) who glow because of their healthy diets, while fighting cancer or other life threatening diseases. Children who eat mostly raw plant food are less likely to be hyperactive or have other behavioral problems that are usually treated with medication. Instead of entertaining their

mouths with food, raw dieters have made food (or the lack of it) their medicine. Because of their alternative eating habits, hygienics and other raw dieters seem to improve nearly any problem they face, including deadly diseases. They believe "*doctors cure disease A by creating disease B.*" Hygienic diets usually consist of live, raw foods and juices. They don't look for "magical" fixes or cures; instead, they change their lifestyles and choices completely.

2) If you **have dieted more than half your life,** you are not alone. We are a nation that is steadily getting fatter, while being obsessed with diets that fail. If you have dieted over and over, your metabolism will be lower than normal and you may also have an under-active thyroid. You are now more fat-efficient than you were before dieting, because your body is tired of starving. Diets encourage and condone binge eating or poor health choices. You are someone who will have to teach your body to trust that you will not diet anymore. Your body will then learn to eat and burn calories rather than storing them. Your dieting has been like a bad marriage that is in need of a divorce. Don't repeat the same mistake over and over. The mistake is DIETING!

3) If you **gain weight around the midsection or get cellulite easily,** your food choices are poor, no matter how small your portions are. Gaining weight in the midsection puts you at a greater risk for diseases of your vital organs. Usually men gain weight on the inside, near their vital organs, while women gain on the outside, on their hips (cellulite). This can be deceiving. Gaining weight in the midsection is harder to detect and more dangerous than weight gain elsewhere. This is also a sign that you have poor insulin balance, which can eventually cause hypoglycemia. This may put you at risk for diabetes, when the insulin spills exhaust. Your meals should be small and frequent, consisting of high fiber and low glycemic foods. Glycemic index is the rate sugar enters bloodstream and its effect on your insulin secretion. You don't have to be "fat" to gain weight in the midsection. It is also a sign of poor tissue quality (tire rim) from poor diet choices or eating one big meal rather than several mini-meals throughout the day. Cellulite does not have to do with weight gain. You can actually lose weight while detecting increasing cellulite. Cellulite has a little to do with genetics but a lot to do with tissue quality. Clean tissue comes from healthy food choices, which smoothes out cellulite better than exercise. There are many theories to cellulite, including poor circulation. Exercise helps circulation. However, high fiber, good fats (EFA oils), and lots of fresh fruits and vegetables (water plus sodium) help bring oxygen to the body's cells regularly. Cellulite creams, massages, and other gimmicks don't work or are only temporary fixes. Cellulite is a manifestation of dirty tissue from impure food.

4) If you are **prone to eating sweets and snacking,** most of your problems will be gynecological, if you are female. Sugar, which I include as a drug, doesn't contain any nutrient value and yet may be considered harmful. I recommend eliminating sugar because it directly affects the endocrine system and inhibits any healing process. The endocrine system consists of all your glands and hormones, all of which are adversely affected by sugar. When you eat too much of sugar, your cortisol, insulin, and estrogen levels become imbalanced, which makes weight loss or detoxing difficult. Eventually cortisol depletion may cause adrenal exhaustion.

Soon insulin depletion may develop into diabetes and estrogen depletion can develop into early menopause. Serotonin (neurotransmitter that relaxes), endorphins (pain, relief), and other feel-good chemicals and hormones become depleted when consuming too much sugar. All cancer patients are advised to omit sugar. Some doctors advise patients to refrain from sugar because it promotes infections. Sugar is also is linked to scar tissue and pain. Eating sugar and junk food triggers the body's "bad" eicosanoids, mini hormone-like substances that help dictate every health action directly related to our health and weight. Eating chocolate releases endorphins (pituitary, reduce pain). This is why people some people "use" chocolate to escape, like a drug. Endorphins react like morphine. Junk food also contains trans-fatty acids, which are worse than saturated fat. These hydrogenated fats are similar to the sweeter alternatives. These fake sugars and trans-fatty acids have the same unhealthy effect on the insulin spill in our bodies that sugar does. They also activate the LDL (low density lipoprotein or "bad fat") level to rise. This means you will experience constant hunger, no matter what. This "sweet-and-snack" habit will add to your problems with weight and leak into your future health issues.

5) If you **prefer large protein meals rather than sweets and snacks,** this can be a problem because of the amount of the saturated fat. Men are dictated by testosterone, which makes them usually prefer protein meals. On the contrary, large protein meals will compromise female hormones. Regardless what protein diet you choose, you can still gain weight if you eat too much protein. You should never consume more than 60 grams of protein a day, unless you are an athlete and divide your meals into six mini-meals. Some have done very well with only 20 grams of protein every other day. Protein can be derived from a number of food sources that are not typically known as a protein foods. Certain combinations of grains and legumes can complete a protein. Consuming large amounts of animal protein can eventually cause some type of chronic illness. It takes a lot of energy to digest protein, particularly animal protein. Eating large amounts of protein is very aging. We are meant to graze all day on small meals of mostly nuts and berries. The meat, long ago, was hunted (activity) and naturally obtained. Modern-day meat is processed with chemicals, dyes, and hormones; it is unnatural! Red meat in particular contains dangerous amounts of phosphates that leech calcium. Our lower intestine (colon) is too long to carry and digest heavy meat meals. The meat usually petrifies because it sits in the intestine too long (ferments) or doesn't have enough energy to entirely digest. This is the *precursor* to many diseases. Some say it is better to have large protein meals rather than sugar. It depends on how you want to die. The bottom line is, just like eating a lot of sugar, eating a lot of meat is very unhealthy. I believe it is one of the major causes or promoters of all serious diseases. When arachidonic acid (fatty acid eicosanoid precursor) is eliminated, women will have less pain when dealing with gynecological problems. Arachidonic acid is found in dairy, eggs, and red meat.

6) If you **eat throughout the day** (unless you are bingeing), you have an advantage over someone who skips breakfast or eats primarily at night. This is the trick to raising the metabolism. But if you eat junk food or large quantities throughout the day, your insulin is over-secreting all day. This can cause put you at risk for diabetes. Weight problem or not, continuous eating prevents the body

from *resting*. Your body's digestion, just like you, needs rest. I never suggest fasting for weight issues. But I do suggest a person fast for *rest* issues. (Fasts should be supervised.) If the body doesn't rest, it can't maintain a healthy weight or rid the body of toxins and free radicals that cause diseases or weight struggles.

7)   If you **eat primarily at night,** you have a probably have a poor metabolism and you're very *fat efficient* (effortlessly clinging to fat). When you fast all day long, your body doesn't want you to lose weight. Instead, it prepares itself for the famine until you feast, so you don't have to starve. Waiting all day to eat late at night causes an insulin overflow when you eat your next meal. This also causes blood sugar drops, edema, and weight struggles. Your body is busy searching and making reserves to counteract this daily fast you're on. Your metabolism lowers every three to four hours, along with your blood sugar. For example, if you were to eat a piece of celery at night, it will use that tiny food source for fat reserves and not for nutrients. If your body has to burn any calories, it will sacrifice muscle, not your fat, because it is in "survival mode". When I compared people who ate one meal at night with people who ate that same nighttime meal plus breakfast and lunch, I found the people with 3 meals lost the same or more weight, than the ones who just ate at night. If you only want to eat one big meal, and perhaps fast the rest of the time, it's best to eat that meal in the first part of the day, not near bedtime when your digestion, metabolism and all your body's chemicals and enzymes are at its lowest performance.

8)   If the "**feast or famine" diet** is your type of eating habit, then you are in the midst of or on your way to an eating disorder. I encourage fasting for health issues only, usually under supervision. Fasting (starving) creates weight struggles. It also causes fat-*efficiency* or effortlessly clinging to fat. Spontaneous and enormous meals are never digested properly because your hormones and enzymes were left dormant during your fast. Starving can cause enervation (draining nerve energy). Bingeing will cause physical damage and mental suffering. Our bodies need a variety but thrive on consistency. Throwing your body in and out of ketosis (fat burning at a high rate) can create the same damage as drug abuse. You will experience hair loss, dental and skeletal problems, digestion difficulties, flabby tissue, and so forth. Your body learns to sacrifice your vital tissue and uses it as a reserve rather than the fat. This is the reason why the feast-famine individual has poor tissue quality, no matter how much he or she exercises. Cellulite is created from poor tissue quality.

9)   Do you get a **coated tongue**? When you are dieting, have you ever noticed that your tongue has a white, thick coating? This is when you are in the state of ketosis, which is the act of burning fat without burning glucose. This changes the acid/alkaline pH balance of your blood and can ultimately lead some to a coma and death. Usually this can occur in diabetics who lack insulin to metabolize carbs, but it can also affect people who starve (low carbs). The symptoms of ketosis are bad breath; a white, coated tongue; and dark urine. Ketosis is an unnatural and unhealthy state that eventually wears out after dieting over and over. The inability to reach the state of ketosis when dieting long term, is a clue to exhausted adrenals. These dieters actually lose more weight when they *eat*, because their body is too exhausted from starving. If your tongue coats easily

between meals, that is usually a sign that you have rarely dieted. A continuously coated tongue, though you're eating normally, can also mean you easily get sick or may have diabetes. High-protein diets have a tendency to put you in this ketosis state, which is an aging state and a burden on your body.

10) If you **practice your addiction or drug of choice when you are under stress,** you no longer just have a diet problem; you also have a mental disorder to supplement your physical addiction. We are creatures of habits. Using food or diets to deal with stress is training your body to abuse food This is much like the Pavlovian conditioning, which is when you condition yourself to do something like it is a reflex . This is because you use food or starving as your survival tool and mechanism to deal with outside circumstances with an "inside job." This is much like a drug addict's behavior. Whatever excuse or problem you use your food or diet to deal with, your bingeing, purging, or starving will top your crisis list. Your addiction will creep its way to the top, willing to outdo any other problem you are facing. The usual signals that tell us we are hungry or full will be rewired to accommodate your addiction. That's when all boundaries are lifted, creating compulsive behavior. This behavior is in need of quick recovery before it may develop into a chronic disease. The physical turns mental, turns deadly.

11) If you **suffer from bloating, headaches, and mood swings frequently,** you may suffer from adrenal exhaustion (too much dieting, drugs, or exercising). Or you may be faced with gynecological problems (triggered by coffee, (caffeine),sugar, smoking, and meat). Ironically, the discomfort and stress of your symptoms will further your adrenal exhaustion and imbalance your other hormones. It's a vicious cycle that is usually symptom-chased by drugs/aids, which aggravate your body and mask the symptoms. Extreme exercisers (usually bulimic or anorexic) will fear their bloating, which encourages them to exercise harder. A possible hypoglycemic reaction from symptom-chasing may also occur. Bloating, headaches, and mood swings are originally warning signs or precursors. Edema (bloating) and headaches can also be symptoms of food allergies or a body full of toxins. Drinking water can cause a diuretic effect that helps reduce edema and clear the lymph nodes of toxins. Coffee (especially with caffeine) and chocolate are major culprits of severe headaches, edema, and mood swings. Chocolate raises the endorphin levels, acting like morphine, numbing the pain. Taking drugstore headache remedies has been known to escalate headache problems. A colon cleanse is advisable. Remember, colon cleansers and enemas flush the friendly bacteria out of the lower intestine. Replenish this with acidophilus (in yogurt). Chronic dieters seem to bloat, particularly in the face. This can be from the kidneys overworking or protein deficiency. Protein, like coffee, initially causes dehydration. Long-term protein diets and coffee users eventually suffer from edema and body fluid imbalance. Some doctors also claim edema is swelling of a lymphatic system in search of protein to create antibodies for infections. They claim edema or bloating is a protein deficiency. On the contrary, I believe in the theory that we eat too much protein, particularly meat. Red meat, as other animal protein, carries dangerous amounts of phosphates. These phosphates, which leech calcium and other additives, create symptoms in the same way as coffee (caffeine) and other stimulants do. These additives also hinder weight loss. Whatever the reason, if you don't address the root of your problems and only treat

the symptoms, then you are allowing the acute diseases to possibly turn chronic. Bloating, headaches, etc., are signals that your body is filled with toxins or food allergies and needs *rest*.

12) If you are **hungry no matter what you eat,** you are most likely a carb addict, which makes an eating disorder very probable. Constant hunger is also a symptom of low blood sugar (hypoglycemia), which can eventually put you at risk for diabetes if you don't change your eating habits. Poor eating habits usually include choosing high-glycemic carbs, which furthers an unending hunger. Using food as your drug of choice when under stress also makes it harder to reach satiation. This stems from chemical imbalances, physically and mentally. Eating the right foods helps correct this. A healthy diet also helps correct your body's signals, so you can reach satisfaction and attain boundaries. You should also address the issues you may be eating over.

13) If you are **light-headed and lack energy** no matter what you eat, you may either have hypoglycemia or adrenal exhaustion. Hypoglycemia is usually due to poor eating habits. Adrenal exhaustion is usually from mental or physical stress (excess exercising or dieting). Continually choosing high glycemic index foods or foods that trigger the LDL level to rise may create a hypoglycemia reaction (insulin surge). Hypoglycemia and adrenal exhausting affect each other, resulting in an exhausted body. Rest without dieting is important. On the other hand, more activity for the sedentary individual seems to encourage circulation and help balance the body's chemicals and hormones. A good colon cleanse may help as well because the body has a priority system. Your body doesn't enter the fat-burning/muscle-building stage until you have digested and eliminated your meal. Heavy protein meals are stressful on the digestive track, leeching energy and minerals. A body full of toxins exhausts easily. If someone doesn't consume enough carbs while eating a protein diet, he or she will also experience a lack of energy. Constantly being lightheaded can mean a very low metabolism or extremely low blood pressure. Proper diet and exercise can usually help in this case. Weakness can also be a sign of anemia. Anemics mistakenly battle their symptoms by eating large amounts of red meat and taking too many iron supplements. Iron can cause constipation and in large amounts can be very toxic. It's best to derive your iron from clean food sources such as greens and black strap molasses. Rather than eating red meat, try green juice. The chlorophyll has a molecular structure similar to hemoglobin and is a good "blood-builder." Greens are filled with essential nutrients, such as vitamin C and P, which are also important in combating anemia. Sunshine is necessary for natural Vitamin D, which helps the calcium and magnesium absorption, enhancing energy. Foods that are easily assimilated give the body time to rest.

14) If you **get colds, allergies, and viral infections easily,** you have a suppressed or compromised immune system. A suppressed or compromised immune system can be a precursor to or symptom of a chronic disease. There is really no absolute "cure" for these symptoms; they sometimes can be referred to as acute. Other times, they're simply cleansing reactions or detoxing symptoms. Nevertheless, they are symptoms or warnings that your body needs rest and detoxification, before it develops a chronic disease. Some chronic diseases can

develop without any warning. A suppressed immune system usually accompanies candidiasis as well. Candidiasis is usually underestimated. Besides yeast infections, most allergies, rashes, itching, athlete's foot, and dry eyes are initial signs of candidiasis. Protein diets are usually suggested for candidiasis because candidiasis is a fungus in the lower intestine that is caused or provoked by sugar. In other words, almost every carb can aggravate or promote candidiasis. On the other hand, long-term protein diets imbalance the pH balance, making the body extremely acidic. This too can provoke candidiasis. Certain carbs that are low in sugar are best, like lemons and greens. The trick is to eat foods low in sugar but can also be able to rest the body. Meat is tiring on your digestive track. Candidiasis can develop into a serious health risk, like a fistula. Severe allergies can be life-threatening as well. There are various theories why there is a rise in children's allergies. Some claim our environment is too sterile because we are afraid of germs or catching viruses. Others claim we are a society that uses too many antibiotics and other drugs. This may be true, but I believe one of the major contributors to allergies is the ingredients in our food. Unnatural and unhealthy fillers are used because it is cheaper. It's hard to read labeling because ingredients are renamed in such a way that you don't recognize them. Natural and artificial flavors can be tricky because they may include all kinds of allergens. Most people are allergic to wheat (gluten) and lactose (milk sugar). This is because these are hard to digest for most of us. I have known people who have endured long, supervised fasts and then reintroduced the foods that they were allergic to, gradually. It worked like a vaccine. This seemed to work for them as long as they remained on a strictly raw diet. Allergies can also be a symptom of pesticide or environmental poisoning (like mold) or parasites within the body. Severe cases of allergies are usually treated with an antihistamine and epinephrine (adrenalin). Obviously this is not a cure, because many sufferers symptoms become worse as they age. Regardless of the cause or treatment, allergies can be deadly and have been known to cause behavioral changes. If you clean your diet up, you will have more energy so your body can fight or cope with these symptoms, hence building the immune system.

15) If you **constantly suffer from cold feet and cold hands** then you are probably dieting (not eating enough) or you have been a continual, chronic dieter. This poor circulation could be a symptom of a number of things. Usually this is a sign of adrenal exhaustion or hypothroidism Diets will only continue to exhaust your body. Adrenalin (epinephrine) is excreted in emergencies. Excess diet stress causes excess adrenalin or cortisol secretion, interfering with weight loss struggles. Eventually, your hormones may become depleted. Epinephrine helps allergies, blood sugar, the heart, and muscles. Cortisol helps with carb and protein metabolism. Cortisol is released at the beginning of the day so we can sleep at night. People under a lot of stress (such as dieters), eventually exhaust their adrenal glands and imbalance their hormones in the same way hypoglycemics may eventually exhaust their pancreas by the over secretion of insulin. Cold feet and hands is also a manifestation of EFA depletion. Essential fatty acids stimulate the mitochondria (cell's motor), which contributes to the thermogenesis of the body. Constantly experiencing cold feet and hands, diet or not, could be a sign of anemia as well. Sunshine helps circulation. Food sources like black strap molasses (iron) and greens (chlorophyll is the best blood-builder) are better than over-exhausting the body with too many supplements.

16) If you **constipate easily or constantly experience diarrhea,** that can be dangerous. Constipation is both the cause and effect of diseases. Almost 90 percent of Americans have a clogged colon. One of the best ways of determining someone's health (and what they eat), is the way they evacuate. Constipation is usually the sign of a poor diet, drug use, or is a precursor to a chronic disease. It can also be the cause of stress or the lack of exercise. Someone who is healthy, or eats well, evacuates at least once a day, preferable two to three times, or after each meal. Your bowel movements should be soft and light in color. You should *never* strain or "push" a bowel movement. Light and loose stools are the usually a sign of too much sugar and junk food. Very light stools are usually a sign of liver problems. Dark stools are usually the sign of too much protein. Heavy bowel movements are usually a sign of a body full of toxins. Light, floating bowel movements are a sign of too much fiber. Diarrhea is usually a sign of too much sugar. For instance, alcoholics suffer from diarrhea because of the sugar content. Constantly experiencing diarrhea is dangerous because it strips your intestines of friendly bacteria and robs your body of electrolytes, which can cause dehydration. High-fiber foods and Aloe vera is best. Occasionally diarrhea is also a side effect of a medication, a sign of allergies, parasites, exposure to a poison, or a precursor to a disease. When the body overheats (as with the flu), it ferments the food, which causes diarrhea. Constipation is the sign of an exhausted body, which is usually due to an illness, consuming too much protein or junk food, or drug use. I don't believe in symptom-chasing constipation, because it is a sign, not an illness itself. It is true that the buildup of toxins can create or contribute to a disease, but your body has to learn to evacuate naturally without relying on laxatives, colonics, or enemas. Remember the body has a priority system. It has to digest and then eliminate before it heals or loses weight. If you fluctuate between constipation and diarrhea, this could be from laxative abuse or the symptoms of IBS (irritable bowel syndrome). Drug users, alcoholics, or people with food disorders (especially bulimics) experience this problem. Because diarrhea or laxative and enema abuse eventually strips the lower intestine of its friendly bacteria, this vicious cycle (constipation/diarrhea) continues and encourages candidiasis. It's best to eat a diet mostly consisting of "broom foods" that sweep the intestines. Broom foods are usually complex carbohydrates or high-fiber foods. Fiber-less foods sit in the intestine, which causes weight gain and diseases. Complex carbohydrates such as vegetables, beans, and whole grains are your best remedy. Foods high in pectin such as cabbage, apples, and citrus fruits are helpful. Raw fruits and vegetables are best because of their added water content along with the fiber. If you don't drink enough liquids, that will cause constipation. Acidophilus, found in yogurt, is best for replenishing the lower intestine.

17) If you are **desire-less and easily depressed,** it is due to a chemical imbalance, physically and mentally. Usually depression initially stems from a nutrient or chemical depletion. Depression is a form of self-pity which can develop into a self-destructive behavior. Using symptom-chasers or drugs of choice perpetuates the depression cycle. Serotonin, the neurotransmitter responsible for our satisfaction, is triggered by tryptophan, which is abundantly found in carbs. The urgency to overload on carbs (usually the wrong kind) can cause a hypoglycemic reaction. Hypoglycemia, in turn, creates a need to supply the low-blood-sugar drop when eating the wrong foods again, furthering the cycle.

Endorphins, dopamine, norepinephrine, and other feel-good brain chemicals are excreted when we experience pleasure while eating junk food, much like using drugs. The withdrawals of junk food, just like drugs, also cause depression and may further create a hypoglycemia reaction. Moderate exercise is a depression remedy that has no ill side effects. During exercise, endorphins and other feel-good chemicals are released. An endorphin is a hormone excreted from the pituitary that causes the exerciser to feel "high" or "in love." However, too much exercise has been known to have the same depleting effect on the body as extreme dieting. Detoxing from a sugar binge causes depression as well. Depression may be an estrogen imbalance. Excess or depleted estrogen levels can cause depression and a low libido. The wrong foods stimulate estrogen imbalance. Balance is the key word here. Rather than using food or excess exercise to deal with depression, learn to confront your issues with good recovery assets like therapy or journals. Sunshine penetrates the pineal gland through the eyes and has been known to be the best remedy for long-term depression. A constant PMS feeling could be a lack of progesterone. There are healthy progesterone enhancers, such as wild yam and chaste berry. Exercise enhances the testosterone to help balance the estrogen and PMS depression.

18) If **diets stopped working for you,** then you have hit "diet bottom" and this may be a good sign to stop dieting. My "bottom" (pun intended) was HUGE before I realized that gimmicks don't work and quick fixes don't last. At this point your body has become diet savvy, learning every trick in the book. Your body is obviously fat efficient because diets don't teach your body to burn calories normally. Initially you may have to be willing to gain *some* weight before you lose any, so your body can trust that you won't diet anymore. Eventually your body will learn to burn fuel the way it should. Hopefully you are at the point that you realize it is not about the food or the diet. You simply have to learn which foods make your body work for you! Foods that are easily digested are then easily eliminated help balance your metabolism. Don't use outside fixes for inside jobs. All the energy wasted on searching for the right diet should be used for addressing the issues that you ate over.

19) If you are an **insomniac or have a hard time sleeping,** then you probably have adrenal exhaustion. This can be caused from the stress of excess dieting, excess exercising, or drug and stimulant use, like smoking and coffee (caffeine). When you are enduring a strict diet, the body has a hard time sleeping. You need very little sleep when you eat a diet of low calories and high quality, such as raw foods. Raw-food dieters only need approximately four to six hours of sleep a night because their food is "clean" and easily assimilated. Eating large protein meals wastes digestion energy, causing the body to tire easily. The live enzymes in raw food give a lighter energy, while sugar and meat react like stimulants, creating a false initial energy that eventually drains the body. Cortisol is released primarily in the morning, making it easier to sleep at night. However, excessive dieting and chronic pain creates stress. Excess stress causes excess cortisol to be released mostly in the evening, which disturbs sleep. Continuous stress eventually depletes the cortisol. This can then develop into adrenal exhaustion. Your body compensates and draws from unusual reserves, causing enervation. This will further sleep difficulty. Antidepressants usually disturb sleep patterns. Stimulants,

drugs, sugar, etc., all add to sleep problems that develop into adrenal exhaustion and enervation. Without starving, choose foods that help the body rest rather than eating a lot of meat or anything that uses too much energy to digest. Eating a big meal before sleep causes nightmares. The inability to sleep causes the aging process to escalate. Rest and sleep have been proven to be the best remedy for all health problems. Women who are unable to carry a pregnancy full-term are advised to get constant bed rest. It is claimed that pregnant women who don't get enough sleep endure harder and longer childbirths. Sleep is not the only way to receive rest. Being free from stress, stimulants, and junk food is also resting. Mental stress is far more draining than most physical stress. A twenty-minute nap between the hours of 10:00 AM and 2:00 PM is a good remedy. One hour of rest or meditation is equal to approximately one half hour of sleep. Sleeping during the day is always disturbed because it interferes with the body's rhythm. Melatonin, the "sleepy" hormone secreted by the pineal gland, is inhibited by sunlight. Good sleeping habits can be developed and reprogrammed as well. Here are some helpful sleep remedies.

A) Go to bed the same time every night.
B) Sleep between the hours of 10:00 PM and 8:00 AM.
C) Engage in anaerobic exercise, which releases HGH (Human Growth Hormone)to help sleep.
D) Meditate before going to bed.
E) Eat a light dinner three to four hours before bedtime.
F) Use the bed exclusively for sleeping rather than for reading or watching TV.
G) Try calcium rather than drugs or stimulants, or try melatonin *occasionally*.

20) If you **feel worse following your exercise routine,** then one of two things may be happening. You may either be suffering from adrenal exhaustion or you may be experiencing "exercise burnout." Either way, you need to rest. Adrenal exhaustion is caused by the continual excretion of excess cortisol. This eventually causes a cortisol depletion. Exercise burnout is usually from doing the same exercise or routine day after day. A body can grow tired of exercise redundancy in the same way food allergies can be caused by eating the same foods every day. Muscles need rest just as much as your mind. Boredom secretes the wrong chemicals and can sometimes hinder the effect the athlete is trying to achieve. Your body fights predictability. Shake up your routine and try fun and spontaneous exercises or sports. This will help your body release endorphins, causing a "high" and a catalyst for other feel-good chemicals to work synergistically. Most of all, take time off from extreme exercise. If you are an avid aerobic athlete, try anaerobic exercises with different muscle groups. Anaerobic exercise releases your HGH which is responsible for your rejuvenation and retains the muscle-building/fat-burning process. Don't ever exercise after a big meal. It takes about six hours to digest a large protein meal and twenty-four hours to burn off what you just ate. There is no such thing as "exercising off" the meal you just ate. You're actually burning off the previous dinner, twenty-four hours ago, while disrupting the dinner you just ate. Exercise one half hour before a light meal and at least three hours after a large meal. It's best to eat a light snack before any exercise and wait at least an hour before exercising. A junky meal before exercise will cause fatigue and a

possible hypoglycemic reaction (bloating). If you usually exercise in the morning, try evenings or vice versa. Exercise is supposed to help depression and make you feel energized. Otherwise, something is wrong.

21) If you **use any drugs, stimulants, over-the-counter remedies or diet aids,** you could be heading for adrenal exhaustion and a chemical depletion in your body. Our bodies can only recognize what we can digest. It has been claimed that items that cannot be digested (e.g. drugs) are *cloned* by our body in order to be recognized. The body does not perform properly while using a diet aid. Most people who use diet aids eventually gain back their weight and more. Whatever method you used for quick weight loss will be the very reason for regaining the weight back. It's simply biology. Naturally detoxing from any drug or stimulant, including coffee (caffeine), has been known to cause a hypoglycemic reaction, inducing fat reserves. Most female problems are usually related to the abuse of stimulants. Caffeine and diet sodas have been linked to bleeding fibroids. It has also been claimed women who smoke have a higher risk of breast, uterine, and ovarian cancer. Apparently women who smoke experience early menopause. Try to think of your skin as your "emergency organ." You can then realize why accelerated aging or wrinkling is the result of the damage we cause inside our bodies. This is especially true of smoking. So imagine what your insides look like. Stimulants cause your cortisol, estrogen, and insulin to work overtime. Excess amounts of these hormones make weight goals impossible. Eventually cortisol depletion may cause adrenal exhaustion. Estrogen depletion may cause early menopause, and insulin depletion may put you at risk for diabetes. There is a payback for every shortcut used and your health (weight) will be sacrificed. Antidepressants have been known to deplete your own serotonin (neurotransmitter that calms) and norepinephrine (a neurotransmitter that causes emotions and stress). Usually people need to change or raise the dosage of their medication because the body builds up a tolerance and eventually compensates for those unnatural hormone triggers. People using antidepressants or medication usually have problems with sleep. Perhaps this could be from the inappropriate release of cortisol in the evening. Or possibly the body may be secreting epinephrine (adrenalin) continuously, triggered by the drugs. Overmedicating yourself, regardless of the medication, can eventually contribute to chronic diseases such as diabetes. Incidentally most over-the-counter drugs such as asthma medicines, cold remedies, and diet aids, carry ephedra, which is a major cause of adrenal exhaustion and kidney problems. Other over-the-counter drugs carry large amounts of alcohol, which can cause female problems or sugar imbalance. Pseudoephedrine, usually used for colds, can cause difficulties for patients that suffer from diabetes, blood pressure, and heart problems. Adrenal exhaustion is usually heightened by the drugs you are using for their symptoms. This can move an acute symptom into a chronic disease such as kidney and liver malfunction. Drugs may have their purpose, but there is never any guarantee that there won't be side effects or paybacks. Nothing is free. You have to weigh the advantages and disadvantages. All stimulants and drugs are supposed to be used for temporary relief, which masks your symptoms without curing the real problem. **You can't buy health. You have to build it!**

QUIZ II: LIFESTYLE QUIZ
Description and Specially Designated Supplement Guide:

Read each lifestyle description. There is *one* lifestyle that best describes you. The lifestyle you choose is the description that seems to dictate or define your choices and circumstances more than any other. Don't pick the lifestyle you desire but rather the lifestyle that describes you and your circumstances and dominates your life. Below each lifestyle description and supplement guide, there is a color. This will be your second quiz and second color. Following this quiz is the third quiz, Body Type Quiz, which will assign a third color. All three of your colors will determine which food plan is best suited for you.

Which lifestyle description best describes you?
Simply circle the color below your description and exercise guide.
Check with your doctor or healthcare provider.

- ☒ Vegetarian?
- ☒ Yo-yo dieter?
- ☒ Highly active or athletic?
- ☒ Sedentary to moderate activity?
- ☒ Over-exhausted, in chronic pain, depressed, or very ill?
- ☒ Burdened with female problems? (PMS, fibroids, perimenopause, endometriosis, yeast infections, bloating, cramping, cycle irregularity, etc.)
- ☒ Overweight, obese, or morbidly obese?
- ☒ Anorexic, bulimic, or extremely underweight?

☒ <u>Vegetarians</u>: Vegetarians don't eat any animal meat. Vegans don't eat any animal products whatsoever. My sister and I respect vegetarians and vegans who eat this way because of concerns about animals (or spirituality). Carnivores eat meat. Herbivores eat plants. Omnivores have the ability to eat both. Theories state that, in the beginning of our evolution, we were strictly herbivores. Later, when our ancestors began to eat meat, our bodies adjusted. Back then we mostly ate a diet of nuts and berries and hunted for meat once in a while. Today's meat is not the same. We eat far too much meat and other types of protein. Although many claim the benefits of meat protein, there are the side effects as well. For instance, meat causes aggression and unnatural growth.

I think it's best for humans to eat a plant diet. There are a number of reasons. First, our teeth weren't made for ripping skin like carnivores'. Our saliva is alkaline, unlike a lion that has acid in its saliva in order to break down the meat immediately. Our body actually needs to train itself to produce hydrochloric acid, which helps digest meat. Unlike carnivores, we get sick at the sight of blood. We also develop ulcers from eating too much animal protein. Our large intestines are quite long, unlike carnivores', leaving meat to putrefy and ferment. It takes at least four to ten hours to digest a meat meal. Sometimes undigested protein is left behind in the intestine for weeks or months, which causes diseases. The growth of tumors is known to be stimulated by saturated fat, derived from animal protein. Red meat in particular contains phosphates (like in soda) that leech calcium. Usually chronic diseases and arthritis are linked to diets high in animal protein. Avid vegetarians, especially vegans, rarely encounter the same diseases heavy meat eaters suffer. Incidentally, it is usually recommended to patients suffering from heart disease, arthritis, or cancer to stay away from red meat. Our cattle (and other animals we eat) are affected by diseases that are passed on to people who eat them. Fish is not inspected properly and is affected by our polluted waters. Farm-raised fish ingest unnatural chemicals. Our animals bred for consumption are either fed unnatural diets they normally don't eat (like corn) for fast weight gain or their diets are pumped up with unnatural ingredients, additives, and hormones. They are also inhumanely placed in small living quarters without any room for movement so they can gain more weight in a short amount of time. Today, when an animal is slaughtered for consumption, it intuitively secretes dangerous "fear" hormones. When a human mother is under stress, she can unintentionally poison her baby by unconsciously secreting harmful substances while breast feeding. Just imagine what kind of hormones the poor animals secrete just before they are brutally slaughtered!

Vegetarians and vegans can derive enough protein from just about any live food. I have found that most of us only need 20 grams of protein every other day, compared to the recommended 50-60 grams per day. Carbohydrates are our true energy source and also contain some protein. Remember it's not the quantity but the quality. Since meat takes too much time and energy to digest, live food is better because it helps the body rest. This makes it easier for the body to find, extract, or make its own B vitamins, iron, and protein for energy. I have witnessed hygienics and fruitarians thrive on *live*, raw food only. They are much healthier, younger, and energetic than most people and are free from medical needs. Children who mostly eat a raw, plant diet are less hyperactive than when they eat foods that aren't in their natural state. People who practice meditation find it easier to lift their chakra level when they refrain from animal protein. For vegans, soy, nut mixtures, and mixing grains with legumes can make a complete protein. Serious vegans don't even use any topical or external animal products.

Unfortunately, most vegetarians and vegans don't eat right. They have the misconception that it is healthy to eat *anything* that doesn't contain animal products, including highly processed protein alternatives. Vegetarians and vegans usually eat far too many carbs and the wrongs ones as well. Any processed food with a lot of unnatural ingredients cause an insulin surge, much like sugar. Overcooking or freezing foods also imbalances your hormones and destroys any vital enzymes. Because vegetarian and vegan diets don't have the correct protein/fat content to block the insulin surge from the carb breakdown, they need to be extra careful about their portions, type of carbs and how often they eat them. It's better to eat pure foods with a lower protein content, such as nuts and avocados, rather than eat highly processed meat substitutes. "Grazing" on pure, whole foods keeps the blood sugar balanced. Everything you need can be supplied by being a strict vegetarian or vegan, but you shouldn't replace animal protein with junk food. Cholesterol problems and fatty production doesn't just come from animal fat. Refined carbs and high-glycemic foods (foods that shoot to the bloodstream faster), enhance the LDL more than most proteins. The good news is that a person eating raw food doesn't need to count fat grams. All the fats in a raw food diet are monounsaturated fats or essential fatty acids. When properly proportioned, the right fat can substitute for protein by blocking insulin. Vegetarians and vegans who mostly eat junk food or highly processed proteins struggle more with weight or edema than individuals who eat mostly animal protein. Vegetarianism is better than most diets, but vegetarians should be very diligent about the kinds of carbs they choose and how they eat them. Contrary to what is usually advised, meat isn't the best way of getting the best energy source, iron, or B vitamins. One of the biggest myths is that anemics need meat, particularly if they feel weak. Not true. Chlorophyll has a similar molecular structure as hemoglobin, making *greens* a better blood-builder. Anemia is also a symptom of a vitamin C deficiency.

Specially Designated Supplements: Sea greens are good protein substitutes (like spirulina) and loaded with the B vitamins, as black strap molasses, are high in iron. Brewer's yeast and bee pollen are an excellent source of energy. Other helpful supplements are B-12, B complex, L-Carnitine (converts stored body fat into energy), L-cysteine (blocks insulin), manganese, bilberry (insulin), copper (red blood cell), alfalfa (blood-builder), wheat germ (B's), barley, and wheatgrass (highest chlorophyll).

Circle this color if *vegetarian* is this is your description: GREEN

~ ~ ~ ~ ~ ~

☒ Yo-yo dieter: This dieter has gained and lost weight over and over for years. Welcome to my life! The yo-yo dieter's metabolism is very low, making it easy to get dizzy and light-headed, with a lack of energy. These symptoms, like those of the extreme athlete, are usually signs of adrenal exhaustion. Adrenaline is produced under excitement or fear. Cortisol is released gradually during the day and less at night, making it easier to sleep. During extreme stress, the adrenal glands, which fluctuate the blood sugar level, are overburdened. This imbalances the hormones, making it harder to lose weight and rest. This also causes bloating and mood swings.

Yo-yo dieters usually have low levels of serotonin and endorphins, which makes them turn to certain carbs or sweets. Most of the yo-yo's body chemicals are completely depleted. The yo-yo dieter might experience the same adrenal exhaustion as an athlete, but he or she doesn't have the athlete's high metabolism or muscle mass, which makes it more difficult to lose weight. When someone diets repeatedly, the body learns to become fat efficient. This happens when our bodies sacrifices vital tissue as a survival technique to save fat for the next starvation. Because the yo-yo dieter's hormones and reserves are usually depleted, the body sometimes leeches necessary minerals from other sources such as hair, teeth, and bones. The yo-yo dieter's set-point (where the weight is maintained, regardless) is usually high, making weight gain inevitable. The yo-yo dieter can develop malnutrition and severe food allergies from diet depletion (lack of food variety). In order for yo-yo dieters to overcome these symptoms, they have to reprogram their bodies to eat, without starving. This may initially cause temporary weight gain before the body learns to burn calories properly. Your body will eventually learn to "trust" that you won't diet anymore, which will give you the results you were seeking, without starvation.

Specially Designated Supplements: multi-vitamin/mineral, vitamin C, calcium, B6 (bloating), lecithin (fat emulsifier), sea greens (blood sugar), chromium (glucose metabolism), L-arginine (decreases body fat), CoQ10 (energy), choline and inositol (helps burn fat), zinc (helps immune and insulin), alfalfa, parsley, Aloe vera juice and acidophilus (digestion), ginger (circulation), B5, astragalus and licorice root (adrenal exhaustion), milk thistle (liver)

Circle this color if *yo-yo dieter* is your description: ORANGE

~ ~ ~ ~ ~ ~

☒ <u>Highly active or athletic</u>: Highly active individuals, particularly athletes, burn a lot of calories and need "clean" energy sources. Their dilemma is that they need fuel without unnecessary toxins that may create fatigue or lactic acid buildup in their muscles (cramping). They also need energy without enervation. The athlete can readily goes into ketosis, which may not be healthy. During ketosis, the body doesn't differentiate what reserve it draws from. So if you are burning more calories than you consume, particularly at a low body weight (fewer reserves), your body is going to sacrifice vital tissue. You can see this in extreme athletes. They look drawn and weathered, as if all the minerals have been drained from their faces. Athletes must constantly replenish their electrolytes (vital mineral compounds that maintain the body's fluid balance). A lot of athletes go through "burnout" stress or "hitting the wall." This is when they suffer from adrenal exhaustion or the opposite: excess cortisol secretions and hormone stress. Sometimes, their norepinephrine and epinephrine (hormones secreted by the adrenal medulla) become depleted, which furthers their exhaustion. Epinephrine helps increase muscle function and helps the blood sugar. Norepinephrine helps balance or regulate blood pressure. Cortisol helps with the carbohydrate and protein metabolism. Some athletes will fluctuate between dehydration and bloating because of the stress on their adrenal glands and endocrine system. Athletes get addicted to the endorphin rush (hormone "high" like morphine), making them push themselves beyond pain.

Doctors usually connect a loss of menstrual cycle to extreme exercise, though the exercise actually helps hormonal balance. Female athletes rarely encounter serious gynecological problems, including female cancer, unless they use steroids, stimulants, and a lot of sugar. If a woman is enervated, she may miss her period, usually because of her diet, not because of her exercise routine. When extreme female athletes complain about missing periods, usually they are depleted of essential fatty acids. When I suggest taking primrose, black currant, borage flaxseed, and fish oils, their periods return.

It is a mistake for athletes to supplement their diets with sugar aids or quick energy snacks without nourishment (empty calories). Far worse are athletes who supplement their routines with fuel aids, stimulants or steroids. Their bodies are already under so much stress that any unnatural stimulant or hormone will put their heart and adrenals under too much pressure. This is why some top athletes are in danger of very serious health problems, which usually begin with adrenal exhaustion. Bigger muscles don't make a better athlete. We are creating too much pressure for these "super-athletes." Society's pressure makes it acceptable to use unnatural means. This is why the athlete's diet and fitness program are their career. Clean carbs (raw) are the most important energy source. Too much meat or sugar can be tiring and makes the body acidic, creating bone fragility (arthritis), hair loss, slow healing, and other health problems.

Specially Designated Supplements: multi-vitamin/mineral, calcium and zinc (helps with cramping), B complex, B5 (stress), vitamin D (bones, heart, muscle), CoQ10 (antioxidant, cell circulation), sea-green and Siberian ginseng (energy), germanium (pain), phosphorus, magnesium and manganese (bones), sodium and potassium (water balance), alfalfa (inflammation), ginger (reduces cramps and spasms), glucosamine, MSM and chondroitin (joints), EFA oils (tissue repair)

Circle this color if *highly active or athlete* is your description: PURPLE

~ ~ ~ ~ ~ ~

☒ Sedentary to moderate activity: A sedentary individual is a person who resists exercise or movement at all costs. These individuals may not have a problem with weight, but they do have health problems due to poor circulation. Sedentary individuals are usually people who have lives that justify their resistance to activity. They *choose* a lifestyle that encompasses their preference for low activity. Usually these people have other addictions they are attending to, like smoking pot, which promotes their sedentary lifestyle. Activity does more than make us fit. It psychologically stimulates the brain for *desire* and *drive.* Sedentary people lack in desire but rely on stimulants for their drive. Exercise naturally raises endorphins ("high" like morphine) and other feel-good chemicals and hormones responsible for metabolism and mental stability.

I would never promote a food plan that enables a sedentary lifestyle, because the Physical Tools need both the food plan and the exercise program to work efficiently. When extremely overweight but active individuals are compared to thin, inactive individuals, the active, overweight individuals are usually healthier. Some diets claim that you don't need to exercise with the proper diet. Not true. My sister and I tried a "twin experiment." We compared ourselves to each other. The one of us who lost weight without exercise was compared to the twin who lost weight with exercise. The one who exercised kept the weight off longer. The one who didn't exercise lost muscle, not just fat. We always called the slim twin who didn't exercise the "fake thinny," because it was temporary weight loss. However, there are eating methods that make it easier for the body to assimilate food without having to burn off calories with movement. Raw food (live enzymes) is the best because it conserves energy that is then used for digestion, elimination, and burning fat.

Individuals who engage in moderate activity are usually people who don't have the time for exercise. These are usually individuals who complain about the "tire rim" around their midsection, even if they do exercise. When they eventually exercise (sometimes to an *extreme*), it will be on certain occasions. People who engage in moderate activity does not need to exercise hard. They need a "clean" diet and consistent activity. It's better to do twenty-minute workout daily rather than sweat for hours on certain occasions.

Specially Designed Supplements: black strap molasses (energy, iron), multi-vitamin/mineral, vitamin D(muscle, bones), B complex (energy), CoQ10 (energy, circulation), Manganese (raises metabolism), lecithin (energy, circulation), acidophilus and Aloe vera juice (digestion), chromium (glucose and metabolism), choline, inositol (helps burn fat), ginger (circulation), milk thistle (liver cleanser), licorice root (energy, blood sugar levels), garlic (lower blood pressure and good for heart), sea greens (for energy and balances blood sugar), cayenne pepper (circulation), DHEA (fatigue), bee pollen (energy, vitamin B)

Circle this color if *sedentary to moderate activity* is your description: BLUE

~ ~ ~ ~ ~ ~

☒ The over-exhausted, depressed, or for the individual that is very ill or has chronic pain: Most people in today's society are burdened with stress and "bite off more than they can chew." This can make someone tired, sick, achy, and very depressed. You have to target every angle of your life in order to "get your life back." It's important to manage your time, be introspective, and make lifestyle changes for your health before these symptoms turn chronic. Depression is a form of self-pity that can turn self-destructive. Depression is usually the result of an unhealthy body, mentally and physically. Instead of targeting the root of the problem, most people usually symptom-chase their exhausted, sick, and depressed body. Find out *why* you are tired, depressed or sick. Are you sleeping enough? Are you doing too much? Are you putting cheap fuel in the vehicle that runs your life? Are you constantly worrying about things you have no control over? There is a whole separate world of alternative medicine and health methods that most people never hear about. These practitioners treat the whole body and the root of the problem, without symptom chasers. They have a far greater success rate than most people realize. I had to diligently search and research this on my own, because society is into quick fixes and putting "Band Aids" on gapping wounds. The overwhelming recovery success rate of alternative medicine won me over. My sister and I now believe that conventional medicine is not the only option. It seems that most doctors symptom-chase by curing disease A by creating disease B. Alternative health methods are finally being revealed to the public, validating their success rate. In many cases proper diets have displayed better results than most drugs for many health problems, including mental illnesses like bipolar disorders, hyperactivity in kids, gynecological problems, fatigue, and many chronic illnesses. This also supports the conclusion that a poor diet agitates pain and illness and may be the cause of diseases as well.

Chronic pain, such as back pain, is more prevalent than ever. I believe it correlates to the weight gain epidemic our nation is experiencing. Usually muscle pain stems from or is heightened by the byproduct of lactic acid from sugar metabolism. (This is diet related.) Joint pain is usually from sugar leeching alkalis and leaving calcium deposits. Patients suffering from arthritis are usually recommended to eliminate sugar and red meat. Pain is a warning sign, not a sickness, but it can contribute to an illness. Symptoms include insomnia, depression, poor circulation, stiffness, moodiness, the possibility of becoming addicted to pain medication, or substance abuse. Continual pain, such as back injuries, causes scar tissue. The buildup of toxins (from a poor diet and drugs) and the absence of exercise worsens pain and builds scar tissue. Sugar, drugs (including pain medications), and a lot of red meat worsens these symptom cycles. A diet high in EFA oils and greens helps lubricate joints and detox the body. Excess cortisol is secreted when experiencing continuous pain. This also makes it hard to sleep and sometimes causes an urge to overindulge in junk food (insulin imbalance). Muscles help hold your skeletal structure in place, which lessens pain. That is why any exercise is better than none. Swimming and stretching are good low-impact activities for people with pain.

Feeding sugar, stimulants, or a lot of red meat to a tired, sick, or depressed body is the worst thing you can do. This causes the body to become acidic, which worsens bone fragility (arthritis) and health problems. There are many complications and restrictions when dealing with the over-exhausted or the very ill. This is because a suppressed immune system is left open to all other diseases. Ill people are in need of rest and yet they are the ones who have a difficult time sleeping. Burdening their bodies with more symptom-chasing drugs makes it worse. If you can't sleep, there is a reason. If you take something for insomnia, you are only addressing the warning sign of something worse going on. Insomnia in the sick or exhausted is usually caused by excess cortisol being released in the evening, rather than the early part of the day. Too much sugar, meat, and stimulants may cause excess insulin, cortisol, and estrogen to secrete. This creates edema, insomnia, depression, constant hunger, and weight issues. Eventually, the insulin surge (hypoglycemia) may develop into diabetes (insulin depletion). Cortisol and estrogen depletion eventually may cause adrenal exhaustion and early menopause. Most drugs initially cause a hyperglycemic reaction that then may develop into a hypoglycemic reaction. "Hyper" means high levels and "hypo" means low levels of blood sugar. Hypoglycemia causes high levels of insulin to secrete (the culprit of diseases) as well as mood swings, bloating, and weight gain. Low levels of serotonin trigger depression and make rest impossible. Sleep is one of the four times we secrete our natural human growth hormone (fat-burning/muscle-building process, rejuvenation). The other three times are during fasting and protein diets (ketosis) and anaerobic exercise. Kids who experience seizures are advised to eat a protein diet. It is believed the insulin that sometimes triggers seizures stays intact when eating a protein diet. This theory also claims the high level of ketosis caused by a protein diet "burns" foreign objects and residue because of the absence of carbs.

Using of drugs or too many supplements will cause the buildup of a tolerance and will act to exhaust a compromised or suppressed immune system. Most over-the-counter drugs such as asthma medicine, antihistamines, cold remedies, and sleep and diet aids contain ephedra or alcohol. This will compromise your endocrine system, particularly if you are female. Cold remedies that carry pseudoephedrine can cause problems for diabetics and patients who suffer blood pressure and heart difficulties. The stimulant or drug might have its advantages, but it may also cause severe adrenal exhaustion and potential kidney and liver malfunctions. The body recognizes everything as a either a food or a poison, including supplements. A tired body recognizes non-foods as foreign objects, which tires the body. When detoxing from drugs or stimulants, a hypoglycemic reaction can happen. This furthers the body's exhaustion, bloating, and anxiety and may trigger many other conditions, particularly while sleeping.

We are the only species that eats when it is sick. Many times the sick or tired person overeats in search of energy or to combat depression. This is someone symptom-chasing these feelings with food. It's not *what* we eat but what we *don't eat* that makes us well! Sick or tired people have low serotonin levels (hormone responsible for fulfillment and satisfaction). Other feel-good brain chemicals and hormones like dopamine and endorphins are also depleted, which creates a greater depression. This is when people turn to foods containing tryptophan (which triggers serotonin) or antidepressants. Antidepressants have been known to have an effect on the adrenals, liver, and immune system. Antidepressants are supposed to trigger the body's serotonin, norepinephrine, and/or epinephrine (adrenal hormones which cause stress/emotions). But eventually they also deplete your own chemicals and hormones, making the depressed and tired individual turn to such things as chocolate, carbs, or substance abuse.

Many depressed or exhausted people are anemic. You should not feed an exhausted body red meat. Instead, try healthy alternatives that give you energy without the tiring effects, like sunshine. Iron should come from food sources like blanched almonds or black strap molasses. Chlorophyll is a powerful blood-builder because it has similar molecular structure to hemoglobin. People who suffer from asthma or allergies (candidiasis) should try omitting dairy, meat, sugar, and usually wheat.

Most importantly, sick people should focus on foods that are easily assimilated and digested. Rest is the key. The body has a priority system. It first digests; then it eliminates, and only after that does your body heal and burn fat. A good colon cleanse frees excess energy used to digest foods that have fermented in the lower intestine. A tired or sick body cannot endure some fad diet, much less overeat. Raw food is usually the best medicine for sick or tired people because there isn't a better medicine than live enzymes. Most tired bodies have allergies. Common allergies are usually a form of candidiasis and are claimed to come from poor digestion and a low immune system, due to exhaustion. When the body is well-rested (detoxed), most allergies disappear. However, a tired or sick body is overwhelmed with excess insulin, the culprit of weight gain and exhaustion. This leaves the body wide open to more diseases. Severe cases of allergies are treated with epinephrine or antihistamines. This is not a cure because most sufferers' symptoms worsen as they age. Allergies have been said to be from our unnatural ingredients, which are confusing because of their misleading labeling. They are cheap fillers. Severe allergies have been linked to hot flashes, aggressive tantrums, or strange behavioral changes. I have known some sufferers who overcame their allergies by fasting long term and then gradually reintroducing the allergens into the body. This worked for them almost like a vaccine, as long as they continued eating a clean and raw-food diet. Some claim our environment is so "germ-phobic" in its excess use of antibiotics that it has created a sensitivity to foods and the environment. I think the rise in allergies proves that most people practice years of corrupted diets and poor eating habits that have created these new symptoms. We then pass these "symptom traits" onto our kids. The more we symptom-chase our tired or sick immune systems with drugs and stimulants, the more tired and sick we become. The drugs and stimulants only mask or numb the symptoms we take them for.

I believe a tired or sick body should be free from drugs and stimulants as much as possible to let the sophisticated body figure out what to do on its own. It's ridiculous to pretend to be a pharmacist to the body, because it is so complicated. What appears to be a deficiency can actually be an overabundance. Most people who take antacids for stomach problems don't realize they may have a lack of acid. Many times natural doctors recommend apple cider vinegar, which can help balance the stomach acid. When taking unnatural remedies, remember nothing is free from side effects or lasts forever. Weigh the advantages and disadvantages and research alternative methods. We think that we must use every drug or supplement to heal our bodies. On the contrary, when the body is clear and rested, it can usually create what it needs or heal on its own. Incidentally, mental work (stress) takes twice as much energy as physical activities. There's a fine line between treating a body and leaving it alone. You need to be completely detoxed in order to listen to your body's intuition.

Specially Designated Supplements: folic acid, black strap molasses (iron, calcium, magnesium), raw garlic (antibiotic effect, immune, blood cleanser), multi-vitamin/mineral, zinc, vitamin C, vitamin E, B complex, B5 (stress), fennel seed (digestion), ginseng (energy), ashwagandha (herb for adrenals), glucosamine, MSM and chondroitin (joints), cayenne pepper, lemon and milk thistle (liver, circulation), ginger (blood cleanser), kombucha (helps combat diseases) and green tea (high anti-oxidants), melatonin (body rhythm, rest) maitake mushroom (immune), lecithin (energy, liver), wheat germ and vitamin E, alfalfa (energy, digestion), chamomile (insomnia, stress), Irish moss, horsetail ((kidneys and bladder), red raspberry leaf (blood tonic), club moss (diuretic), chickweed herb (healing agent), echinacea and astragalus (immune), goldenseal and red clover (like antibiotic), gotu kola (depression), fennel seed (gas), apple pectin, ginger (bowels, candidiasis, nausea), kava kava (depression, urinary tract), licorice root (adrenal, depression), saw palmetto (stimulates appetite), skullcap (sleep), tea tree (gargle for colds, topical for sores, and candidiasis), Aloe vera juice and acidophilus (digestion, candidiasis), CoQ10 (anti-aging, cardiovascular), white willow (natural "aspirin"), St John's Wort (antiviral properties), ginkgo biloba and peppermint (depression), digestive enzymes and colon cleanser

Circle this color if *over-exhausted, depressed, or very ill* is your description: WHITE

~ ~ ~ ~ ~ ~

☒ Female problems—PMS, perimenopause, endometriosis, fibroids, bloat, cramping, yeast infections: Estrogen, the female hormone, is stored in fat. This is why females with gynecological problems usually have a hard time with weight. A surplus of estrogen and a deficiency of progesterone (which balances the estrogen) causes PMS, edema, painful cramping, weight gain, irregular cycles, and depression. Sometimes the hormone imbalance leads to other health issues such as endometriosis and fibroids, sometimes cancer. Excess estrogen triggers insulin spills (hypoglycemia), which causes bloating and irritability. (Lemon helps edema.) An estrogen surplus also creates unbearable food cravings. The blood sugar levels are imbalanced as well, because all the hormones work synergistically. How do women usually deal with these symptoms? By eating sweets or taking medicine. Women usually prefer chocolate for several reasons. Chocolate raises endorphin levels (reduces pain and induces positive emotions) and triggers serotonin (neurotransmitter and hormone that satisfies and calms). This can cause an addiction to sweets, which worsens gynecological problems. Certain sweets mimic or triggers excess estrogen, as do certain drugs. Meat, dairy, and eggs contain arachidonic acid (fatty acid eicosanoid precursor), which induces cramping pain and PMS.

Too much sugar or estrogen causes candidiasis. Gynecological problems and candidiasis go hand in hand. Candidiasis is a fungus in the lower intestine brought on or enhanced by sugar and/or antibiotics. It's also a sign of a very weak immune system and a precursor to a possible chronic disease. Women think candidiasis is simply a yeast infection and treat it by symptom-chasing it with popular over-the-counter medications or prescription drugs. The yeast infection is a warning sign that your immune system needs rest and your body needs a clean diet. Although protein diets are usually recommended for candidiasis, this can also offset the alkalinity of the body, making it too acidic. Acidity can agitate candidiasis and other health problems. Candidiasis can sometimes manifest as a rash, athlete's foot, dry eyes, itchiness, infection, irritations, or allergies. It can become as extreme as a fistula.

Estrogen excess has been the blame for the rise in endometriosis, fibroids, cycle irregularity, excessive bleeding, and some female cancers. Estrogen is abundant in some of our foods as well. For instance, products like soy carry phytoestrogens (plant estrogen). This plant estrogen is very good for you in moderation. Phytoestrogens can help women through menopause or bone loss when they experience a depletion of estrogen. During perimenopause, phytoestrogen in moderation can bind with your own excess estrogen and help balance it. There are also various toxic forms of estrogen that are formed artificially. These are very harmful to women and men. When you microwave something in plastic, harmful estrogen residue is excreted. Some claim smoking pot causes an unnatural estrogen surplus. All poisons and pesticides found in our food and water leave an estrogen-based residue, emasculating all male animal species as well.

Women rarely connect their problems with weight, bloating, depression, candidiasis, memory loss, or abdominal pain to their imbalanced hormones. This is why they simply continue to symptom-chase disease A and cause disease B. Incidentally, women athletes rarely encounter serious gynecological problems (with the exception of possibly missing "cycles" due to diet, stress, or stimulants). The testosterone levels are increased during exercise, helping the estrogen balance. Testosterone is responsible for an increased libido, which is the opposite effect when there is estrogen dominance. Taking synthetic hormones or steroids can put you at risk for serious gynecological complications or problems such as fibroids, tumors, or cancer.

A lot of women use birth control pills, which put the body into a state of fake pregnancy. This can eventually develop into early menopause. Smoking and other stimulants also cause early menopause. Women who eat a lot of sugar or use stimulants usually have severe perimenopausal symptoms. Symptoms of perimenopause can be experienced ten years before menopause. Perimenopause is the opposite of menopause. It happens when there is a surplus of estrogen in the body, which is one of the main culprits of cramping, bleeding, fibroids, and tumors. Continually secreting excess estrogen eventually develops into early menopause. Women who eat live, raw foods and don't rely on birth control pills continue their periods longer than most without harsh symptoms. They attribute their "disease-less" body and sound memory to the mere fact of maintaining their regular cycle. A woman's cycle helps release toxins as well. During perimenopause, if you want to help maintain your natural rhythm and original cycles, which ensures better health, try researching bioidentical hormones. Some are sold at various health food stores. Certain bioidentical hormones can help with some side effects of female problems as well. Osteoporosis is inevitable when there are gynecological problems, because of the estrogen imbalance, calcium loss, and vitamin B deficiency. Animal protein, such as red meat, carries phosphates that leech calcium. Calcium deficiency is the root of all diseases. Dairy products are not really your best source of calcium because of the difficulties they cause with digestion. Your best sources of calcium are from soy, leafy greens, blanched almonds, and black strap molasses. Fasting on fresh green juices with flax oil a few days prior to a painful cycle has been successful for many sufferers.

Specially Designated Supplements: lemon, calcium, vitamin E, B complex, primrose, black currant, borage and grapeseed oil (EFA), flaxseed, hempseed and fish oils (Omega 3), Don Quai, soy, phytoestrogen and black cohosh (estrogen), natural progesterone cream, chaste berry and wild Yam (progesterone precursors), B6 (bloating), sea greens (hormone balance), alfalfa (hormone balance), licorice root (both estrogen and progesterone, depression), Omega 3 (tissue healing), black strap molasses (calcium and iron), bioidentical hormones

Circle this color if *female problems* are your description: ORANGE

~ ~ ~ ~ ~ ~

☒ The overweight, obese, or morbidly obese: I've never known an extremely overweight person who took kindly to the term "obese," let alone "*fat.*" Rude or not, this is a serious condition. If you don't know if this term applies to you but you or others have questioned it, then you should confront it before your poor health confronts you. It's really difficult to put a real number on what true obesity is. People's bodies have different structures, genetic make-ups and proportions of muscle mass. Supposedly, anything 20 pounds under normal weight is underweight. *Overweight* is considered 20-25 pounds above normal weight. *Obese* is defined as 30 pounds or more over normal weight. Using body mass index (BMI), 25 pounds or above is considered overweight; 30 or higher is considered obese; and 40 or higher is extremely overweight. Someone who is 100 pounds overweight is considered morbidly obese. Compared to our weight gain epidemic, those numbers appear very low. Obviously, if your weight prevents you from living life like others, including breathing properly, then you are on your way to being obese. Exceptions aside, this extra weight is usually the cause of all your medical problems. Yes, some medical problems and medications cause weight gain, but the original problems usually originated from poor eating habits. You are most likely hypoglycemic or diabetic. Type II diabetes, once considered an "adult disease," is now prevalent among children as young as ten years old. This is usually diet related. Therefore, it can be corrected with early detection and diligent health choices. Obesity is usually a combination of genetic predisposition and learned behavior (poor choices). Regardless of the reason for the excess weight, obesity becomes a disease and the behavior associated with it is considered compulsive overeating. (This will be discussed further in Chapter Nine.)

For some overweight individuals, simple education and changing poor habits can help. However, compulsive overeating is not about the food. It's about the underlining issues: imbalanced hormones and missing chemicals (from a poor diet) that cause and continue a self-destructive lifestyle. The overeating and weight-gain cycle is hard to break because of the mental stress—feelings of hopelessness and isolation. Obese individuals have a food addiction much like a drug addict. For example, endorphins (hormones that react like morphine) are released when one overindulges. Dopamine (neurotransmitter that causes a"high" sensation) is released in anticipation of eating the food. Hormones like leptin and PYY336 give us signals that we are full. Both hormones are dormant or depleted in the overweight individual. (Leptin located in fat cells also helps increase energy.) On the other hand, obese individuals have an overabundance of the hormone ghrenlin, which signals hunger in the brain and sometimes tells the brain to supply the body with extra fat. There's a link between sleep deprivation and obesity. The hormone ghrenlin over secretes around 11:00 PM, giving way to "midnight munches." Other hormones, such as leptin, don't work properly when the body doesn't receive enough sleep.

Sleep deprivation causes cravings for salty and sugary foods as well. Serotonin comes from tryptophan and helps satiation. It is triggered by carbohydrates, like grains. Obese individuals turn to food in order to comfort their missing chemicals. Chocolate raises endorphin levels as well. When you are overweight, cortisol (the stress hormone) over-secretes, causing more weight gain. Obese individuals usually have a depleted level of norepinephrine (hormone in adrenals), which causes a lack of energy and desire as well. These symptoms cause the obese individual to return to the only behavioral pattern he or she knows: eating to numb the pain and escape shame.

The worst thing you can say to someone obese is to simply diet. As if that person didn't know! That makes him or her feel weak and ignorant, which is not the case. Most overweight individuals have struggled with weight since puberty. Once they started to starve (dieting), that promoted their binge habits. Starving causes fat efficiency, or easily clinging to fat. Once someone is overweight, the body retains that memory and every fat cell in the body is screaming for more food to fulfill that "blueprint." Like a drug, it takes more food each time to reach satiation. Eventually, there is no feeling of fulfillment, which causes a destructive behavioral pattern of eating until becoming sick or unconscious. Obese people lose control over their own behavior. Willpower has nothing to do with it. They need help. Diets are the worst remedy. That's the only time obese individuals develop a poor metabolism. If an obese person has rarely dieted, that person's metabolism is still in good shape. He or she will respond well to a diet of hearty meals, without any deprivation. Obese individuals should avoid trigger foods and trigger circumstances that will set off their compulsive behavior. They must reevaluate their relationship with food and stop using it like a drug. They need replacements for both binge foods and escape methods. There is always a replacement. Don't use outside fixes (diets) for an inside job (issues). Target your food plan with a recovery program. Gastric bypass and other surgical weight loss means are considered controversial. The risks are high and the guarantee is not one hundred percent. I know people who opted for the surgery and regained their weight. There is a 1 percent chance of complications, including death. There seems to be recent claims that hormone balance is restored, mysteriously, after the surgery. For instance, ghrenlin (appetite hormone) and PYY336 (hormone signal's you feel full) have been known to return to normal in patients who have undergone gastric bypass.

Specially Designated Supplements: vitamin C (metabolism), CoQ10 (energy), L-Glutamine (lessens carb craving), L-Carnitine (fat deposits), L-Phenylalanine (appetite suppressant), L-Tyrosine (antidepressant and less appetite), potassium (energy and sodium balance), fennel (removes fat, appetite suppressant), pectin (slows absorbing after meals-good for diabetes), guar gum (curb appetite), oat bran and rice bran (lowers cholesterol), psyllium seed (intestine cleaner), maitake mushroom and copper (diabetes), cayenne and Aloe vera (digestion), bilberry (insulin), juniper berries (diuretic, blood sugar), parsley (digestion, thyroid, bloating), red clover (appetite suppressant), garlic (lowers blood pressure, digestion)

Circle this color if *overweight or obesity* is your description: RED

~ ~ ~ ~ ~ ~

☒ Anorexia, bulimia, or severely underweight: These individuals are much like the exhausted and very ill individuals because they are so depleted of vital nutrients. Unlike the exhausted and very ill, who need to rest their digestive tracts, the anorexic and bulimic must become accustomed to eating food consistently. The brain chemicals are misguided and the hormones are imbalanced. Although I always emphasize that it's not about the food or the numbers on the scale, a food plan is necessary to help take the obsession away and to replenish the missing chemicals that trigger the disease. The worse thing you can tell anorexics and bulimics is they need to gain weight in order to get well. Those are the wrong words. (Further details are Chapter Nine.) Incidentally, it is impossible to gain excess weight if you eat healthy. The object is to obtain a healthy body so it can function properly. This creates less stress, mentally and physically. Their fear of fat isn't real. The fat and body misperception is caused by imbalanced chemicals in the brain, sometimes triggered by certain foods or the lack of food. Usually anorexics have an abundance of serotonin, which creates anxiety about food. Bulimics usually have a hormone imbalance as well, such a lack of CCK, a hormone that signals fulfillment. I would tell someone who wants to gain weight the same thing I would tell someone who wants to lose weight: Use a food plan that allows the body weight to adjust organically. Anaerobic exercise is better than eating junk food, for someone who wants to gain weight. Junk food causes flabby tissue or cellulite, even without weight gain. Someone considered underweight is 20 pounds or more below normal weight. Hollywood makes being underweight seem the norm. If you are naturally underweight without drugs or starving, then your health is usually good to above normal. If you have a sudden and enormous amount of weight loss, that is a health concern. It is sometimes the symptom of parasites or poisoning, a precursor to a serious disease, or a sign of an eating disorder.

Specially Designated Supplements: brewers yeast, bee pollen, EFA oils, flax seed, primrose, black current, borage, fish oil, folic acid, black strap molasses (iron, calcium, magnesium),sea greens (B source and helps blood sugar), raw garlic (antibiotic effect, boosts immune, blood cleanser), multi-vitamin/mineral, zinc, vitamin C, vitamin E, B complex, B12 (increases appetite, helps hair growth and quality), B5 (stress), fennel seed (digestion), lecithin (energy, liver), wheat germ and alfalfa (energy, digestion), chamomile (insomnia/stress), Irish moss, horsetail (kidneys and bladder), red raspberry leaf (blood tonic), chickweed (healing agent), echinacea and astragalus (immune), goldenseal and red clover (like antibiotic), skullcap (sleep), tea tree (gargle for colds, topical for sores, and candidiasis), Aloe vera juice and acidophilus (digestion, candidiasis), CoQ10 (anti-aging, cardiovascular), St John's Wort (antiviral properties), ginger root, and peppermint (appetite stimulants), bioidentical hormones.

Circle this color if *anorexia, bulimia, or severely underweight* is your description: BLUE

~ ~ ~ ~ ~ ~

✋ Please note that certain supplements may cancel another supplement's effect—or worse, interfere with your medication. Always check with your healthcare provider no matter how natural or innocent a supplement may appear. In addition, I do not endorse taking mega amounts of supplements. In some instances, herbs have had some questionable results. At one time my refrigerator looked like aisle seven at the health food store. My hope was to replenish ALL depleted nutrients with 5,000 supplements, hoping that would cure my FAT. It only complicated my health and left me with expensive urine. If needed, some of these supplements (below the lifestyle description) may work well under certain circumstances. Hygienics or raw-food dieters do well without any supplements. Though I try not to repeat anything daily, my standard supplements are:

Garlic, cayenne pepper, lemon, garlic, sea greens (chlorella, kelp, spirulina), flaxseed, green tea, Aloe vera juice, tea tree oil, and barley grass.

Quiz III: BODY TYPE QUIZ:

What body type are you?

What workout and sport is best for your body type?

My sister Shane and I were supposedly born with an ectomorphic body structure: tall and thin. (It's been so long we barely remember). However, years of yo-yo dieting made us fluctuate between mesomorphic and endomorphic. There were brief moments that we were ectomorphs (for a five-minute photo shoot), but we would binge right back into our usual "endo-meso" body type. Motivational techniques (such as Mental Tools) were helpful. They helped us learn to accept our bodies' transition, instead of trying to starve our way back to an ectomorphic body type.

There are basically three types of body structures. Some individuals may fit exactly into one of the three; others might be a crossover combination of two or all three of the body types. Most people are prone to *one* body type with several attributes of another. The three major body types are endomorphic, mesomorphic, and ectomorphic. Realizing your body type makes it easy to achieve a healthy set point as well as your weight goal. The preferred exercise guide is below each body type. After deciding which body type best describes you, circle the color below your body type description. This will be the third color you have chosen and the last of the three Physical Tools Quizzes. When you finish with this quiz, continue to the next chapter, Chapter Four: Eco Anti-Diets, to determine your food plan. Your three colors will help you decide which food plan (Eco Anti-Diet), is best suited for you according to your colors.

Circle the color below the body type (and exercise guide) that best describes your structure.

☝ *Check with your doctor or healthcare provider.*

1) <u>Endomorphic</u> is a body type that basically has a heavy body structure. Usually endomorphs are short and stocky, sometimes curvy. Their bone structure is usually "thick." More times than not, they have slower metabolisms and a lack of energy. They tend to gain weight easily and in the shape of an apple. The weight gain is usually on the inside near their vital organs, which usually means poor insulin balance or response. Because of this, they have more weight-related diseases than the other two body types. Their problems with weight usually begin at puberty or younger. Endomorphs blame their family disease history because they think it's all about genes. They usually accept their body structure but continue poor eating habits. It is a mistake for endomorphs to desire an ectomorphic body type. Their genetic make-up will fight this goal. In the process, endomorphs gain more weight from their diet failures and become fat efficient through unrealistic diet habits.

Endomorphs are usually people who overeat or starve. Normal eating habits are not the norm. Endomorphs can be very healthy and fit if they follow a healthy lifestyle. Competing with ectomorphs will further the cycle of starving and bingeing. Diet deprivation is the worst thing an endomorph can do. This will cause the body to bounce back to its set point, plus gain more weight following every diet to compensate for starving.

Workout and sport preference: Endomorphs would do best with both anaerobic (without breath) and aerobic (with breath) exercises. The aerobic exercises enhance the fat-burning/muscle-building process. The anaerobic exercise focuses on muscle mass, which raises the metabolism. Anaerobic exercises release the CCK hormone which makes you feel full. It also releases HGH, which also triggers the fat-burning/muscle-building process. Endomorphs who hit a plateau need to switch exercises and shake up their routines. Try aerobic exercise one day and hardcore resistance training the next. Our muscles have a memory. Just as our bodies can learn to out-trick an unvaried diet, our bodies can also grow tired of the same exercise day after day. A lot of trainers prefer resting a muscle group for twenty-four hours. This is why trainers prefer switching exercise programs and target specific body areas on alternated days. Good examples of sports for endomorphs are cross-country skiing, power walking, and stair climbing.

Circle this color if an *endomorphic body type* best describes you: RED

~ ~ ~ ~ ~ ~

2) Mesomorphic is a body type that is basically somewhere between endomorphic and ectomorphic. *Meso* is borrowed from the Greek language, pertaining to "the middle." Of the three body types, mesomorphs tend to be more athletic. A mesomorphic body type will often be of a medium build and medium height and will usually have a muscular frame, more often than not. Mesomorphs can be considered "thick," but are not fat. They are usually athletically inclined and appear sturdy. Mesomorphs gain weight easier than ectomorphs, but not as easily as the endomorphs. They gain weight on the outside of their bodies, such as the hips and thighs, or gain it evenly, unlike the endomorphs. Their weight gain could possibly appear pear-shaped or be evenly distributed, hence thick. Because mesomorphs usually retain good muscle mass, their metabolisms are higher than the endomorphs. Mesomorphs' insulin response can go either way. Mesomorphs can eat large meals without worrying, if eating proper foods. The mesomorphs who are prone to eat high-glycemic foods (foods that shoot to the bloodstream too fast), refined carbohydrates, trans-fatty acids, or foods that trigger LDL tend to struggle with weight gain, no matter how active they are. This is when a mesomorph can become bulky; muscle is built beneath their fat.

Workout and sport preference: *Mesomorphs do best with aerobic exercises or certain anaerobic exercises such as sprinting. Keep in mind that some claim anaerobic exercises use up your reserves before you burn fat. That is why aerobic is very important to achieve a lean, well-defined body. Again, mesomorphs will never achieve (nor should they try to achieve) an ectomorphic body type. When mesomorphs starve below their set point (their normal weight point), I consider this a "fake skinny" because it will be impossible to maintain. Mesomorphs regain lost weight (and more) when they return to normal eating. Good examples of sport exercises for mesopmorphs are court sports, bicycle racing, or mountain biking and sprinting stairs.*

Circle this color if an *extremely muscular mesomorphic body type* best describes you: GREEN

Circle this color if a *soft mesomorphic body type* best describes you: ORANGE

~ ~ ~ ~ ~ ~

3) <u>Ectomorphic</u> is a body type that is basically a slim body structure. Ectomorphs are usually tall with a small-to-medium bone structure and a good or high metabolism. They usually have a healthy insulin balance or response (the ability break down carbohydrates). Ectomorphs don't gain weight easily and they don't have much of an appetite. Ectomorphs sometimes complain that they need to gain weight. This may sound cruel to someone who struggles with weight gain, but it can be just as frustrating. Ectomorphs' health and genetic health history are usually fair to good. In some cases, ectomorphs can transfer into another body type if they continuously practice poor eating habits. This will cause excess insulin spills, which makes weight gain inevitable. Usually ectomorphs graze continuously and eat what they want. If someone is thin because of starvation, that doesn't make that person ectomorphic. Starving is temporary weight loss. An ectomorphic body type is naturally thin. You can usually identify an ectomorph by a small wrist and long fingers. When ectomorphs gain weight, they have the luxury of relying on their genetic memory, which makes weight loss easy, returning them to their normal body weight in no time. There are exceptions. Some ectomorphs who are entering perimenopause or are dealing with post-pregnancy or gynecological problems can suddenly gain weight. However, most ectomorphs struggle to gain weight. When they do gain weight, it seems to be mostly in their midsection. Ectomorphs who eat junk food to gain weight are usually the ones with a "spare tire" around their waist area or cellulite. This is because poor food choices make poor tissue quality. Junk food is never distributed evenly throughout the body. Cellulite may have nothing to do with excess weight. It's usually the result of poor tissue quality (and circulation) from food toxins and substances (such as stimulants).

An ectomorph's diet should be as healthy as the other two body types. Just because you are thin does not mean you have a "free ticket" to poor health choices. When health is the goal, the weight will naturally adjust to what it is supposed to be. Overeating or eating fatting foods creates flabby tissue or sometimes weight loss, especially when you are sickly. Unhealthy, slim bodies can't gain weight in the same way an unhealthy overweight body can't lose weight. Gaining weight is a normal or "allergic" symptom to poor health choices and habits. If someone has very poor health habits and remains slim, other symptoms of poor health will manifest (such dental problems, hair loss, skin eruptions, frail nails, or problems with the vital organs). Continual poor health choices will not go unseen. It's best to target your overall health.

Workout and sport preference: Ectomorphs do well with anaerobic exercises, particularly isometrics and weight training. Anaerobic exercises release human growth hormones, helping them sleep and build muscle tissue. Exercise (with a healthy food plan) is the proper way of gaining weight (clean tissue). Good examples of sport exercises for ectomorphs are resistance training, yoga, and stretching classes.

Circle this color if a *muscular ectomorphic body type* best describes you: PURPLE

Circle this color if an *underweight or soft ectomorphic body type* best describes you: BLUE

☞ *Exercise options for all body types:*
(Chapter Ten: Barbicise)

CHAPTER 4:
THE ECO ANTI-DIETS

Which came first: the diet or the binge? Don't know; I ate them both.

The Eco Anti-Diet is a food plan that is NOT a diet. A diet is a fixed food plan (one-size-fits-all) that consists of some form of deprivation and depletion. It usually includes a gimmick, fix, or shortcut that eventually backfires. Diets make you *fat* because they don't teach you or your body how to eat. Eventually, diets make your body fat efficient, which means you gain more weight faster and easier than when you began. Do you notice that thin people are always eating and never diet? This is because continuous "grazing" raises the metabolism. The body's vital chemicals and hormones are disturbed—even destroyed—through depleting diets. Starving lowers the metabolism and blood sugar, creating an insatiable urge to binge and sabotage the diet. If you don't eat enough food or sufficient nutrients, your body will shut down, age, and refuse to lose weight. Our bodies are meant to eat. Normally, we should be satisfied and eat a variety of foods.

A *food plan*, unlike a diet, is able to adjust according to your health, preference, and circumstances. Your Eco Anti-Diet food plan is a food plan that is ecologically friendly (mostly raw, live food without animal meat) and made specifically for you and your situation. Eco Anti-Diets may not be the same from one month to the next. The Eco Anti-Diet food plans also include allowed/disallowed treats to prevent depravation. If you are unable to completely refrain from animal meat or sugar, these treats allow you to wean yourself off them slowly. The Eco Anti-Diets are a simple guideline that doesn't include symptom-chasing (focusing on weight only). HEALTH is the goal. This will enable your body to be in top, efficient shape chemically and hormonally so it can utilize, eliminate, and *burn* the food the way it should. Eco Anti-Diets are rejuvenating and, therefore, anti-aging. Automatically, your byproduct will be weight loss and looking younger. It's important to commit to your Eco Anti-Diet, because it takes the *control, guesswork, and obsession* out of our daily activities. This means there is FREEDOM when you commit to these simple steps and hope that you'll achieve your goal: *health*, which creates the by-product of a beautiful and fit body.

Goal (health) = Byproduct (beauty and fitness)

There is no calorie or fat-gram counting with any of the Eco Anti-Diets. Instead, "intuitive portion rationing" is used because every person has a different appetite at different times. Low calories create a low metabolism and therefore a fat-efficient body. A calorie is not a calorie. A calorie in the laboratory is not the same as a calorie ingested. Substances that contain *no* calories can cause insulin over-secretion, which creates further weight loss difficulties. "No-fat" diets create extreme hunger and an insulin overflow, which sabotages your diet and weight loss. Your foods cause hormone and chemical reactions in your body. Fat has many purposes; it satiates our appetite, triggers vital hormones (that boost metabolism), and blocks insulin. The fats advised in these Eco Anti-Diets (monounsaturated and essential fatty acids) actually lower or replace the "bad" fats (LDL) and raise the "good" fats (HDL). Certain fats are essential for our bodies' thermogenesis. Our bodies are dictated by hormones, unlike a Petri dish. That is why I stress health as your goal, not the diet or weight loss. The byproduct will be the weight loss if you make sure the foods you eat will help—not harm—your body's hormone levels and chemical reactions.

These are the seven separate Eco Anti-Diet food plans. Your food plan is determined by the three colors you obtained from your three quizzes (21 Questions, Lifestyle Quiz, and Body Type Quiz).

<u>DIRECTIONS</u>: HOW TO DETERMINE WHICH ECO-ANTI DIET (food plan) IS BEST FOR YOU:

1) Gather all three colors suggested for you according to your quizzes (21 Questions, Lifestyle Quiz, and Body Type Quiz). Each color correlates to a specific Eco Anti-Diet. The combination of all three of your colors will give you *your very own* Eco Anti-Diet. Your Eco Anti-Diet is the one best suited for you according to all three of your quizzes.

2) Write one X per color that was suggested for you under the column that matches your color. You should have three X's under the three colors suggested from your previous quizzes. You will have a total of three X's, one per color.

3) At the bottom of the color columns is a "total" for your colors. Look at your X's for each color column. If you have two or more X's for one color total, *that is your custom made color.*

4) If you have three different X's (in three different color columns) and no majority, your color will automatically be WHITE.

Example I:
*Cindy chose PURPLE for her 21 Questions (answered **Yes** to 14 of the questions, which means fairly poor health),*
chose ORANGE for her Lifestyle Quiz (yo-yo dieter), and
chose ORANGE for her Body Type Quiz (mesomorphic, soft).

QUIZZES:	RED	BLUE	YELLOW	PURPLE	ORANGE	GREEN	WHITE
21 Questions:				X			
Lifestyle Quiz:					X		
Body Type Quiz:					X		
Total:				1	2		

Cindy's Total has 1 PURPLE and 2 ORANGES. ORANGE is the only color repeated.
Cindy's custom-made color is ORANGE because ORANGE has the majority of X's (two or more) in her total.

Example II:
Tom chose GREEN for his 21 Questions,
chose BLUE for his Lifestyle Quiz, and
chose PURPLE for his Body Type Quiz.

QUIZZES:	RED	BLUE	YELLOW	PURPLE	ORANGE	GREEN	WHITE
21 Questions:						X	
Lifestyle Quiz:		X					
Body Type Quiz:				X			
Total:		1		1		1	

Tom's Total has: 1 BLUE, 1 PURPLE, and 1 GREEN. Because he has three different X's for his total (or three different colors), he is automatically the color WHITE. Anyone who has three different X's (in three different color columns) and no majority will automatically be WHITE.

Mark Your Own Color Chart:

Quizzes:	RED	BLUE	YELLOW	PURPLE	ORANGE	GREEN	WHITE
21 Questions:							
Lifestyle Def:							
Body Type:							
Total:							

Your total has a majority (two or more) X's of _____ color.
This makes your color _____ , which is your own custom-made color.
   —OR—
Your total has three different X's (in three different color columns) with no majority. Automatically, you are **WHITE,** which is your custom-made color.

YOUR CUSTOM-MADE FOOD PLAN

ECO ANTI-DIETS: These are the seven Eco Anti-Diet food plans choices.

Find your custom-made color below. Right beside your color is your own Eco Anti-Diet.
The color doesn't have any hidden message.
The only object of the color is to direct you to your own Eco Anti-Diet.

✦ RED   **Eco Anti-Diet 1**: *The Curb–Carb Corrector*
✦ BLUE   **Eco Anti-Diet 2**: *The Veg Metabolizer*
✦ YELLOW   **Eco Anti-Diet 3**: *The Garden Tonic*
✦ PURPLE   **Eco Anti-Diet 4**: *The Switch 'n' Twist*
✦ ORANGE   **Eco Anti-Diet 5**: *The Rock 'n' Rotate*
✦ GREEN   **Eco Anti-Diet 6**: *The Appetite Alternator*
✦ WHITE   **Eco Anti-Diet 7**: *The Trio Mix*

✦   **ECO ANTI-DIET 1: The Curb-Carb Corrector** *(Red)*

The Curb-Carb Corrector is a food plan that consists of three meals and two snacks. Eco Anti-Diet 1 is best for people who have an imbalance of insulin from diet abuse or ongoing protein diets. All protein diets rely on the gimmick to use protein, not carbs, for energy, thus creating a low insulin secretion. Insulin secretes during the breakdown of *carbohydrates*. Food plans with little or no carbs create a lazy or dormant pancreas, further impairing the process of carb breakdown. Dieters who use these food plans, particularly extreme dieters, have poor insulin response or balance. This creates a poor reaction to foods with a high glycemic index (foods that raise the blood sugar at a fast rate, affecting the insulin balance). These dieters may also experience hypoglycemic episodes (edema, moodiness, constant hunger, easy weight gain) when they introduce *regular* carbohydrates back in their diets. High-protein diets are toxic, aging, and unnatural. We are meant to eat a variety of carbohydrates—mostly complex carbohydrates (fruits, vegetables, and whole grains and beans). Eco Anti-Diet 1 helps keep the insulin secretion in tact, while slowly incorporating carbs back into the diet. Although Eco Anti-Diet-1 is higher in protein, you should focus on omitting or at least limiting animal meat. Your goal is to train your body to burn "clean" energy from carbs, not meat, which rejuvenates your body. You should let the body *learn* to use carbs the way we are meant to: as energy (to burn calories). It's very important to drink a lot of water on any diet that limits or omits carbs. It is recommended to *drink eight eight-ounce glasses of water per day* two hours after a meal and one half hour before a meal. Keep in mind water can have a diuretic affect (just like meat).

Try squeezing a little lemon into your water. The lemon's minerals will help retain the electrolytes and replenish your body. A squeeze of orange changes the molecular structure of the water, so it is a little more "soft" or "clean." It is the *natural* sodium in fruits and vegetable that helps plump up skin so it appears rejuvenated.

Pick one out of each category

Breakfast Choices
Protein: 4-8 oz. low-fat dairy yogurt, eggs—1 yolk and 2 whites, protein powder (preferably whey) or 4-6 oz. tofu
Fat: 2-4 oz. nuts/seeds, 2 Tbsp. flaxseed oil or EFA oil, sunflower seeds, almonds, nut-butter, or hempseed (high EFA)
Fruit: handful of berries, 1/3 melon, 1/2 grapefruit or apple

Snack
Protein: 1-4 oz. low-fat dairy, 2-4 oz. tofu, or protein powder (preferably whey)
Fat: nuts, 2 oz. seeds, 1/3 or avocado
Fruit: berries, plum or apple

Lunch Choices
Protein: 4-6 oz. tuna substitute, chicken/turkey substitute, tofu or rice protein
Fat: 2-3 oz. seeds, 1/2 avocado 3 Tbsp. or oil (monounsaturated like olive oil).
Vegetable/Fruit: 2 cups steamed vegetable such as broccoli, cauliflower, mushrooms, zucchini; vegetable salad including all greens, onions, tomatoes (w/o carrots, peas, or corn); or fruit salad including melon, apples, berries, and cherries

Snack
Protein: 1-4 oz. low-fat dairy, 2-4 oz. tofu or rice products, or protein powder (preferably whey)
Fat: nuts, seeds (2oz), or avocado (1/3)
Vegetable/Fruit: berries/green apple or vegetable slices (no carrots)

Dinner Choices
Protein: fish substitute, chicken/turkey substitute, 4-6 oz. tofu or rice protein
Fat: 2-4 Tbsp. monounsaturated oil, 1/2 avocado, or 1-2 oz. sliced olives
Vegetable: 2 cups steamed vegetables (w/o corn, peas, carrots) or a large salad (w/o carrots)

Notes

1) Eliminate sugar and high-glycemic carbs. It will take at least 4-10 days for your body to acclimate to a "low insulin zone." It takes 21 days to excrete sugar out of your system. Sugar is addictive and is linked to pain, arthritis, scar tissue, infections, and slow healing. Continue this menu until you lose any edema effect and carb cravings. This way of eating can help prevent possible hypoglycemic reactions. After 21 days, slowly incorporate all varieties of fresh fruits and vegetables.

2) Consume no pasta or flour. Your grains and breads can be included gradually after 3-4 weeks. Only eat whole grains (slow cooking) or sprouted breads such as sprouted sweet bread or whole, multi-grain breads.

3) Use "broom foods." These are foods with fiber that "sweep" your system (especially live, raw food, such as fresh fruit and vegetables).

4) Don't weigh or measure your meals after 21 days. Use "portion intuition," using the palm of your hand for each serving size. Use your palm to create three different portions: one protein and two carbs. Don't have more than three different foods on your plate.

5) It is preferred to have meat or fish substitutes rather than any animal meat. It's best not to have more than one high-protein serving per meal. Your proteins can vary as well. For instance, instead of tofu there is tempeh. Fish is supposed to be "magical" because of the essential fatty acid, Omega 3. Flaxseed, walnuts, and EFA supplements are a better form of Omega 3. Apparently there is the fish controversy about mercury content and poor fish inspection and regulation. Our polluted waters are a proven problem. If you feel the need to choose fish, limit fish high in mercury, such as tuna or shark. Shellfish (filter feeders) are common sources of food poisoning. Wild fish such as salmon (from Alaska or Montana) is better than farm-raised fish. It's preferable to eat no more than 9-12 oz. per week. There are better protein alternatives. Regardless, make sure the protein content is close to the carb-gram count. If you insist on animal meat being your source of protein, eliminate red meat altogether and supplement your meals with digestive enzymes and a colon cleanse every few months to help aid the heavy digestion. Eventually wean yourself off of all animal meat so you can achieve optimum health and cleaner calorie usage.

6) All low carb/protein diets create a lack of energy. Make sure the few carbs you do have are mostly raw, fresh fruit and vegetables, as opposed to the "zero-carb-zero-nutrient" snacks. The live enzymes will give you the lift you need.

7) Do not use stimulants. You are already putting extra strain your digestive tract by eating heavy protein, particularly animal protein.

✦ **ECO ANTI-DIET 2: The Veg Metabolizer** *(Blue)*

The Veg Metabolizer is a food plan that focuses on *balancing* important hormones and *restoring* critical brain chemicals. This is done by the frequency and portions of the food plan. This diet is best for vegans or people who want vary their nutrient sources. Protein should be primarily plant-derived (without animal products), so the body can be clear of toxins and heavy digestion. It is better to have a lower protein content that is whole and pure, like from nuts and avocados, than highly processed protein alternatives. Instead of relying on a high protein content to block the insulin of the carb breakdown, the Veg Metabolizer's "grazing" techniques (small mini-meals throughout the day) will help maintain the metabolism and insulin balance. Many experts have claimed that our bodies have never changed since the caveman days. Our ancestors would "graze" in the summers, never leaving more than three hours apart between meals. In the winters, their bodies automatically knew to store fat because of the sparse food. Our bodies eventually learned to save, store, and make fat by secreting extra insulin (for every sparse meal) when we didn't graze within three hours. It's the same today. If you eat large meals more than three hours apart (protein or not), your body switches into "winter mode." This usually creates extra insulin secretion for the next meal, allowing the body to make fat easier. The Veg Metabolizer plan teaches your body to be able to eat *a lot* of calories without gaining weight by using the "grazing" technique our bodies have always known. This also keeps the muscle-building/fat-burning process in tact.

To make a complete protein you:
✓ combine beans with: brown rice, corn, nuts, seeds, or wheat
✓ or mix brown rice with: beans, nuts, seeds, or wheat
✓ or cornmeal fortified with the amino acid L-lysine

Protein and alternatives: It is usually recommended to have 50-60 grams of protein a day. It has been debated and proven that we can survive on 20 grams every other day or less! Protein is derived from many sources other than animals. Instead of meat try soy, rice, wheat, nuts, or "complete protein" combinations like grains with beans. Select from a variety of different proteins. The body needs variety in order to obtain all the vitamins and minerals needed.

Carbohydrates: Try choosing fruits and vegetables before incorporating breads and grains for the initial three weeks. Always select fruits that are in season (in the front of the produce section). In the first three weeks, make apples, grapefruits, berries, and melons your fruit choices. Gradually incorporate sweet fruit after the first three weeks. Primarily eat complex carbohydrates like raw/steamed vegetables with some whole grains, beans, or sprouted bread. Omit or limit pasta and flour. Try spelt, oat, rye, or a vegetable alternative. Mostly use "broom foods, in particular raw foods.," foods with fiber that will "sweep" through your system, Potatoes have a bad rap because they are a high-glycemic food. They are filled with vitamins and eight essential amino acids (complete protein). Try yams or red potatoes (lower insulin) and block the insulin (high glycemic index) with grated cheese or a yogurt/avocado topping. Select from a variety of carbohydrates to obtain all the vitamins and minerals you need.

Fats: Nuts, seeds, olives, avocados, EFA oils, and monounsaturated fats should be your primary fats.

Eliminate or strictly limit: Trans fatty fats, sugar (and alternatives), caffeine, soda, salt, refined carbs, and animal products. Meat, sugar, coffee (caffeine) and other stimulants have been proven to spike insulin or disrupt hormones in some way, which will sabotage your health and weight goal.

Alternatives: In place of the eliminated foods, try flaxseed oil, nut butters, black strap molasses, fruit sweeteners, cinnamon, vanilla, sparkling water with fresh squeezed juices, green tea, licorice root, herbs, sprouted sweet bread with soy, nuts, added and rice replacements. Also, try using apple cider vinegar (helps pH and digestion), lemon ,flax seed oil, herb spices or sun-dried tomatoes on your salads, instead of salt.

High- and low-glycemic index foods: the relative potency of carbohydrates and their propensity to raise and stabilize blood sugar. This means high-glycemic foods affect our blood sugar and insulin.

High glycemic index— dried fruit, bananas, mangos, corn, peas, carrots, potatoes.

Low glycemic index—apples, grapefruit, melon, berries, plums, all leafy greens, cauliflower, broccoli, yams, nuts, seeds, avocado.

Do not omit all high-glycemic index foods. High Glycemic foods are not necessarily bad for you. Some are very good for you, especially compared to some acceptable "low-glycemic foods." Do, however, watch how you eat these foods— when you eat them and how much. When you are healthy and in shape, you

*won't have a "reaction" to high-glycemic foods (details in Chapter Twelve).
High-glycemic fruits and vegetables are fine to eat sparingly, following 2–3 weeks
of eating low-glycemic foods.*

1) Eat at least 6-8 mini-meals per day, never allowing more than 2 hours between meals.
2) Eat one protein alternative with one fresh fruit or vegetable per meal for most of the mini-meals.
3) Eat no more than 3 different variety servings at no more than 2 mini-meals.
4) Eat heaviest or largest mini-meal during the first half of day.
5) Eat high-glycemic index foods during the first half of day or with protein that is high in nitrogen (dairy, eggs, tofu).
6) Eat fruit meals before 2:00 to 3:00 PM.
7) Eat *sprouted* breads and *whole* grains (usually before 4:00 PM with protein).
8) Eat variety of proteins and carbs throughout the day. Try not to repeat the same protein or carb.
9) Use "portion intuition," using the palm of your hand as one serving.

The object is to replace large meals, eaten a few times a day, with many mini-meals, eaten continuously throughout the day. Learn delayed gratification and remember your next meal is only 2 hours or less away. It is impossible to have true hunger if you eat small mini-meals 6-8 times a day.

✦   **ECO ANTI-DIET 3: The Garden Tonic** *(Yellow)*

This is a live/raw, detoxing, and healing food plan. The Garden Tonic is a food plan that is meant exclusively for health. It is a completely raw plant-food diet consisting of just fruits, vegetables, avocados, nuts, and seeds. Overcooking and freezing foods destroys enzymes and nutrients. This food plan is meant to rest, clean, detox and heal your body. A healthy body is free to adjust to the appropriate weight. This is the simplest food plan because it's a "pick 'n' eat" plan.

Eat 6-8 raw-food meals every 2 hours as follows:
1) Five of your meals should be whole fruits and vegetables.
2) One to three of your meals can be fresh juice. Drink 6-8 oz. every 2 hours.

Juice choices: (fresh, w/o additives)
    Carrot, beet, leafy greens, apple (or combo),
    Coconut
    Grapefruit and lemon,

Green powder (usually green grasses with others and sea greens—"superfoods") preferably with fresh citrus or apple juice

Fresh, diluted fruit juice of your choice with sparkling water

3) All five meals should include <u>raw</u> fruits or vegetables, avocado, or nuts and seeds.

4) One to two small fruits (1/4 to 1/2 melon) per meal during the first half of the day

   Fruit choices:

   Oranges, grapefruit, apples, plums, berries, or melon (cantaloupe or honeydew)

5) Primarily eat sub-acid or citrus fruits (as in above choices)

6) Include dried fruit, bananas, and other sweet fruit sparingly after a month or two of eating raw food.

7) Vegetables are preferred for the second half of the day (no more than 3 carrots per day and 2 per meal, except for juice).

8) Eat a variety of vegetables that includes greens. "Monoing" (eating one type) vegetables are fine, but not preferred.

9) Have ½ -1 avocado or no more than 2-3 ounces of nuts and seeds per meal. (4-6 oz. if nuts are sprouted).

10) Food combining is preferred but not exclusive:

   Fruits are preferably eaten alone.

   Melons are eaten separately.

   Dried fruit is eaten separately.

   Fruits and vegetable are eaten at different meals.

   It's best to add your avocados, nuts, and seeds with your vegetables.

   It's best not to mix avocados with seeds or nuts.

11) Diabetics and hypoglycemics should limit juice replacements to one meal, preferably fresh, green juice with spirulina. Every meal should be primarily vegetables, apples, grapefruits, berries, and honeydew melon. Each meal should be supplemented by 1/2 avocado or 2-3 oz. of seeds or nuts (preferably sprouted).

12) For those who need warm food in cold weather, try warm juice (like apple), fresh vegetable soup, or steamed vegetables.

Notes

I find blending vegetables with onions, garlic, tomatoes, and avocado in a food chopper or blender makes a tasty but very clean salad. Eating this way curbs hunger. Meat, sugar, and stimulants (and some spices) create ongoing cravings.

As soon as your meals become less raw and more perverted, then it's better to add protein rather than alter or overeat your raw cleansing foods. It's better to have a small portion of imperfect food rather than too much of diet food. The object of the Garden Tonic is to incorporate "clean" meals in order to heal, rest, detox, and be free from cravings caused by stimulants, overcooking, and fragmented foods.

Fruit that is in season is usually in the front of the produce section and is usually on sale. Don't buy fruit that is not in season. Fruit that is not in season is picked prematurely in order to be shipped from exotic locations. Apples, oranges, and lemons are available year round. Berries are best in spring, and melons are best in summer. Apples' prime season is fall. Peaches and cherries are very seasonal and should only be eaten from about June to August. Grapefruits are best at the end of summer through spring. If a fruit is expensive, that usually means it's not in season and not very tasty.

Finally, my sister and I are at the point that we have "turned raw." We eat live, raw food not only because it is ecologically friendly but because of the health benefits we receive. These benefits are much more than superficial. Eating this way saved our lives. Our eating disorders and poor food choices were killing us. Live, raw food (plant food only) nourished us while *lifting* our food addiction. Feeding our bodies raw medicine adjusted our diet-abused bodies. It takes time to gradually wean off "perverted" foods. You must eliminate animal products and sugar for at least three months before even considering a completely raw diet. Our raw diet has given us our "second chance." I do not recommend a completely raw diet, unless supervised. You should gradually teach the body to accept pure and uncooked foods.

Raw-food plans are our favorite because of the "survivors" we've witnessed. These survivors saved their lives without doctors, drugs, or surgery by radically changing their eating habits. There are groups around the world, that refer to themselves as hygienics, who simply eat *raw* (details in Chapter Two). Hygienics contradict the claim that fasters suffer bad breath. They view fasting as a cleansing process, including the smell of the breath. The pick-and-eat diet is the perfect diet. There are so many variations of the term *raw food*. Some raw dieters claim foods cooked under 105-120 degrees is considered raw. There are those who claim raw cheese and kefir (yogurt culture) is also considered raw. Some raw-food restaurants offer foods with various herbs, oils, spices, and low-cooked foods. However, the raw hygienics that I refer to eat nothing but natural plant foods—*live and raw*—in certain food combinations. They do not add any spices, herbs, oils, supplements, cooked foods, or "altered" foods—nothing but raw fruit, vegetables, and nuts and seeds that are mostly sprouted.

Most "militant" hygienics began eating this way because they faced a serious medical condition. At one time they were facing death and lost faith in doctors, drugs, and surgery. Or their doctors gave up on them. Some of these "patients" were minutes away from ordering their caskets and turned their lives around 180 degrees with a raw diet. A lot of these "patients" began with a low-sugar juicing regimen in order to detox and heal. The juices were primarily made from green vegetables, beets, carrots, green apples, and coconut. These foods nourished their bodies just enough to "starve" their diseases away. Gradually, they incorporated other whole fruits and vegetables, avocados, nuts, seeds (usually sprouted). In order to sustain an *alkaline* diet, they would mostly use avocados, sprouted seeds, occasional nuts, and spirulina for their protein. They showed great results instantly or some recovered totally, and they look fantastic! Live enzymes are the fountain of youth. Their skin's collagen is plumped up, which reduces wrinkles. Their eyes are clear and sparkling. Their bodies are tight from clean tissue. They are vitalized from the energy of live, raw foods and rested because the foods are easily digested. It takes a certain type of person to be completely *raw*. It's a lifestyle not a temporary gimmick diet.

Unfortunately most of us *abuse* foods in order to socialize, seduce, and medicate ourselves. Food, for most of us, is mouth entertainment. Raw-food dieters use it to *live*. They literally eat to live. They enjoy their food because they associate it with all the benefits that their raw food gives them. Their taste buds are not perverted, unlike most of ours, so simple foods taste sweet and juicy. People who eat raw foods have a spiritual philosophy about life. They are grateful and enjoy simplicity, while taking responsibility for any obstacles in their lives instead of thinking of themselves as victims. I have also witnessed individuals who maintained a diet exclusively of fruit or juice. There have been others who ate a diet solely consisting of almonds and oranges. Think that's impossible? I think it's impossible that most people eat nothing but chemically altered foods and stimulants! That's a miracle of survival! Incidentally, raw-food dieters don't need to worry about the high calorie content or the considerable amount of fat. (Their foods are cholesterol-free and contain no saturated fat.) Their food is easily assimilated, which leaves energy to heal and burn calories and body fat. If someone wants to eat a strictly raw diet, it's best to research or study about it at a "raw institution," as we did. These institutions specialize in this and can guide and monitor your health, while supervising your diet.

✦   **ECO ANTI-DIET 4: The Switch 'n' Twist** *(Purple)*

The Switch 'n' Twist is the combination of two Eco Anti-Diets that are rotated every other day. This diet rotates between Eco Anti-Diet 1 (Curb-Carb Corrector) and Eco Anti-Diet 2 (Veg Metabolizer).

Eco Anti-Diet 4 (Switch 'n' Twist) = Eco Anti-Diet 1 (Curb-Carb Corrector) + Eco Anti-Diet 2 (Veg Metabolizer).

	Eco Anti-Diet 1 (Curb-Carb Corrector)	1st Day
	Eco Anti-Diet 2 (Veg Metabolizer)	2nd Day
Eco Anti-Diet 4	Eco Anti-Diet 1 (Curb-Carb Corrector)	3rd Day
Switch 'n' Twist	Eco Anti-Diet 2 (Veg Metabolizer)	4th Day
is:	Eco Anti-Diet 1 (Curb-Carb Corrector)	5th Day
	Eco Anti-Diet 2 (Veg Metabolizer)	6th Day, etc.

The Switch 'n' Twist is a food plan that offers a wide variety. Variety gives us better vitamin and mineral sources. The same type of protein, carbohydrate, and fat, day in and day out, can create food allergies. The Switch 'n' Twist helps balance the insulin. Switching from a low-carb plan (Curb-Carb Corrector) to a high-carb plan (Veg Metabolizer) will prevent the body from learning the "trick" to any diet. Athletes "carb load" before an event, switching from a protein diet to a carb diet for extra energy. It's always good to shake up your food plan.

✦   **ECO ANTI-DIET 5: The Rock 'n' Rotate** *(Orange)*

The Rock 'n' Rotate plan is the combination of two Eco Anti-Diets rotated every other day. It rotates between Eco Anti-Diet 1 (Curb-Carb Corrector) and Eco Anti-Diet 3 (Garden Tonic).

Eco Anti-Diet 5 (Rock 'n' Rotate) = Eco Anti-Diet 1 (Curb-Carb Corrector) + Eco Anti-Diet 3 (Garden Tonic).

	Eco Anti-Diet 1 (Curb-Carb Corrector)	1st Day
	Eco Anti-Diet 3 (Garden Tonic)	2nd Day
Eco Anti-Diet 5	Eco Anti-Diet 1 (Curb-Carb Corrector)	3rd Day
Rock 'n' Rotate	Eco Anti-Diet 3 (Garden Tonic)	4th Day
is:	Eco Anti-Diet 1 (Curb-Carb Corrector)	5th Day
	Eco Anti-Diet 3 (Garden Tonic)	6th Day, etc.

Rock 'n' Rotate is a food plan that rotates your eating habits from one extreme (low carb) to the other extreme (all carb and no protein). When diets no longer work, the body is crying for variety and rest. Eco Anti-Diet 1 (Curb-Carb Corrector) will help block the insulin, while Eco Anti-Diet 3 (The Garden Tonic) will help rest and clean the body. Heavy protein every day can be very toxic and tiring on the body (aging). People who lack energy regardless of what they do or eat feel best on this food plan. This is because Rock 'n' Rotate rests the body for one day (without depletion or enervation) and then feeds the body the next.

✦ ECO ANTI-DIET 6: The Appetite Alternator *(Green)*

The Appetite Alternator is the combination of two Eco Anti-Diets rotated every other day. It rotates between Eco Anti-Diet 2 (Veg Metabolizer) and Eco Anti-Diet 3 (Garden Tonic).
Eco Anti-Diet 6 (Appetite Alternator) = Eco Anti-Diet 2 (Veg Metabolizer) + Eco Anti-Diet 3 (Garden Tonic).

	Eco Anti-Diet 2 (Veg Metabolizer)	1st Day
	Eco Anti-Diet 3 (Garden Tonic)	2nd Day
Eco Anti-Diet 6	Eco Anti-Diet 2 (Veg Metabolizer)	3rd Day
Appetite	Eco Anti-Diet 3 (Garden Tonic)	4th Day
Alternator is:	Eco Anti-Diet 2 (Veg Metabolizer)	5th Day
	Eco Anti-Diet 3 (Garden Tonic)	6th Day, etc.

The Appetite Alternator is a food plan that concentrates on balancing the hormones and chemicals one day and resting the next. People who need to fast (to rest and detox) but shouldn't do so long-term (usually because of adrenal exhaustion or blood sugar problems) should try this food plan. The Appetite Alternator is low in high-protein foods on both of the alternating days. Too much protein, particularly in animal products, is very tiring on the digestive system and causes health problems. The Appetite Alternator is one step closer to an exclusively raw diet, which is rejuvenating and healing. People seem to use spices and alter their foods because they've become accustomed to eating the same foods day in and day out. This corrupts our tastes buds, eventually making the diet more about spices or overcooked food rather than meals that benefit us. When you eat raw every other day (The Garden Tonic), food tastes sweeter because you have "cleaned out" on that day. It's not what we eat that makes us healthy, but rather what we don't eat. Eco Anti-Diet-6, The Appetite Alternator, trains the body to enjoy simple and less "perverted" foods. It's not a "feast-or-famine" food plan, but rather an "energize-or-rest" food plan. All bodies need rest and variation.

✦ **ECO ANTI-DIET 7: The Trio Mix** *(White)*

The Trio Mix is the combination of three Eco Anti-Diets rotated in a certain order. It rotates between Eco Anti-Diet 1 (Curb-Carb Corrector), Eco Anti-Diet 2 (Veg Metabolizer), and Eco Anti-Diet 3 (Garden Tonic) in the specific order suggested. The Trio Mix uses Eco Anti-Diet 1 (Curb-Carb Corrector) as the main Eco Anti-Diet and rotates each of the other two Eco Anti-Diets: Eco Anti-Diet-2 (Veg Metabolizer) and Eco Anti-Diet 3 (Garden Tonic).

Eco Anti-Diet-7 (Trio Mix) =
    Eco Anti-Diet-1 (Curb-Carb Corrector)
+   Eco Anti-Diet-2 (Veg Metabolizer)
+   Eco Anti-Diet-3 (Garden Tonic)

	Eco Anti-Diet-1 (Curb-Carb Corrector)	1st Day
	Eco Anti-Diet-2 (Veg Metabolizer)	2nd Day
	Eco Anti-Diet-1 (Curb-Carb Corrector)	3rd Day
Eco Anti-Diet 7	Eco Anti-Diet-3 (Garden Tonic)	4th Day
Trio Mix is:	*(repeat the same order)*	
(in this order)	Eco Anti-Diet-1 (Curb-Carb Corrector)	5th Day
	Eco Anti-Diet-2 (Veg Metabolizer)	6th Day
	Eco Anti-Diet-1 (Curb-Carb Corrector)	7th Day
	Eco Anti-Diet-3 (Garden Tonic)	8th Day, etc.

The Trio Mix is a food plan that can be good for *anyone*. Regardless of your health or diet problems, this food plan targets all areas of all health problems. Although all three Eco Anti-Diets are in this food plan, it is Eco Anti-Diet 1, The Curb-Carb Corrector, which is rotated every other day with the other two. That means you will eat raw (Eco Anti-Diet-3, The Garden Tonic), every fourth day, not sooner. This food plan may help food allergies, adrenal exhaustion, and diet boredom. Long-term dieters usually sabotage their diets because the body and the mind get bored with ritualistic or daily food plans. The Trio Mix makes this different for the person who gets stuck or obsessed about a certain food, food group or diet. The body becomes diet savvy if you don't incorporate a variety of foods and shake up the way you eat them. If you explore all types of foods, your body will respond very well. How else can we discover or solve a deficiency without trying other foods and food plans?

Eco Anti-Diet Notes:

✓ *All Vegans can follow any of the Eco Anti-Diets without sacrificing their way of life. Wherever it suggests dairy, eggs, cheese, or other animal products, Vegans can substituted soy, rice, grains, beans, nut proteins, or any other non-animal protein replacements.*

✓ ***Sample menus*** *are in Chapter Twelve for all the Eco Anti-Diets.*

✓ *Make sure all meals are eaten in a quiet environment, away from distractions. (e.g. TV, highly emotional conversations, and video games). Be sure to sit down for each meal, rather than eat on the run (in the car, making dinner, etc.). When you enjoy and respect your meals, your food works for you and digests properly. Snacking at a movie theater is not a planned meal; it's entertaining your mouth. Instead, practice to be aware of your eating habits and portions. Eating in front of a mirror has been proven to help people make conscious and better meal choices.*

✓ *There is no such thing as "blowing" your Eco Anti-Diet. The Eco Anti-Diets are guidelines that help you attain your goal without the need to binge. I never suggest "perfect" dieting. This is about progress, not perfection. Just for today, make sure your food plan is better than yesterday. Each day you will be closer to a toxin-free body so your body can perform better. Moreover, I encourage allowed/disallowed treats (further discussed in Chapter Five, Mental Tools). Allowed/disallowed meals are an occasional treat (not on your food plan) that replaces one of the meals on your food plan. If you have a sudden craving for a sugar treat or animal protein, allowed/disallowed treats will help you gradually wean yourself off of bad habits. If your allowed/disallowed treat is preplanned for a certain time, in a certain amount, it will lift the shame, compulsion, and obsession that usually drives dieters to sabotage their diets. The motive is to learn to eat with some type of commitment and refrain from bingeing, without feeling deprived. The weight will eventually drop off.*

✓ *Only weigh and measure your food in the first twenty-one days. Gradually begin using portion intuition with the help of the palm of your hand. Do not weigh or measure yourself, as well. There are some who insist on monitoring their fat percentage. A popular method to determine body fat is the fat-percentage method, using the water or pinch test. Others use BMI (body mass index). Still many claim this is fairly inaccurate because it does not consider your body type. The latest preference is to measure the waist area. This will determine your health risks. However, all these measuring methods can still be obsessive. (Further details of these instructions are in Chapter Teh.) It's not about the weight and food (symptom). You want to learn to commit to your Eco Anti-Diet, which will release the obsession. The Mental Tools in Chapter Five will help you figure out what you are eating over. The byproduct will be the appropriate weight loss.*

✓ *Eco Anti-Diet 1 is the only low-carb food plan that endorses high-protein alternatives. My sister and I do not eat animal products. We do not endorse eating animal meat whatsoever. However, certain individuals have a harder time omitting animal products, including poultry and fish. For them it is best to gradually omit (limit) animal meat from their diets. Remember, our object is health, and through our experience and research, animal protein (especially red meat) has been linked to many serious medical problems that eventually hinder weight loss.*

✓ *Eco Anti-Diet 3 should never be chosen by itself. Fasting is not recommended, unless supervised. (Fasting long term is considered fasting four or more days in a row.) Eco Anti-Diet 3 is not for people with weight problems or eating disorders, unless they incorporate it with one of the other Eco Anti-Diets on the alternate days. A daily raw-food diet is a lifestyle that must be introduced gradually, after attaining long-term recovery. Combining Eco Anti-Diet 3 with the other Eco Anti-Diets, allows the body to clear and clean itself so you are able to heal and achieve the proper weight you are meant to be.*

✓ *Eat no later than three or four hours before bedtime. Sleeping with a stomach full of food causes digestion problems, which further disturbs your sleep (causes nightmares).*

✓ *Don't drink liquids with meals. When you drink liquids with a meal, it disrupts the digestive enzymes. If you eat a meal of at least one raw food, such as a fruit or vegetable, you don't need to drink any liquids. Always drink water (at least eight eight-ounce glasses per day two hours after a meal and one half hour before. If your food plan has at least one live, raw food at every meal, you don't need to drink eight glasses of water a day, unless you need to.*

✓ *It's best to omit or at least limit use of alcohol and stimulants (like caffeine and sugar). It's silly to try to determine the carb or calorie content of "drugs." The body recognizes all indigestible substances as a poison. The body then "clones" the poison. The symptom of this "cloning" gives the stimulant effect, which wears off or puts strain on our bodies. Our bodies are dictated by hormones. All indigestible substances affect our bodily functions. Caffeine is used as a stimulant, appetite depressant, and diuretic. This may eventually cause hypoglycemia. When you drink coffee,(especially with caffeine), the insulin overflows, searching for glucose to burn. If you must drink coffee, add cream or soy milk to help block the insulin surge. But in the long run, all stimulants may eventually exhaust your adrenals and other bodily functions, which cause weight loss difficulties. That is why I stress health first, not weight loss.*

✓ *Pregnant women should always check with their doctors and not be restricted to any rigid food plan. The excess insulin spillage causes edema and* constant cravings. Just because a pregnant woman may crave something sweet and sour does not mean she has to turn to pickles and ice-cream. There is always a healthy alternative for every craving. Pregnant women should use their intuition and remember they are also eating nutrients for their child. It is a myth to think pregnant women have to eat for two. The normal weight gain expectancy is only about twenty-five to thirty pounds, which is equal to approximately an extra couple hundred calories per day. Many pregnant women can't believe how much their appetite increases. Usually they forget that the absence of their medication (like antidepressants) and stimulants also causes the appetite to increase. I have noticed that pregnant women who rest, eat "clean," and exercise (low impact) up until they give birth have the easiest child births.

CHAPTER 5:
MENTAL TOOLS

What are you eating over, or what's eating you?

Everyone said I appeared "profoundly introspective." Whether it was at church, a lecture, or with others and discussing their hardships, I was busy obsessing. Outside conversations would be numbed by my constant chant of my new *diet. My "diet mantra" was the only wheel turning in my head twenty-four seven.*

You can't have a successful food plan without addressing the issues you eat over. Unresolved issues will sabotage your diet. It's also ridiculous addressing issues while "intoxicated" (still eating over them). When we are "high" from our binges, we are just like a drunk who is intoxicated. It takes twenty-one days for sugar to detox from our systems, and it takes about six to twelve weeks for our hormones and brain chemicals to return to normal. So the right foods need to compliment a good recovery program, just like a good recovery program should compliment a committed food plan. Recovery is a term that simply means free from obsession and compulsive behavior. A recovery plan contains techniques that help you refrain from destructive habits. The Physical Tools help establish a healthy food plan and food choices so your body can react and respond accordingly. Foods can stimulate, enhance, or deplete important brain chemicals and hormones. In order for the Mental Tools to work best, you need Physical Tools as a supplement to create a balance physically and mentally. In other words, the Physical and Mental Tools need to work synergistically. The Mental Tools are reinforcement for the Physical Tools (your food plan). It is useless to have the "perfect diet" if you continue to sabotage it. These motivational techniques will make it easier to commit to your food plan, confront the issues you eat over, and replace the foods and situations that are triggers for diet sabotage. These motivational techniques will help you change your life choices and free yourself from destructive, obsessive, or compulsive patterns.

       7 Mental Tools: motivational techniques that....

+   Help you learn to commit,
  <u>confront, and replace triggers (foods and situations)</u>

=   **FREEDOM**: How to lose the obsession over your food and body

Denial and dishonesty are the reasons people continue to make the same mistakes. (Making the same mistake continuously, when you have a twin, is like déjà vu squared.) Denial makes it easier to be a victim. There is no responsibility when people choose to be victims. Rather than working on themselves, they can blame their diet or other outside circumstances. (Blaming my twin was like blaming myself—didn't work!). *In secrets lie sickness*. When people are unable to be honest and cling to denial, they are *unwilling* to change. Unwillingness is a sign that they are setting themselves up to repeat their mistakes. This is *premeditated* behavior. Insanity is described as doing the same thing over and over and expecting different results. What do you think you've been doing when you continually buy into diets and diet aids?

There are three ways of looking at ourselves: one, the way we see ourselves, two, the way others see us, and three, the way we really are. (Four ways if you have a twin.) Food addicts (or any addict) use "magical" thinking to live in the past or future—never in the moment. They are either obsessed about their image without being able to truly introspect, or their denial and self-absorption leaves them with extremely distorted perceptions. Only through humility and willingness do we achieve some perspective on how we really are. The following seven techniques outline a process that helps develop our true selves and confidence. A sick person will confuse confidence and humility with grandiosity and insecurity. These Mental Tools help guide us to become the people we were meant to be. They will help someone live in the *now* gratefully, not in yesterday or tomorrow.

To begin a good self-help program, you need to learn two very important things: <u>*Commitment and Sacrifice*</u>. Most (food) addicts confuse commitment with obsession and sacrifice with deprivation. This is not what I mean by *commitment* and *sacrifice*. Regardless of how rigid and disciplined the diet or the dieter is, there is always some point when dieters break their word. That is why you first need to learn to commit in small ways. This way you build trust with yourself. First, commit to a simple, easy food plan. *Writing* down the commitment, is part of the Mental Tools. The Physical and Mental Tools should constantly change, sometimes daily. Circumstances, growth, and health will make change necessary. This is a daily ongoing process, rather than living for the end results. Your food plan and motivational techniques won't be perfect but should progress daily. Without commitment there will be *no* success at all. The ability to follow through has obviously been a struggle that leaks into all parts of the addict's life. Commitment is an exercise we need to practice and improve every day. These simple commitment exercises will teach you to follow through and finish what you set out to do. Sacrifice is not about deprivation. It is about learning to surrender old ways, including bad habits, unhealthy thinking, and ritualistic patterns. You need to let go of comfortable and familiar habits that brought you to this dilemma. Without sacrifice, commitments are impossible. In order to commit, we need to sacrifice old ways of bartering with fate (reckless living). In order for a commitment to stick, you may need to sacrifice (give up) "slippery" food, people, places, and things. These "slippery" things make you slip right back to old ways, including old eating habits. It's important to sacrifice, or avoid these foods and situations, so you can focus on your commitment. It's easier to *commit and sacrifice* when you do it one day at a time.

The Mental Tools will also help you learn to *confront* uncomfortable situations with easy writing exercises. The Mental Tools consists of trigger replacements for foods and situations that should be avoided. These techniques help prevent compulsive behavior. Having a physical and mental plan will give you *freedom* from your own self-will and obsession.

The object of the Mental Tools is to learn to put "deposits in the bank," ready for an "emergency withdrawal." Food addicts repeatedly make the mistake of setting themselves up physically and mentally. *Environment is stronger than willpower.* Every choice you make is a blueprint for future patterns. Applying and sustaining these Mental Tools makes it easier, so that you're not open for *compulsive* "set-ups." The Mental Tools eventually make it easier to make better choices, rather than giving in to the same uncontrollable urges. Most of all, the Mental Tools help make your life manageable. Act—don't react.

The Mental Tools are broken up into seven daily, simple motivational techniques:

1) <u>Buddy or sponsor</u> support system
2) <u>Daily journal</u> of food plan and feelings
3) <u>Trigger list:</u> foods, people, places, and things to *avoid that day*
4) <u>Replacement list:</u> replacing the triggers
5) <u>Leverage list:</u> the disadvantages of sabotage and the advantages of abstinence
6) <u>Gratitude list:</u> five daily gratitude affirmations
7) <u>Connect and contribute</u>: giving, helping, and sharing which manifests success

1) **<u>The buddy or sponsor system</u>:** Find a buddy or sponsor to share your recovery and food plan with.

This support system allows the food addict to share their experiences, strength, and hope with another addict (preferably food addict) with the same goals. (A sponsor from any twelve-step program is helpful as well.) The buddy or sponsor cannot be a spouse or family member but must be somewhat available for daily contact with you. If you can't see the buddy in person, use the phone or email. A buddy or sponsor system is important because you need to learn to commit to another person. It's best if this buddy or sponsor shares the same addiction as you, or at least the same recovery program. You don't owe this person anything except the willingness to work together for a healthy and manageable lifestyle. When you have a responsibility to another person (commitment), it will make the rest of the food and recovery program easier to commit to. Depending on the buddy or sponsor, it's best if you can share your other six exercises with that person as well. Your buddy or sponsor is not your teacher, parent, or food cop. He or she is there to listen while you share your feelings, progress, commitments, doubts, and slip-ups. Usually, it's better to choose someone who's recovered more than you.

One-on-one therapy is helpful, but sharing with another addict seems to make it easier to open up and not feel so unique. (Sponsors are also recovering addicts.) Most addicts feel they have "unique-itis," feeling they are different and alone. You aren't paying the sponsor or buddy for a service. The buddy also recovers through what you share with him or her. You can have several buddies or sponsors as well. This helps availability so that you can preferably speak with someone every day. I had several buddies and sponsors. Some were solely for my food program; others were for my assignments. Don't feel obligated to a buddy or sponsor if you feel uncomfortable or feel you need to move on. Don't try to impress the buddy or sponsor. Buddies are not there to judge you or give their opinion. Your buddy or sponsor is there so you can learn to be *accountable*. This way it's easier to honestly open up, *share* feelings, and refrain from isolation. It secures commitment.

Example I: Cindy shares her food plan with a few buddies and shares her feelings and assignments with a sponsor. She uses the phone or the internet if she can't be with them in person. Cindy has a great support system.

~ ~ ~ ~ ~ ~

2) **Daily journal:** Keep a daily journal and divide it into two sections: a) food plan and b) feelings.

Prepare a writing journal that will be divided into two categories: food plan and feelings. The journal is a daily writing exercise that changes every day. No two days should be the same because we are looking for progress, not perfection.

a)   The first section of your journal involves your *food plan*. First write down every meal and snack that you commit to for that day. This will include your Eco Anti-Diet food plan, which you figured out from the questionnaire and quizzes in Chapter Three. It may also include allowed/

disallowed eating. This is when you PLAN a "taboo" treat, at a certain time, in a certain amount. These treats are not normally on your food plan. Suppose you have a relentless craving. Rather than "blowing your diet," have this occasional treat in place of a meal. This may include a sugar treat or animal protein that you are gradually omitting or at least limiting. Allowed/disallowed foods should never be trigger foods: Those should be avoided. Trigger foods, further discussed in assignment 3, are foods that cause non-stop bingeing. Let's say it's a holiday. You are in the mood for holiday treats. You may plan to have a certain treat (not a trigger), such as pudding in a small and normal portion. If you feel you need a certain allowed/disallowed meal or treat daily, it may develop into a trigger food, especially if you eat it compulsively (unplanned, non-stop bingeing). The motive should be to learn to eat normally (not compulsively) *without dieting*. You shouldn't attach feelings of guilt to certain foods. This will further the urge to punish yourself by sabotaging the rest of your food plan. Instead, without denying yourself, plan this allowed/disallowed meal or treat at a certain time, in a certain amount. The planning and commitment lifts the obsession and urge for a non-stop binge. This is where your sponsor or buddy comes in handy. You should commit your food plan to one of them and include any possible allowed/disallowed meal or treat. Verbally committing to someone else will also help differentiate between an occasional treat or a trigger food. When you keep your to word, it helps alleviate compulsive behavior. Commitment helps manage the obsession that creates the insanity (feeling out of control). Your meals may begin larger than normal or a with a few allowed/disallowed treats. The important thing in the *beginning* is to keep to your word and commit without eating trigger foods (creating a non-stop urge). You can still enjoy your food without "living to eat." If you associate every holiday or event with food rewards, it becomes harder to break the food/body obsession. It's best to write your food plan and allowed/disallowed treats *before* you eat them. However, if you happen to eat before you commit to your meals on paper, follow your meal with a written, detailed account of what you ate. It's more important to be accountable rather than rigid. Knowing everything you eat has to be written down prevents compulsive behavior. Your Eco Anti-Diet is a guideline that teaches you how to eat. It's not about perfection. It's about progress. Makes sure today you are better than yesterday and tomorrow will be better than today, one day at a time. If you can't speak with your sponsor or buddy, leave your food plan commitment in his or her message box or email. First write down your food plan and then commit to it with your buddy or sponsor.

b)   The other section of the journal involves your *feelings*. You should write down all the feelings you have kept secret or have eaten over. Most people are in denial at this stage. You will use a *pen* rather than a *fork* to deal with your issues. This new way of opening up may be uncomfortable at first. You may feel sad, silly, annoyed, or angry. These feelings are *real* and normal. Embrace them. This prevents you from using outside sources to escape from these inside feelings. Refrain from writing solely about food and body image. You have already spent too much time obsessing over these issues. The object is to free yourself from body and food obsession. Your food and body obsessions aren't real. They are symptoms of the real issues you have avoided for years. Writing down your experiences and feelings can be a relief. It's as if you are "detoxing" yourself of unhealthy secrets. You are getting rid of all the *crap* that was "constipated" in your deep emotions. Make sure this part of your journal is safe and private except for possibly sharing this with something like a sponsor. Refrain from "people pleasing" or validating your feelings with your sponsor. If you find you are writing about the same thing every day, then you are starting to obsess over it. Learn to move on and be open to all feelings rather than one person, place. or thing. You may include the same subject, as long as the feelings change. It's a daily growth development. Just go with the flow.

Example II: Cindy's Journal

a) *Foods: Just for today, I will commit to Eco Anti-Diet 5 (Rock 'n' Rotate), consisting of these foods…Today, at my sister's wedding, I will commit to replacing one meal with an allowed/disallowed snack, which will consist of one small piece of my sister's wedding cake and a glass of Champaign.*

b) *Feelings: The wedding buffet made me feel overwhelmed and anxious. Mom made me feel guilty. I don't want her to try to control me. My boyfriend didn't call me, which made me feel lonely and obsessive. I called my sponsor so I wouldn't eat over him. I didn't weigh or measure myself today, which is getting easier. Sometimes it's a struggle, but today I feel great that I didn't use food or my boyfriend to fix my frustration or escape my depression.*

~ ~ ~ ~ ~ ~

3) **Trigger list:** Write a daily list that is divided into two categories: a) trigger foods to avoid and b) trigger people, places, and things to avoid.

This is also a writing exercise that is divided into two categories: trigger foods to avoid and trigger people, places, and things to avoid. Write the triggers just for that day, one day at a time. Every day your triggers may or may not change. Gradually, you will have fewer triggers. Eventually, you will be free from compulsive behavior.

a) *Trigger Foods* are any foods that give you the feeling of being out of control. They are foods that seem to trigger a *non-stop* eating behavior. Initially, all foods seemed to be a trigger for me. Every day I would write down the foods to avoid. When you realize that there is *no* negotiation with these foods, it gives you a sense of freedom. Just for *today*, write the foods that you obsess over. This will help you let go of things you want to control.

Rather than postponing your new diet, postpone your trigger foods until tomorrow. Every time you practice delaying your triggers, you are releasing yourself from compulsive behavior and obsession. One day at a time, it becomes easier. Eventually, trigger foods won't be able to trigger you. This list will be like a homemade rehab for your mind. It's the insanity, not the food, that takes our minds hostage. Writing down the triggers becomes a relief and makes the food less powerful. People always ask me how I can deal with trigger foods, people, places, or things. This is how I did it. My homemade rehab prevented me from setting myself up for compulsive eating or behavior.

b) *Trigger people, places, or things* can "set you off" eating compulsively (bingeing, purging, obsessing, etc.). This is not an excuse to avoid responsibilities or things that need confrontation. An example of a trigger situation to avoid is weighing and measuring yourself or your food. In the beginning, both Shane and I had to avoid certain people, places, or things so that we could concentrate on recovery. It's not their fault or yours. Your feelings may be especially sensitive because you are no longer "numbing" yourself with food. It may feel different. Don't avoid the feelings. Instead write, share, and talk about these feelings. Sometimes you may need to confront someone. Regardless of what you do, don't avoid your feelings. Instead try avoiding the unhealthy situations that cause triggers. You need a healthy environment where you can recover from old habits. *Environment is stronger than willpower.*

For the extremely sick person, rehabs work well because everyone is surrounded by healthy people with mutual motives. You may need to avoid someone who has been your past "binge buddy," sharing your mutual addiction or habits. Your trigger list may not necessarily change for a while, but it should be reviewed daily. Simply write down any person, place, or thing that draws you back to your addiction and bad habits. This could be an object, situation, circumstance, or possibly an event. For instance, an anorexic may feel compulsive when she buys a swimsuit. The triggers may include the swimsuit as well as shopping. Remember, this is a one-day-at-time program. An alcoholic may be able to be a bartender when he's achieved long-term sobriety, but not in the beginning of his recovery. It's the same for a food addict or body-obsessed individual. Surround yourself with a healthy environment.

Example III: Cindy's Trigger List
a) *Trigger foods: ice cream, chips with sour cream dip, chocolate-nut candy bars, cinnamon rolls, pancakes with whip cream, soda, hot dogs*
b) *Trigger people, places, and things: my ex-boyfriend, the yogurt shop (ice cream), joining a gym, going to the weekend beach parties.*

~ ~ ~ ~ ~ ~

4) <u>The replacement list</u>: Write a daily list that is divided into two categories: a) replacing trigger foods and b) replacing trigger people, places, and things.

This is a list that follows and replaces the trigger list. Again, this may not change daily, but it should be reviewed daily. Like the trigger list, the replacement list is divided into two sections: replacements for food and replacements for people, places, and things. You are essentially replacing unhealthy rewards and poor environments.

a) First work on the food replacements. Write down enjoyable but healthy alternatives that you normally don't think about when eating compulsively. These foods should be safe enough to store in your home or are simple enough to make. Basically these are foods that are good for you and enjoyable enough to replace a trigger food. Remember your goal is to enjoy eating healthy meals without compulsive behavior. The weight will drop off as the byproduct of continuous healthy behavior. Trigger replacements are not the same as allowed/disallowed meals. Trigger replacements are *healthy* alternatives to your trigger foods. They help prevent the urge to binge and may be incorporated into your daily food plan. Although allowed/disallowed meals are also planned at a certain time and in a certain amount, they are an occasional treat that is not on your food plan. Trigger replacements are *totally* health-generated. This will help you reprogram yourself to learn to *eat to live*, rather than *live to eat*. We can also train ourselves to enjoy foods that are good for us. By planning ahead, we can learn to replace the triggers that release the shame and obsession. Shame evolves to sabotage. A planned replacement gives a feeling of earning the meal. My triggers were cheese and sweets. Initially, I invented clever replacements for my habitual triggers. I ate them without feeling deprived. I found that yogurt with black strap molasses, nuts, and raisins replaced the desire for cheese and sweets, all in one. It was healthy as well. The replacement list must be practical. If you say *never* to your usual trigger foods, without some type of compromise, you *will* return to them. The compromise is the replacement. The trigger replacements *can* (if necessary) be incorporated into your Eco Anti-Diet food plan. Don't leave an open space for your deleted trigger foods or it's open season for a set-up to go back to them. This is to simply teach yourself that there are other enjoyable foods outside of your binge food routine.

b) Replacing trigger people, places or things is similar to food replacement. You simply find healthy alternatives to trigger people, places or things. It's a good idea, in the beginning, to refrain from or limit magazine ads or watching a lot of television. It's a new experience to refrain from succumbing to every desire, so don't put "slippery" ideas in your subconscious for now. You should discriminate by choosing what your subconscious absorbs. Do not abuse this opportunity by replacing one unhealthy situation with another escape. Escaping will lead you right back to compulsive behavior. Again, do not avoid the feelings—just certain environments that are triggers. The replacement should help you confront those feelings you are avoiding. Sometimes, watching a movie, reading a book, or shopping can still be a method of escaping those feelings. Replace a trigger person, place, or thing with something applicable that will invest in your growth. A person's replacement could be visiting a sponsor or therapist. Therapy should never be a negative dumping session. Recovery is about getting in touch with your feelings. Learn to be less affected without giving away your power (giving up). There is a big difference between giving up and surrender. Giving up is laced with bitter regret. Surrender is feeling of relief while embracing trust and gratitude. Try replacing a trigger event with a charity event or group therapy. Shopping is another escape from investing in your recovery (yourself). Those activities sustain a self-absorbed body obsession that eventually develops into shame. Addictive behavior will follow. You may want to replace a certain restaurant that serves trigger foods. Restaurants were difficult for me and had to be totally avoided in the beginning. If I was obligated to socialize at a restaurant, I would suggest an exotic restaurant that served weird and unappealing food. A lot of restaurants now cater to vegetarians and even vegans. Perhaps you may need to replace a restaurant with a compulsive overeaters' meeting. You will feel good that you are investing in your recovery.

Example IV: Cindy's Replacement List

Triggers	Replacement
<u>Foods</u>	
ice cream	blended or whipped frozen fruit or frozen yogurt with fruit
potato chips and sour cream dip	sea-vegetable chips and avocado/bean dip
chocolate-nut candy bars	trail mix with carob chips
cinnamon rolls	sprouted cinnamon sweet bread w/o flour, yeast, sugar
pancakes	homemade French toast (sprouted) topped with berries
whipped cream	whipped cream cheese or soy whip w/o sugar
soda	sparkling cider or juice with carbonated water
hot dogs	tofu dogs on sprouted buns
<u>People, Places, and Things</u>	
ex-boyfriend	replaced ex's photos with pictures of puppies and kittens
yogurt (ice cream) shop	juice bar
joining a gym	join a women's or specialty gym with a friend
weekend beach party	recovery retreat, athletic event, camping, or charity event

~ ~ ~ ~ ~ ~

5) **Leverage list:** Write a daily list divided into two categories: the disadvantages of sabotage and the advantages of abstinence.

On one side of the list, write down all the disadvantages to being "drunk" with your "drug of choice." This will include your mental pain, health problems, and the havoc your poor eating habits has created. You need to remind yourself of what is was like when you were "intoxicated" and the insanity that went along with it. On the other side of the list, write down all the benefits of abstinence (freedom from bingeing, purging, dieting, etc.).

In order to change, you need to dissect your old habits and understand that they *don't work*. If you are still getting something out of your drug of choice, then you won't change. Leverage is moving away from insanity and pain and moving toward peace and fulfillment. Have you ever noticed most success stories come from a point of leverage? Successful people are driven from both a positive and negative side. They move away from pain or have a reminder of something they don't want to return to (poverty, pain, etc.)., They are also focused on something they want or aspire to. I am so impressed by Olympic athletes who overcome an unusual circumstance, such as a handicap or tragedy that they use to propel themselves to the top. If we don't remind ourselves of the pain, we will soon return to it. However, if we concentrate on the pain rather than a "carrot" in front of us, we will return to pain like a bad affirmation. We need to teach ourselves that there is hope at the other end of pain.

It's been said that if people were to watch themselves on a tape, acting "drunk," they'd be less likely to return to that behavior. This is what leverage is for. Remember when your teacher or parent would tell you to write down all the advantages or disadvantages to something you were choosing? This is somewhat the same. Following a binge, I would ask myself why I couldn't remember the pain. Why did I solely remember the "high," which didn't compare to the pain? Part of the addictive nature (physically and mentally) is to forget the pain. Brain chemicals such as dopamine and serotonin, or hormones such as endorphins (love) and norepinephrine (fight or flight), are released when we experience a "high." The mere memory of using our drug of choice causes dopamine to secrete. This creates a memory of the "high," to be greater than any pain from the drug of choice. Mentally, we've trained ourselves. This is much like a Pavlovian conditioning (act or move by learned impulse). When certain feelings surface, we automatically turn to our drug of choice and use it for our survival mechanism. That is why it is important to reprogram your mind. Remind yourself that these symptoms will surface when you are detoxing. Detoxing causes cravings and withdrawals. Create new *tools* that will help prevent going back to the pain. You need to make an effort to write these down. During your "insane" moments (of cravings and withdrawals), your memory won't allow you remember this pain. Therefore, you need to write it down in black and white, daily! The painful memories may have been forgotten through "blackouts" and denial, but they will eventually be lifted or have little effect. This is why your pain list may change, daily perhaps.

On the other side of the leverage list are the advantages to being "abstinent" or "sober." You simply write what abstinence means to you, what it has brought you, or how it's helped you achieve your goals. This too can change. This is not a Christmas list. It's not about expectations or goals. It's about how the sanity, trust, gratitude, peace, and freedom have helped manage your life. Simply put, write the pain of your destructive and compulsive behavior on one side and the benefits of abstinence (abstaining from destructive behavior) on the other side. **Don't run from pain. Use it as leverage!**

As I've mentioned, this is not a superficial list. Don't write about a car you've lost or a guy you would want to date, if you lost weight. You can however, write about the money wasted on your drug of choice or how refraining from isolation has brought you new friends. My pain leverage was the memory of waking up bloated and loathing myself. Although my physical health was poor, my mental state was worse. That was enough for me. On the other side was relief from obsession. Because we are dictated by feelings, that's what you should focus on and write about. This list should include adjectives and adverbs, rather than nouns. This list can change when the feelings change.

Leverage: What it was like before "abstinence" (painful feelings) and what freedom from obsession feels like.

Example V: Cindy's Leverage List

<u>*What it was like when I was bingeing*</u>: *I was extremely out of control. My life was completely obsessed with binge foods and places to eat them or transmitting them into a love addiction. I hated myself. Eventually, I didn't want to be around my "binge buddies." I isolated because I was embarrassed, ashamed, and felt hopeless. I'd always swear to another diet the next day. It was easy to swear off food forever when I was stuffed and sick to my stomach! I couldn't move or breathe properly.*

<u>*What it is like now that I am abstinent one day at a time*</u>: *I finally trust myself. There is a sense of relief and hope. I am free from the prison I made by obsessing over my food and body weight. I focus on other goals now that I have time away from worrying about food and diets. I feel energetic and I'm able to sleep normally. I don't worry about numbers on the scale, because everyday I have progressed. I have faith and I've learned to let go of "control." Maybe I'm not perfect, but for once, that's okay.*

~ ~ ~ ~ ~ ~

6) **Gratitude list**: Every day, affirm five simple things to be grateful for. (Each day is different.)

This is a daily exercise that can be written or verbally affirmed. It's best to do this first thing in the morning. Humility goes hand in hand with gratitude. Gratitude is important for the addict because most addicts are blinded by bitter cynicism. They see the glass as half empty and think no one understands them. You take things for granted when you are ungrateful. My mother taught me that there is *no such thing* as being lucky or having continuously bad luck. There's only the ability to be open to seize a good opportunity in front of you. When you are negative, you are unable to see good opportunities, even if they are right in front of you. Negativity prevents you from living in the *now*. There are clues to continuous bad luck. Continuous bad luck happens to people who stay victims and want to blame their circumstances without taking any responsibility. Without gratitude, we can't find "sobriety," love, success, or peace. Because I grew up in a dysfunctional family, I operated best in a crisis mode. I seemed to attract crises, because that was when I would perform at my peak. Usually an addict's life is consumed with problem solving, because the addict is addicted to the highs of a crisis. Recovery is moving past the crisis and learning from it without blame so that you don't repeat it. This exercise seems simple or unimportant. On the contrary, gratitude is the gateway to life-change.

Everyday you are to **choose five things** you are grateful for. I'm not talking about superficial things or obvious things. I'm talking about simple pleasures we take for granted. When we are stuck in our food or body obsession, we never notice the greatest gifts of all. It could be as simple as noticing a bird singing outside your window, a clear sunny day, or a nice hot bath. When I was using my drug of choice, I never noticed anything unless it had to do with food or weight. Again, the gratitude list should be different every day. The object is enjoy the moment and to be aware of all the simple things we take for granted. This exercise actually causes the secretion of vital brain chemicals and helps balance hormones. Good affirmations and a positive mind have been proven to help a person physically and mentally.

Example VI: Cindy's Gratitude List
Every morning Cindy writes or says:
1) *I am grateful for my best friend's support.*
2) *I am grateful for a beautiful sunshine morning.*
3) *I am grateful for the opportunity to visit my ill grandmother.*
4) *I am grateful for the sweet smell of the flowers outside my window.*
5) *I am grateful for my kitty, who loves me unconditionally.*

~ ~ ~ ~ ~ ~

7) **Connect and contribute**: Daily simple and easy assignment It's not the quantity of what you give, but the quality. Meaning it' better to be sincere and simple rather than grand and righteous. What is your motive? Where is your heart?

Choose one of the following: a) one selfless deed or b) one group therapy or c) one spiritual gathering

When we are wrapped up with our self-absorbed diet and image obsession, we never bother connecting with others, unless they feed our obsession. During our obsession, we *use* or abuse people, rather than connecting with them. If we don't connect we isolate from everything but our disease. Relapses occur when we focus exclusively on ourselves.

As long as your main focus is on yourself, your obsession will be, too. It waits patiently, smoldering inside, until suddenly it blows up in your face! Have you ever noticed people who always complain about nothing? Although you may want to show them what a real problem is, they are so wrapped up in themselves they don't care. Addicts complain about everything except their addiction. The best way to "get out of yourself" is to reach out to someone else. But first you need to invest in yourself so you have something to offer. Incidentally, don't get confused with making contributions and people pleasing. People pleasers are people who have their own agendas. Their motive is their image. People pleasers don't get gratification from giving or doing for others unless it is duly noticed. They usually need to complain or announce their good deeds. People pleasers are insecure people who feel like they must "buy" their love. It's unhealthy to behave as a people pleaser or to be involved with one (further details in Chapter Nine). They enjoy being the martyr, victim, or the hero. I've noticed these people actually brag that they are people pleasers. Then again, that is their very nature: to be so self-absorbed they don't realize that's not something to brag about. Contribution, on the other hand, is about reaching out to others. This helps us realize we are not alone and not so different. Connecting and contribution helps lift the obsession so you can focus on something or someone else. For this exercise, there is a choice of three connect and contribute activities to do. Although any one of the three is to be done daily, the group therapy is suggested once a week. The three choices of connect and contribute exercises are a selfless deed, a group therapy meeting, or a spiritual gathering.

a) <u>One selfless deed</u>: This deed is simple and easy but should be anonymous, hence *selfless*. What I mean by *anonymous* is simply unannounced. Don't wear it on your sleeve. This small, simple deed should be without any benefit except feeling good about contributing. It could be as simple as planting a tree for the environment, helping a woman cross the street, or picking up trash in a park. It's extremely honorable to be a part of any charity or charitable event, as well. Just make sure for this exercise, that the motive is pure and not for your ego. If you love animals, as I do, there are numerous shelters and adoption agencies that could use your help. Helping an animal is practicing contribution with unconditional love, *especially* when you don't own the animal. Practicing vegetarianism for the sake of animals is a daily contribution to animals! A lot of people anthropomorphize their own pets (make the pet an extension of themselves). Owning a pet is rewarding because the pet is a part of you. Making your pet a family member is practicing unconditional love. Moreover, adopting a *rescued* animal, rather than buying a purebred, is notably honorable. Helping any animal that you don't own is the highest form of charity.

This exercise will help you reach out, anonymously or to anonymous people, places, and things without trying to benefit from it personally. Your main motive is to help or benefit someone or something that is not attached to your ego. This will build your confidence, character, and outlook on life. The gift is yours when you learn to connect and contribute!

b) <u>Group therapy meeting:</u> This may entail a twelve-step meeting, outreach rehab meetings, some self-help seminars or classes, etc. The reason I prefer group therapy as opposed to one on one therapy is because you connect and contribute with other suffering addicts. By connecting this way (sharing your experiences, strengths, and hopes), you are contributing to others' recovery (hope, inspiration, motivation). This sharing process keeps everyone on the same level. It very inspiring to be involved in a therapy group that shares their courage, life stories, and support. It's very similar to a spiritual experience. For the person who goes through daily battles with addiction, one or more group therapy per week is best. It also helps you to learn to connect and contribute. (Further details about therapy and recovery programs are in Chapter Nine.)

c) <u>Spiritual gathering:</u> When I heard that any type of addiction was a sign of being "spiritually bankrupted," that was an insult to my personal spiritual quest. Well, think about it. All addictions are about *control,* and needing complete control means a lack of faith. I don't preach any type of religious preference at all. I've met some people who do not have a specific religion but lead a very spiritual life. They are beautiful people who enjoyed giving, helping, and sharing. True spirituality seems to be the way someone lives (by example), not what that person preaches. I think there's a spiritual quality to anyone who reaches out (connects and contributes) and shares non-judgmental love and empathy. It sounds simple but seems to be rare, even in the name of religion. Most people who attain lasting abstinence or recovery incorporate some type of spiritual program with their therapy. The spiritual paths that are not dictated by fear, guilt, and shame seem to be the most successful. They found what we addicts were looking for in our drug of choice: fulfillment, which is found in simplicity, not in outside circumstances. It's important for those who found their whole recovery through their beliefs to continuously attend spiritual gatherings. It surrounds them with the inspiration that they need to sustain their recovery. However, if you attend church just because it is an obligated tradition, that does not count. This is not about a spiritual image or impression. You need to experience internal spiritual awakenings that help with gratitude, trust, and obsession. The spirituality helps lift destructive self-will through surrender. Spirituality is a feeling and not an event. A spiritual gathering could be as simple as a meditation group. Whatever it is, it should usually be done with others, not alone.

Example VII: Cindy's Connection and Contribution
Monday: Took my neighbors' trash out because they were sick.
Tuesday: Went to twelve step meeting.
Wednesday: Fed a stray cat.
Thursday: Returned my grocery bags to be recycled.
Friday: Went to meditation group.
Saturday: Donated five dollars to children's fund (usually spent on junk food).
Sunday: Brought snacks to the church meeting.

~ ~ ~ ~ ~ ~

For best results, it is necessary to do these assignments daily for six to twelve weeks or when your food plan becomes "slippery." Once you have obtained a healthy relationship with your food and issues, you can choose to do these exercises when it feels necessary. I do many of these exercises automatically. I've cultivated good habits that reinforce commitment to my food plan and separate my eating habits from the way I deal with issues.

This completes the Mental Tools, which supplement your Physical Tools. I've been asked numerous times what my "trick" was for losing weight. Or how I freed myself from obsession and destructive behaviors. The Physical and Mental Tools are my methods. It took years of researching and experimenting to arrive at these Tools. I took every successful method from every food and recovery plan and made my own daily formula. If it can work for my sister and me, it can work for you!

Note: I do not endorse any specific religion or discuss my own spiritual path. My sister and I are unqualified to do so. I do believe, however, a successful recovery program entails some type of spirituality.

CHAPTER 6:
DOES THIS CHAPTER MAKE ME LOOK FAT?

The Fat Conspiracy
All American… "Baseball, Tofu Dogs, and Fat-Free Apple Pie"

<u>Food</u>: **Fat is where it's at!**
<u>Body</u>: **It's not your fault!**

I spent many a nights on my usual midnight rounds at the convenient stores, loading up on all of my four basic food groups: fat, grease, sugar, and oil. I'd usually ask the cashier if he happened to know the number of fat grams in my dozen donuts, packages of cookies, dozen candy bars, few bags of chips, a liter of soda and a stick gum. It was <u>exhausting</u> trying to figure it out, especially because many of the midnight cashiers could not speak English. I think they thought I was trying to rip the store off. I would have paid the cashier more if he would have helped me condone some of those fat grams.

☞ *Food: Fat is where it's at!*

Fat doesn't make you fat. Hormonal imbalances do. Fat is a soft greasy solid substance occurring in organic tissue or a natural oil substance in animal bodies, deposited under the skin or around certain organs. It's the main constituent of animal and vegetable fat. It's also one of the four main nutrients needed to maintain life, meaning it's natural to have or eat fat. Unfortunately fat has been "coined" as a dirty word for what we see or what we eat. People in other countries, such as France, eat a considerable amount of fat without worrying about counting fat grams. The French are also known for being very thin and healthy. As I stated, fat does not make fat. Moreover, certain types of fat help you to lose weight and boost your metabolism. Hormonal imbalance makes you fat, because without fat—especially essential fatty acids—your body is unable to function accordingly. Fat triggers the good eicosanoids (mini-hormones that dictate every action, including lowering blood fat and cholesterol). Essential fatty acids are the "building blocks" of eicosanoids and also responsible for thermogenesis (body-heat metabolism) in the body. Without EFA's, your cells' motors, the mitochondria, cannot work properly. This is a main reason why anorexics have poor circulation and difficulty acclimating to cold weather. Estrogen, the female hormone, is stored in fat, which makes it very difficult for women to lose weight. Without EFA oils, anorexics usually miss their periods. Most anorexics don't realize essential fatty acids are needed for fuel, yet it are *never* stored as *fat*. Fat makes us feel full. Fat also blocks the excess excretion of insulin, which is another hormone responsible for weight gain. We need fats—especially "good" fats (HDL, or high density lipoproteins) that help lower or replace the "bad" fats (LDL, or low density lipoproteins). Without fat, the body secretes too much insulin, which triggers the adrenal glands to secrete excess cortisol, another hormone that contributes to weight gain. Eventually, this can cause adrenal exhaustion.

The less fat you eat, the more the body clings to it. Fat is needed for all your bodily functions. Food fat may end up in fat stores on your body, but first it needs to be digested, absorbed, and transported to its cellular destinations. All fat is not the same, just as all calories are not the same. We cannot live without certain fats. Essential fatty acids are just that— essential. They are part of the polyunsaturated groups known as Omega 3's and Omega 6's. Omega 9 is not essential. You must supply the body with Omega 3's, found in fish oils and flaxseed, and Omega 6, which is found in seeds and grains. Because we have more starches than we need in our diet, we have too much Omega 6 and we are lacking in Omega 3, more than any other EFA. Our ratio of Omega 3 to Omega 6 should be higher.

The human body can synthesize all fatty acids from the food we eat except for two very important polyunsaturated fats: Omega 6 and Omega 3. Widely distributed in plant and fish oils, both of these fatty acids serve as raw materials from which the body makes hormone-like substances that regulate many bodily functions, including blood pressure, immune response, blood clotting, lipid levels, inflammation from injury. Though they are very important, too many fatty acids, *essential* or not, can cause health problems.

This is how it works. Every cell has fat-like substances that help control and enhance tissue and blood building, hormone production, and nervous system function. Fat (lipids) is composed of building blocks called fatty acids. There are three major categories of fatty acids: saturated, monounsaturated, and polyunsaturated. These are chemical classifications based on the number of hydrogen atoms in the chemical structure of a given fatty acid molecule. Monounsaturated fats, like in olive and canola oil, actually reduce the LDL, or "bad" cholesterol. It is recommended to have about 20 percent of monounsaturated or polyunsaturated fats (nut and vegetable oils) in your diet. Raw diets have far more fat consumption, only because their diet is PURE and natural consisting of only avocados, nut, and seed fats and they don't face any problems with weight, cholesterol, or health problems relating to fat.

Saturated fat is where the problems begin. These fats are mostly found in animal products such as meat and cheese. Excess saturated fat clogs arteries and may cause heart disease and obesity. Our liver needs saturated fat to manufacture cholesterol. Excessive intake of saturated fat raises your "bad" cholesterol and can be deadly. Saturated and unsaturated fats are found in all foods. Saturated fats are the least healthy and are usually solid at room temperature (butter, for example). Saturated fats are also found in coconut and palm oil, which happen to be liquid at room temperature. Chemically speaking, saturated fat is filled to capacity with hydrogen. Unsaturated fats are liquid at room temperature, such as vegetable oils.

Monounsaturated fat has one (mono) hydrogen bond missing on the fatty acid chain. Monounsaturated fats found in olive, canola, or grapeseed oil reduce the amount of LDL in the bloodstream. Monos do not cause heart disease the way saturated fats do, and they may even help fight cancer. Other monounsaturated fat sources include peanuts, avocados, olives, and other vegetable and nut oils.

Polyunsaturated fats have two or more points of unsaturation (multiple hydrogen bonds). This is preferable because when there is only one hydrogen bond it will try to pick up another bond, which can cause cellular damage. These fats are found in oils, such as sunflower, safflower, sesame, and flax oil. Polyunsaturated fat is the chief source of the essential fatty acids necessary for proper cell membrane function and many other metabolic and glandular process.

Trans fatty acids or hydrogenated fats are good polyunsaturated fats converted into a hybrid by partial hydrogenation. An example is corn oil made into margarine. In laboratories, this "invention" proved to be lower in cholesterol. These fake fats usually cause more harm by affecting the hormone insulin to over-secrete. These fats should be completely avoided. Careful packing has made it hard for the consumer to determine if there are trans fatty acids in the labeling. For instance, corn syrup; it is a "cheaper" ingredient than trans fats, at the expense of the consumer.

There are two types of lipids: triglycerides and phospholipids (cholesterol). Triglycerides are food fats and represent 95 percent of all fat in the body. They are transported to fat depots, like the breasts and muscles, where they are stored. Cholesterol is a soft, waxy substance manufactured in the body and plays an important role in brain and nerve cells. Cholesterol is found in animal-based foods as well as in the human body and is considered the best predicator of a person's chance of suffering from cardiovascular disease. If you have high cholesterol you will usually also have high triglycerides, but only high cholesterol is fatal.

Within the body, fats travel around, mixing with the particles called lipoproteins (or, collectively, cholesterol). The two different kinds of lipoproteins are called high density (HDL) and low density lipoprotein (LDL). Lipoproteins are water soluble, protein-covered bundles that transport cholesterol through the blood and are synthesized in the liver and intestines. HDL is considered the good cholesterol simply because it cleans the bad cholesterol out of the arteries. LDL is the bad cholesterol that makes up 93 percent of the cholesterol in the body, but it is also necessary for the proper function of many of the body's primary systems. It is only considered bad because the remaining 7 percent of LDL's accumulate and cause damage in your arteries.

Breakdown of FAT FACTS

✓ Lipids are fats that are composed of building blocks called fatty acids. Every cell has fat-like substances that help control and enhance tissue and blood building, hormone production, and nervous system function. All lipids basically fall into two categories: triglycerides and phospholipids (cholesterol). Triglycerides are responsible for the fat in your body. Phospholipids are cholesterol and lecithin. They are fats that are vital to cell membranes, nerve fibers, bio salts, and are also a precursor to sex hormones.

✓ Triglycerides are dietary fats and oils used as fuel or energy and the storage form of fat (carried in blood). Triglycerides make up 95 percent of the fat in the body, and 95 percent of your dietary fat is also triglycerides (especially if you are eating animal protein). They are good insulators.

✓ Cholesterol (or phospholipids) makes all cell membranes and hormones. It is a waxy fatty acid carried in the blood. Seven percent of cholesterol is found in the blood. The remaining 93 percent is located in the body. Twenty percent of cholesterol comes from your diet; the rest is from the body. Cholesterol forms all hormones, such as estrogen, cortisol, and the mini-hormones called eicosanoids. When people are told they have high cholesterol, that refers to the cholesterol deposits in the arteries. Cholesterol may rise when fasting, because the body needs to break down stored fat for energy. Lecithin is a phosphatide high in essential fatty acids that keep cholesterol in check, along with choline.

✓ Saturated and unsaturated fats are in all foods, just in different ratios. Saturated fats are solid at room temperature, like in butter and meat. They are usually found in animal sources. Coconut and palm kernel oil are high in saturated fat and are liquid at room temperature, as is vegetable oil. Unsaturated fats are basically mono or polyunsaturated fats. They are liquid at room temperature and include vegetable or nut oils. Unsaturated fats reduce serum (blood) cholesterol. Fats and oils contain nine calories per gram: twice as many as carbs or protein. The body can convert unsaturated fats into saturated, but it can not convert saturated into unsaturated.

✓ Mono-unsaturated fats reduce LDL in blood. Good sources for these are olive or canola oil. Both oils are mainly mono-unsaturated (about 65 percent), a little polyunsaturated oil (30 percent) and very little saturated (5 percent). They have neutral eicosanoids and have no effect on insulin levels. This is why they are considered a good fat. Both olive and canola oil are also excellent for cooking. Canola oil is better for cooking at higher temperatures. Peanuts are high in fats and are very good for you. The fat in peanuts slows down the absorption of carbs into the body.

✓ Polyunsaturated vegetable oil is the chief source of essential fatty acids (EFA), which include linoleic, linolenic, and arachidonic. Examples are sunflower, safflower, sesame, and flax oil. Cooking usually distorts EFA's, so it's better to cook with olive oil.

✓ Trans fatty acids or hydrogenated fats are a good polyunsaturated fat that is converted into a hybrid by partial hydrogenation. In this process, the double carbon bonds turn to an unnatural configuration that creates or promotes bad eicosanoids. Margarine (hydrogenated from corn oil) doesn't contain cholesterol, yet it creates high cholesterol from the excess insulin spills. Hydrogenated fats are not as bad as partially hydrogenated fats.

✓ HDL and LDL are also referred to as good and bad cholesterol. They are lipoproteins that carry the fat (triglycerides), or cholesterol, in the blood. Contrary to what people believe, LDL is very important because it carries the fat to build cells but can leave excess on the artery walls. HDL is considered good because it cleans up excess fat and carries it to the liver to make bile. However, that's all it does. We need both, but we need to watch the ratio so your cholesterol is not high in the blood. High cholesterol is the excess left over, and usually means high triglycerides. High cholesterol is more deadly. LDL carries all linoleic acid foods. The natural ratio of HDL to LDL is three to five.

✓ EFA's, your essential fatty acids, are necessary for life and cannot be made in the body. These are polyunsaturates that are important for structural and regulatory body functions. You need to get your EFA from your diet. There are eight essential fatty acids, divided into two main classes: the Omega 3's and Omega 6's. Omega 9 is not essential. The ratio of Omega 3 to Omega 6 in our food should be one to one. However, our soil today is so depleted that there is a lack of Omega 6 in our grains and other foods. Still, because we eat too many starches, we need to add more Omega 3 than Omega 6.

✓ Omega 3 (linolenic acid) is high in fatty acids, EPA (considered good), DHA, and ALA. This includes all fish oils, walnut oil, canola oil, wheat germ oil, primrose, flax oil, and beans. Omega 3 is responsible for lowering cholesterol by 30 percent. It also helps fight heart disease and thins blood. Omega 3 oils are always used and never stored as fat.

✓ Omega 6 (linoleic acid) is high in linoleic acid, which can be found in most foods, and arachidonic acid, which is also responsible for contributing to bad eicosanoids. You need all EFA's, however, it's the ratio of all oils and foods that determine your health. Omega 6 diets are carried by LDL. Still, Omega 6 is the most important because it ends up forming good eicosanoids (depending on insulin restriction). Omega 3 has little effect creating good eicosanoids. Omega 6 helps blood clot. Omega 9 (not an EFA) is oleic acid, found in most oils and foods such as primrose, flax, avocado, olive, nuts, etc. Hemp oil has the perfect ratio of EFA oils.

✓ Linoleic acid is an essential fatty acid found in most foods and is considered the only true EFA! It is found in the Omega 6 class and with proper diet and portions is converted into GLA.

✓ GLA (Omega 6) and EPA (Omega 3) are the two most important fatty acids because they are solely responsible for forming all the good eicosanoids. GLA is naturally found in slow-cooked oatmeal, mother's milk, borage, primrose, and black currant oil. It can also be activated by linoleic acid (Omega 6) with the help of EPA (Omega 3) in order to make good eicosanoids. Alcoholics and other addicts generally have a hard time making GLA. Though GLA fights all infections, it is the easiest to destroy.

✓ ALA is an Omega 3 class fatty acid that acts like aspirin. It kills both good and bad eicosanoids, making it undesirable. Other Omega 3's help save the good eicosanoids. Examples of Omega 3: flaxseed, canola, walnut, corn soy oils, and black currant.

✓ VLDL is a lipoprotein made by the liver that usually carries (or is composed of) triglycerides. It is used for energy. VLDL leaves cholesterol deposits behind which it then converts into LDL.

✓ Eicosanoids (super hormones that affect all hormones) are the mini-hormones in every cell, formed by fatty acids. They're the "molecular glue" that holds the human body together. Discovered in the mid 1970s. There are hundreds of them. They were formally recognized with the Nobel Prize in 1983). There are five main families of these super-hormones: prostaglandin, thromboxanes, leukotrienes, lipoxins, and hydroxylated fatty acids. Prostaglandins were discovered in the 1930's, and because they were the first eicosanoids to be discovered in the prostate gland, the medical books still incorrectly refer to all eicosanoids as prostaglandin. They are made from Omega 3 (LNA) and Omega 6 (GLA). EFA's are the building blocks of eicosanoids. Once an EFA is oxidized, it can be made into eicosanoids.

✓   Glycogen is a hormone formed from cholesterol that was affected by good eicosanoids. It is a tasteless polysaccharide (or hormone), which is the main carb used for energy stored in the liver or muscles. It cannot be used for energy with excess insulin. Glycogen is formed with the help EPA. Glycogen prevents production of arachidonic acid.

✓   Insulin is a hormone twin of glycogen, formed from cholesterol that was affected by bad eicosanoids. When there are excess carbohydrates, it raises the blood glucose. The pancreas secretes the hormone insulin into the bloodstream to lower the levels of blood glucose. In correct amounts, insulin helps glucose to be used as energy. Insulin is a storage hormone that converts this glucose into fat with an over-release. This over-secretion can also happen with stress, age, disease, trans-fatty acids, high VLDL, hyperinsulinemia, ALA, etc. Insulin helps build extra cholesterol in the body, making it unnecessary to retrieve any from the bloodstream, furthering high LDL. Insulin activates linoleic acid and then makes it into arachidonic acid. That can also create bad eicosanoids. The Islets of Langerhans are special cells within the pancreas that secrete insulin.

Tips that prevent insulin surplus: exercise, the HGH (human growth hormone), sleep, protein diets with arginine, fasts and anaerobic exercise, proper food and correct portions, lack of stress, genetics, low weight, good muscle tone, low glycemic index, fiber, low calories or many mini-meals without more than two hours in-between.

✓   Glycemic index is the rate sugar is released into the blood. High glycemic index means the sugar enters the blood quickly. This is bad. Low glycemic index is when the sugar gradually enters the blood. This means lower insulin spills. Fruit is low compared to refined carbohydrates. Juices, however, can produce a higher glycemic reaction because they lack fiber. Some fruits are higher on the index than others, such as bananas, which are higher than honeydew melon. Some vegetables are higher than others, like carrots are higher than leafy greens. Ice cream is a low glycemic food (compared to frozen non-fat yogurt) because the protein/fat overrides the sugar. High glycemic foods stimulate the LPL (fat storing enzyme) and elevate the serotonin, which can create weight gain.

✓   Mitochondria are responsible for the thermogenesis within the cell. Glycogen moves the fat from the blood to the mitochondria. Insulin prevents this and keeps the fat in the blood, to be stored as fat.

✓   Ketosis is an abnormal metabolic rate that forces the body to use fat in a rapid breakdown, causing abnormal biochemicals called ketone bodies. Insufficient carbohydrates in the liver (twenty-four hours worth) and low carbs in the diet force the body to break down fat for energy. Ketones are incompletely burned fats that are disbursed for energy without completely being burned. The body tries to rid itself of these ketones through urination, causing more water weight loss than fat. The body also gathers fats faster after ending ketosis. Ketosis blunts serotonin. Ketosis is not exactly like diabetes, but is somewhat like it. (Called ketoacidosis, it also breaks down fat for energy because the glucose is unable to be used with the proper insulin.)

Solution: It is better to allow the essential fatty acids to be activated into good eicosanoids by eating foods in a ratio that eliminates excess insulin spills. It's best to replace your "junky" fats (saturated and trans fatty acids) with good fats (essentials–correct ratio and monounsaturated fats).

☞ *Body: It's not your fault!*

In the morning after a binge comes the dreaded "pre-fat-bloat" hangover. I'd start my diet-day with a thorough search for the perfect scale to weigh myself. It was hard to read my home drugstore scales through all the crumbs. Gym scales were crowed with people waiting in line. Hospitals did not allow me to strip down for their scales. Then I found the perfect answer: truck stop scales! It was embarrassing holding up truck drivers, trying to weigh in their cargo. Those scales were accurate but depressing. I weighed about the same as the truck cargo. It was a good excuse to binge again. At least I learned to forgo the weigh-in before my new diet...tomorrow.

Fat is needed for a variety of bodily functions. It's our primary form of energy storage. Fat pads the body and it also surrounds and cushions our vital organs. The fat under your skin insulates your body from temperature extremes, and some dietary fat enhances the food we eat.

As a nation, we are more obsessed with food, diets, and weight loss than any other country. About 25 million Americans own health club memberships and over 3 billion dollars were spent on home exercise equipment in the last year alone. And yet we continue to get fatter as a nation.

The normal weight and height for an average woman is about 5'4, 140 pounds. Most of today's top models are about 5'10" tall and weigh about 110 pounds. They represent about 2 percent of the population and yet we use them as "guidelines." We will pick up a magazine with a thin celebrity so we can find out what her diet is. How ridiculous! You don't know how they became slim. There are all kinds of tricks the super rich and famous use that normal people don't know about. And they want to keep it that way. They are paid to sell a diet, not an expensive procedure or chemical that they don't want people to know about. Perhaps some assume that, by purchasing unrealistic photos of models with their pseudo diet, "osmosis" will occur. It's not a conspiracy or the fault of the media.

We are buying into their sales pitch because we are in selective denial. Yet, obesity is now outpacing smoking as the fastest growing fatal disease. We all pay for this, whether we are fat or not. Medical complications are directly connected to obesity. Weight-related diseases are affecting our over-extended hospitals and inflated insurance programs. *Obesity* is defined as increased body weight due to an excessive accumulation of fat. Defining someone by scales or charts is too relative. The most accurate way to determine your true weight is to figure out your total body fat percentage. This is done by taking your body weight and dividing it into your total fat weight, which gives you your body fat percentage. Normal recommended ratios are about 10- 13% for men (athletes 6-7%) and 15- 23% for women (athletes 10-13%).

Nevertheless, if you are questioning yourself about obesity, then you have a problem with weight. An extra ten pounds of weight puts stress on every part of your body. Every fat cell secretes excess insulin. If you are overweight, it is easier to gain more weight and harder to lose weight. Once you've gained weight, you've entered the *fat dilemma!* Your set-point is lower; it's harder to get under a certain weight regardless of what you do. And yet you feel hungry all the time. What little weight you do lose (which is harder every diet) comes back faster with a little extra for dessert. Large people usually deal with our judgmental society. Overweight people are always presented as "the fat funny one," "the lazy one," perhaps even "the sneaky one." Fashion, restaurants, airplane seating, amusement parks: everything seems to cater to slim people only. It's as if overweight people don't exist. Over half the nation is overweight and yet we treat those people as if they are the minority. Overweight people are discriminated against for jobs in all vocations. Insurance reasons might be the excuse, but a thin drug addict will usually get hired over someone who is "fat." Our kids, who are going to be the only generation who won't outlive their parents, are suffering with adult diseases. Furthermore, as kids they, too, usually endure the cruel remarks made by other kids or even adults. Telling them they aren't fat isn't going to help. Getting the junk food out of the schools and having more outdoor activities, rather than computer games or TV, will help.

Large people don't become large simple because they love food. Nor is it because they have a "bad metabolism." On the contrary, usually overweight individuals have very good metabolisms because they eat a lot of food, which boosts the metabolism. I feel ambivalent about women who "embrace their fat." Although it takes courage to go against what the superficial world accepts, the weight is affecting them physically and mentally. When someone is overweight, I simply ask myself, "What's eating them?" or "Why are they eating?" Extra weight means extra issues. Denial will only carry you so far.

It's easier to combat fat if you know what you are up against and that it's not your fault. It has nothing at this point to do with willpower. You are fighting chemicals and hormones that make it much harder to lose weight and easier to gain more weight. It's no different than a drug addict detoxing off of drugs. Your own body's chemicals are equally as strong, causing withdrawal symptoms as bad as any alcoholic or drug addict. These are what you are up against if you're "**FAT**":

IT'S NOT YOUR FAULT!!!

☞ There are excess insulin spills from all fat cells, which creates weight gain.

☞ Most overweight individuals suffer from hypoglycemia and are at risk for diabetes. Hypoglycemia is when blood sugar drops, creating constant hunger, bloating, depression, lack of energy, and easy weight gain.

☞ When you are overweight, the adrenal glands work overtime (adrenal exhaustion). This usually causes extra cortisol to be released (extra weight).

☞ While you are overweight, the serotonin level lowers, making you depressed and hungry; this can cause a "sweet tooth." (Tryptophan in carbs is a precursor for serotonin.)

☞ The hormone leptin is responsible for weight management, increasing energy, and decreasing appetite. It's located in all fat cells but is dormant in overweight people.

☞ The hormone ghrenlin (hunger mechanism), located in the stomach, causes hunger and is overabundant in overweight individuals. Ghrenlin also is responsible for creating extra fat.

☞ The hormone PYY336, which signals we are full when we have eaten, is absent in overweight individuals.

☞ In women, the estrogen works synergistically with insulin. Estrogen is stored in fat. Excess estrogen causes a "sweet tooth." Estrogen causes edema, making it impossible to enter the fat-burning/muscle-building process.

☞ Most overweight individuals gain their weight in the midsection or in an apple shape because of their imbalance of insulin, which puts a strain on the vital organs.

☞ Excess weight taxes the lungs.

☞ Excess weight causes sleep disturbances, and sleep deprivation is directly linked to obesity.

☞ Sleep deprivation causes the malfunction of hormones that are vital for weight loss, such as ghrenlin (hunger hormone), which increases near midnight.

☞ When unable to sleep eight hours per night, the body is overwhelmed with cravings for salty and sugary foods.

☞ There is also extra lactic acid and residue from a poor diet, making it extremely difficult to exercise

☞ Weight gain causes hormonal imbalances. Women experience hair loss while growing facial hair. Men will gain fatty tissue in their chests, along with other problems women endure.

☞ The overweight body is depleted in their reserves. Sugar, meat, and chemicals deplete your reserves. This causes the liver to malfunction. Hair loss, dental problems, and bone malfunctions will manifest as well.

☞ The overweight body tissue is so *dirty* (toxins) that cellulite is inevitable.

☞ It takes twenty-one days to excrete sugar from your system—thirty to ninety days for sugar addicts. During this time, the excretion causes unbearable cravings for twenty-hours after ingesting sugar.

☞ Certain foods like chocolate raises endorphin levels, making cravings like those of a drug addict.

☞ The addiction physiologically causes brain chemicals, like the neurotransmitter dopamine, to excrete a "high" feeling from the mere thought of the food you are craving (Pavlovian).

☞ The mental agony, guilt, and anxiety of eating foods your body *forces* you to releases more cortisol, affecting insulin.

☞ This furthers any depression, depleting your own serotonin while excreting other poisonous chemicals from mental stress.

☞ Your own brain chemicals, like serotonin, are so depleted that your only quick source of serotonin is instant junk food (relief).

☞ Your food (your enemy) is your only friend and medicine to "fix" the physical and mental anxiety and depression. Food and overeating become your survival tool and mechanism, creating an unstoppable pattern of addiction.

☞ Being alarmed with poor health and having low self-worth, the overweight individual is forced to *diet*.

☞ Diets deplete your own serotonin and can't make new or necessary serotonin due to the lack of calories and carb content. Thus depression sets in.

☞ Diets also create a sluggish metabolism, especially after continuous dieting, which makes it hard to lose weight while eating barely anything. Your body *fights* any starving whatsoever!

☞ Depression and the stress of extra weight causes excess cortisol and leaves the body "stuck" with edema (bloating).

☞ Diets make all of your vital chemicals and hormones react poorly. Then it becomes impossible to try a restrictive diet again, regardless of the diet or person who is dieting.

☞ The diet is sabotaged out of pure frustration, depletion, feeling ill from detoxifying, and all the powerful chemicals and hormones working diligently *against* your willpower!

☞ You are forced to binge to retrieve the serotonin and familiar feeling of medicating yourself, to escape self-loathing.

☞ Without bingeing, you are prone to gaining at least five pounds more than when you started the diet.

💣 THE CYCLE CONTINUES!

As soon as you realize it is not your fault, you will realize you can do something about it. These are not excuses but are reasons for the "insanity." You CAN make your life more manageable with the right tools and frame of mind. To remain a "victim" of low self-worth will only perpetuate using your survival mechanism, furthering the addiction. Chemically speaking, you are up against powerful drugs that the body is either excreting or depleted of, making it impossible to think straight. Hormonally, you are extremely unbalanced. This encourages a habit of relieving your symptoms with food, which is the problem to begin with. Mentally, everyone has made you think that you lack willpower when, in fact, most people never have to endure what overweight people go through both physically and mentally. You can take responsibility and move from being the victim to recovery. You do this by letting go of diets and deprivation altogether. You teach yourself about the foods that will satisfy you while increasing your levels of good brain chemicals and important hormones. These new delicious and healthy foods will help you learn to eat to live, not live to eat. A spiritual and mental program is also necessary to compliment the food plan so you can figure out what you are eating over and teach yourself how to express your feelings instead of denying them.

Gastric bypass or any weight loss surgery is a personal choice. I have witnessed some success stories of some individuals who were given a head-start toward changing their lives. Sadly though, there are many people who would not change their eating habits and stretched their stomachs back out to their original size again after surgery, which caused them to gain all of their weight back. Please don't fool yourself into thinking that gastric bypass in not a very serious procedure, because it is—just like all other surgeries. It doesn't fix an eating disorder. Fixing the outside appearance does not fix the inside issue, which is why they were eating. If you have had bad habits for years, trying to fix them overnight instead of working to "earn" your health is another part of the disease. You can't buy health. Building a cell is building health. Every day that you work to "earn" your health, you blueprint a new pattern that stays with you mentally and physically.

Simply put, fat is a symptom of a problem, not the cause of it or the reason for it. Don't symptom-chase by dieting. Your body is dictated by hormones. Learning about your body and how certain foods work synergistically with your body's chemicals and hormones will make you an active participant in getting well and healthy (losing weight). You must realize, though, that your goal is HEALTH, and then the byproduct will be weight loss. We are not meant to be fat. If we work synergistically with nature, then nature's laws will guide us to our goals.

CHAPTER 7:
ADJUSTING THE METABOLISM

There was a time that my metabolism didn't exist. I feared passing any bakery in case I accidentally "inhaled" some calories from the mere smell of a pastry.

Metabolism: Physical and chemical processes necessary to sustain life, including the production of cellular energy and synthesis of biological substances. It's the chemical processes in a living organism by which food is used for tissue growth or energy production

This chapter is dedicated to the metabolism because it's always the dieter's dilemma. I was only jealous of one thing about my sister: her metabolism. It was better than mine, but eventually we both shared "malfunctioning" metabolisms. I think that, during one of our out-of-control binges, we ate our thyroids.

Why does it seem slim people eat and eat? How is it that French people eat large amounts of fatty foods and remain slim? Why are overweight people the *only ones* eating diet food? Think of it this way: Our bodies are so sophisticated; they can ingest just about anything and either use it, store it, or eliminate it. Years ago, the Egyptians were so afraid of being poisoned that they added a little arsenic to their diets every day so their bodies would be immune to it. It was the same way with the French. For years, French tradition allowed cream sauces and other fatty foods. Their bodies developed enzymes and other chemicals that handle these fatty foods. It's the same way with our bodies and diets. If you have dieted for years, your body has acclimated to low calories, low fat, and poor nutrition. It adapts by lowing your metabolism and by raising your set point. The set point remains at a certain weight, so no matter what you do, it won't budge. It has reached a plateau. Your body also seems to gain weight without ingesting many calories. You have become fat efficient.

How do most people remedy this? They adopt a stricter diet. What does this do? It lowers the metabolism and raises your set point. Your body responds the same way to excess exercising as it does to excess dieting. Following approximately forty-five minutes of hard aerobic exercise, the body switches to pulling from its reserves (glycogen). If you deplete these reserves, the body looks for handy fuel, such as vital tissue rather than fat, because the body is entering enervation and stress. This usually causes excess cortisol to be released, which triggers excess insulin spills. This may further cause a hypoglycemic reaction (bloating, exhaustion, hunger). Your body refuses to enter the fat-burning/muscle/building process while under this edema and stress. Subsequently your body compensates by lowering the metabolism and raising the set point.

☞ *What is a high or low metabolism?*

There are some experts who claim there is no such thing as a low or high metabolism, simply because there are no numbers that define what *high* or *low* is. It's a term that is loosely used to rate how well you burn calories or use carbs.

☞ *How do you raise the metabolism or "speed it up"?*

1) Calories (The more calories you eat the raises the metabolism).

2) Movement (Any type of movement raises the metabolism).

3) Eat frequently, every three hours or less.(Not eating within three hours lowers the metabolism).

☞ *How do you repair a "damaged" metabolism?*

1) Don't starve or diet. This lowers the metabolism and raises the set point.

2) Don't exercise excessively.

☞ *What are some helpful tips to "boost" the metabolism?*

1) Eat small, frequent mini-meals throughout the day, every three hours or less. Divide high-calorie foods into small mini-meals.

2) Refrain from all sugar, stimulants, and "false" metabolism boosters. Coffee, (especially caffeine), cigarettes, and energy boosters disrupt your hormones (thyroid, metabolism), which causes excess insulin spills. This can cause a hypoglycemic reaction, which also affects the metabolism.

3) Eat foods high in fiber: "broom" foods that *work* your digestive system and thus work your metabolism.

4) Focus on anaerobic exercise rather than aerobic. Anaerobic exercise develops the muscles without exhausting your adrenal glands. Muscle weighs more than fat. Anaerobic exercise causes the secretion of HGH (human growth hormone), which automatically puts you into the fat-burning/muscle-building process. Your body naturally raises the metabolism when muscle weight increases.

5) Put a "peak" in your exercise routine as well. Instead of long distance running, try short sprints that will raise the heart rate and shake up your exercise routine. This also "breaks" your weight plateau.

6) Rest. Meditate and relax. Exercise should be done once daily. Then rest the body so it can heal, accumulate energy, and store reserves.

☞ *Why does someone have a low metabolism?*

A low metabolism can be the result of a number of things. Using too many over the counter drugs, too many stimulants, or too much exercise all contribute to it. When someone eats large meals with long intervals in-between, it causes hormonal imbalances that lower the metabolism. And let's not forget stress or depression. All these factors and more can lead to a low metabolism. Our bodies have not changed since the caveman days when we grazed constantly, every three hours or less. When you wait more than three hours between meals, your insulin usually over-secretes with the next meal. This prevents the body from entering the fat-burning/muscle building process. Adrenal exhaustion, candidiasis, or hypothyroidism can also cause metabolic disturbances. Hypothyroidism is the underproduction of the thyroid hormone. The thyroid is a large gland in the neck that secretes hormones that regulate growth and development through the rate of metabolism. Keep in mind that all hormones work synergistically.

☞ *What are the symptoms of hypothyroidism?*

Cold temperature intolerance, fatigue, slow heart rate, weight gain, painful periods, weakness, yellow skin, hair loss, depression, and more.

☞ *How can you tell if you suffer from metabolic problems or hypothyroidism? (Check with doctor.)*

Try a thyroid self-test: In the morning, place a thermometer under your arm and hold it there for fifteen minutes. Keep very calm, preferably in bed while very still.; 97.6 degrees or lower may indicate an under-active thyroid. If temperature is continuous for more than a week, then you may suffer from an under-active thyroid; check with doctor.

☞ *What helps remedy a metabolism or poor thyroid function?*

✓ Kelp
✓ B5 and B complex
✓ L-Tyrosine
✓ Brewer's yeast
✓ EFA oils
✓ Black cohosh
✓ Black goldenseal
✓ Distilled water
✓ Proper foods that boost metabolism: foods high in fiber and iron (black strap molasses, dark greens, raw milk, eggs, and dried fruit).

☞ *What should be avoided?*

✓ Refined foods, fluoride, and sulfa drugs or antihistamines.

"FIX" *your* METABOLISM WITH *extra* FOOD

☞ If you are dieting without losing weight or you gain weight while eating a normal diet, try this:

✓ Divide your normal daily diet into 6-8 mini-meals. Add extra calories to your diet in the following manner:

✓ Add approximately 25 calories (example:1/4 of an apple) of the same food to 3-4 of your meals, every other meal. For instance, take the 100 calorie apple, split it in four pieces and have one piece four times within your eight mini meals.

✓ Make sure the 25 calories added to every other meal (75-100 calories/day) are from a clean protein or a raw vegetable or fruit.

✓ Make sure the 25 calories added to every other meal (75-100 calories/day) is one type of food for the day (example: 1 apple per day), but....

✓ Make sure the 25 calories added to every other meal (75-100 calories/day) changes every other day (example: apple one day, a piece of tofu the next, etc).

✓ On the fifth day, add 25 calories to *each* meal in the same way as stated above. This will mean you are adding 150-200 calories per day, divided into 25 calories per meal (example: 1 ½-2 apples per day or tofu, divided up evenly into each meal).

✓ On the tenth day, add 25 *more* calories to each meal. This will mean you adding 300-400 calories per day, divided into 50 calories per meal. Vary and mix your added calories in that day, unlike before (example: apple *and* tofu per day, divided up evenly into each meal).

✓ By the fourteenth day, if your metabolism is normal, return to your normal diet habits. If you seem to manifest signs of a poor metabolism ,start over with day one.

This technique tricks the metabolism because you are sneaking the extra (but clean) calories in gradually—per meal, per day. By the tenth day, you have added 300-400 calories to your diet per day. If you gradually add several calories, evenly distributed, to your normal diet, it speeds up the metabolism.

~ ~ ~ ~ ~ ~

Above all, don't symptom-chase a low metabolism. Find the reason your metabolism is low and target that problem first. These are all helpful hints for a sluggish metabolism, but they won't cure the reason you have one. If you are a chronic dieter or you refuse any activity, all the tricks in the world won't break Mother Nature's laws. If you have exhausted adrenal glands, continuous candidiasis, or any female problems, your other hormones, such as cortisol and estrogen, work synergistically with your thyroid gland, eventually causing further malfunctions. Target problems synergistically and treat your body as a *whole*. Bad health in one area will surely leak into another.

Exercise tips that boost your metabolism:

1) Spilt your exercise routine into three different times of the day: morning, noon, and night. Make two of the three workouts aerobic and one of the three workouts anaerobic.

2) Or try 5-10 minutes of "peaking" exercise after each mini-meal. *Peaking* is going beyond your normal speed or endurance and raising the heart rate. You should eat 6-8 mini-meals

3)   Or delay aerobic workout sessions until the evening.

It usually takes 45 minutes to reach the fat-burning/muscle building stage. Exercising beyond 45 minutes can be enervating and sometimes causes the exerciser to "hit a wall," or plateau. If you exercise more than necessary, you can cause your plans to backfire and you may also exhaust your adrenal glands.

Chapter 8:
THE CHOCOLATE FETISH: *FOOD, SEX, AND LOVE*

Rate your date!
Is your lover into <u>you</u>?
(A "hot fudge sundae" or a "rotten egg"?)

As far as my sister and I were concerned, food, sex, and love were enmeshed. Our biggest love affair was with FOOD! All of our boyfriends were jealous of the noises my sis and I made in the kitchen, rather than in the bedroom.

Rate your Date! Relationship questionnaire:

Simply circle Yes or No beside each question:

1. In your relationship, is the subject of long-term commitment or marriage avoided?　Yes　No

2. Do you discourage your lover from fantasizing?　Yes　No

3. Would you leave the relationship if your mate gained a lot weight?　Yes　No

4. When your mate receives compliments from the opposite sex, do you feel insecure?　Yes　No

5. Do you need constant attention and compliments from your lover?　Yes　No

6. Do you get jealous of your ex's lovers or lover's ex's?　Yes　No

7. Do you wait for calls from your lover rather than initiating the call yourself?　Yes　No

8. Are you the one in charge who needs control of the relationship?   Yes   No

9. Are you opposed to your lover having a boy's night out or a girl's night out?   Yes   No

10. Would you prevent your lover from having a best friend of the opposite sex?   Yes   No

11. Are you attracted to mates who are unavailable (married, "cold," addicts, disloyal)?   Yes   No

12. Would you stand up your friends at the last minute if your lover called spontaneously?   Yes   No

13. Did you have a poor relationship with your parent of the opposite sex?   Yes   No

14. If you were dumped by your lover, are you the revengeful type (rather than moving on)?   Yes   No

15. Are you attracted to lovers you have to chase?   Yes   No

16. Do you expect your lover to rescue you and solve your problems (credit card debts, car payments, etc.)   Yes   No

17. Do you expect more than you receive in your relationship?   Yes   No

18. Do you generalize characteristics of the opposite sex? ("All men are the same.")   Yes   No

19. Do you consider your mate more like a friend than a lover?   Yes   No

20. Do find yourself losing your appetite when you are with your lover?   Yes   No

21. Do you complain that all men just want to have sex?   Yes   No

Is Your Lover into You?
(A "hot fudge sundae" or a "rotten egg"?)

1. Does your lover emphasize that he or she doesn't want to ruin his or her friendship with you?   Yes   No

2. Does your lover call you last minute for a date?   Yes   No

3. Does your lover have a need to get high or drunk when you are out on a date?   Yes   No

4. Does your lover make you wait for phone calls (late or forgotten)?   Yes   No

5. Does your lover get nervous when speaking about commitments, relationships. or the future?   Yes   No

6. Does your lover make future promises but put off immediate commitments?   Yes   No

7. Is your lover moody and disinterested in you at times, but he or she makes up for it at other times?   Yes   No

8. Is your lover too busy to see or call you regularly?   Yes   No

9. Does your lover want space, time, and freedom before getting serious and figuring out what he or she wants?   Yes   No

10. Did you make the first move on your lover?   Yes   No

Ladies, have you ever noticed how women tend to drown themselves in chocolate when they've been dumped? It's frustrating to see the guy in a broken relationship be able to move on, making an *easy* transition from one woman to another without indulging in food. How many of us spent tons of money in therapy trying to rebuild our self-esteem, while the "creep" simply moved down to the next phone number in his little black book. I hated myself for having feelings for my "creep" when he obviously had none for me. *Finally*, I learned to stop comparing my mate with my twin's (or girlfriend's), which made it made easier to accept men and respect our differences.

This chapter combines years of my research through observation (as a voyeur), studies (with perverts), and personal experiences (obviously pathetic). It's not a coincidence that my sister and I worked as models and had a major food problem, because both are connected in more ways than one.

Since the beginning of time, men have been the hunters (gathering the food) and women have been the nurturers (taking care of the cave and the children). No matter how modern we feel, our roles haven't changes much from our ancestors'. In early times, women had to endure long, hard, foodless winters. This is one theory why it's always been natural for women to crave foods that are fattening, such as high-glycemic foods that raise the blood sugar faster. This induces higher levels of LDL (low density lipoprotein, the bad cholesterol). This historic biology is the reason women's bodies are fat efficient. Men (hunters) usually crave protein because they are dictated by testosterone. Women biologically store fat on the outside of their bodies, while men usually store it on the inside. The biological purpose of women's fat was both physical attraction and better reserve storage to bear children. Through the ages, women have maintained their innate nature as caretakers, using *food* as the main instrument. Subsequently, culture and traditions pass on generations of celebrating with food. A family dinner is the most intimate and endearing event that a family group can share. It could even be considered from a woman's viewpoint as the foreplay of exploring a relationship.

Science plays a big part in the love affair that woman have with food, particularly chocolate. A lot of women have a fetish for chocolate and can replace their feelings for a man with this little piece of forbidden dessert. Certain foods stimulate woman in the same area of the brain where sex and alcohol stimulants men. Women also respond to serotonin more easily than men. It is in the foods we crave and activates certain feel-good brain chemicals. Tryptophan, an amino acid abundant in carbohydrates (like grains, legumes, and seeds) is the precursor to serotonin, a brain chemical and hormone that is responsible for making us feel calm, happy, and fulfilled mentally and physically. That is why women prefer carbs to protein. When women suffer from depression, PMS, stress, and relationship difficulties, they use these foods to fix a feeling. Diet deprivation or exhaustion can also cause women to turn to chocolate or other high-sugar carbs for "relief." Chocolate increases endorphins (hormones that create a "high" or euphoria). Although chocolate has been given a thumbs up for having flavonoids and antioxidants, it still carries some questionable ingredients like theobromine. Theobromine is an alkaloid closely related to caffeine. Chocolate has also been referred to as an aphrodisiac. No wonder it's estimated that we individually eat approximately twelve pounds of chocolate a year! Regardless of the reason, women respond better to a box of chocolates than men do. Women also respond better to antidepressants, which trigger serotonin and/or norepinephrine (hormones and neurotransmitters). This further affects their sleep, emotions, and adrenals.

Women should refrain from competing, completing, or comparing ourselves with men because we are wired entirely differently. We interpret almost everything—especially food, love, and sex—as if we are from two different planets. Generally speaking, men usually use the left side of the brain. They deal with love, stress, and problem solving intellectually, simply, or quickly. Men fall in love with a woman through visual images and fantasize when they are away. Women, on the other hand, use their whole brains to make a decision, usually taking longer to decide. Women use the right side (feelings and intuition) to guide their own intellect. This causes a need for discussion and possibly over-analyzing. I have been accused of diarrhea of the mouth. Now I know why. Some claim gay men or very sensitive men are also able to tap into the right side of their brains, making it easier for them to empathize with women's feelings. Recovery seems to be a struggle for women or men who primarily use the right side of the brain. This is because they emotionalize the addiction and connect it with their self-worth. When you emotionalize the addiction, you are *attaching* your feelings to a drug. These enmeshed feelings seem to *dictate* as well as *define* the addict. Have you ever noticed that highly creative individuals are constantly polarized between feelings of shame and grandiosity? They are controlled by their emotional addiction, not their intuition or actions. These right-brain addicts prefer "magical" thinking rather than rationalization, thus making recovery grim. Addiction seems to be prevalent among *artists*, who primarily use the right side of the brain.

Women fall in love with the way men make them *feel* when they are with them. Women need men to share their feelings. Our feelings actually manifest a "glow" when we fall in love. Because we are predominately dictated by the way we *feel*, as opposed to what we see, we connect (or sometimes replace) the same feelings that food gives us with sex and love. Basically, we fall in love with these feelings. We use treats as substitutes for love and feelings. This is why we lose our appetites when we fall in love. When men forget to call us, omit gifts on special occasions, or don't want to discuss love or difficulties, we feel unloved. It's as if they are showing us that we are unworthy. When men stray, we feel completely betrayed. Men are not so complicated. You pretty much know where men stand because they are very direct. They can separate food, sex, love, and several mates without guilt, because they don't emotionalize things the way we do. A man's innate nature is to be a hunter who is visually stimulated. It is said that an average man thinks about sex approximately once every three minutes. (That's about the same amount of times I think about food and diets.) It's easier for men to disconnect their feelings for their mates while straying. This can be considered double standard, because men interpret humiliation and disloyalty differently than women do. A man's choice of his ideal woman usually has nothing to do with intelligence. It's been proven that, the higher the woman's IQ, the harder it is for her to hook up. I'm in no way condoning or promoting a certain behavior. I'm just objectively pointing out a man's basic nature and the way they interpret love, which is far different than a woman's. Because men don't respond the same way as women do, men often feel that women are testing and grading them. Sometimes men find themselves in a no-win situation. Women will sometimes ask loaded questions such as, "Does this dress make me look fat?" or "Did you find her attractive?" How does the guy answer this? Ladies, let's be honest. No answer would suffice. We really want to be validated and supported. Let's face it: Any answer will make us overreact because we sense a lack of reaction or mutual feeling. We usually ask a rhetorical question that is meant to generate empathy for our feelings.

Women also deal with stress differently than men because of our different hormones. Men are predominately dictated by male hormone testosterone, which usually causes them to physically act out—more like an external release. Before you know it, they forgot about their issue, have moved on, or quickly deny it. Men would rather pout *alone* in their bear cave and be done with it. Women, on the other hand, release their frustration by initiating a dissecting discussion without a need for resolution. Women eventually internalize their stress, which may affect their adrenal glands (cortisol), blood sugar, and insulin levels. This can trigger a hypoglycemic reaction, which causes further depression or mood swings. Naturally, we want to help balance our blood sugar drop by turning to foods with sugar. The cycle of depression continues, causing our feelings to "smolder." Women really do have a *biological* need to "talk it out."

As women, we emotionalize everything that is said to us or has personal connotation. If a man tells us, or even hints, that we are gaining weight, we attach those feelings to our self-worth. We actually define ourselves not only by how we look, but by how it is conveyed to us. Men are just the opposite. Rarely will a man emotionally attach himself to feelings about his appearance or feelings of love. Women can continue a relationship by phone, unlike men, because we are in love with the feeling of being in love. Men have a hard time with the telephone because it lacks a physical connection. We are the ones who wait for phone calls and are hurt if they don't call us. Perhaps a man's *ego* can be provoked, but rarely will issues be about his appearance or feelings of love. I've learned to separate my dates from my "phone dumping", (complaining about various issues). That's what's great about having girlfriends or understanding gay male friends.

As I've mentioned, men communicate with quick and simple solutions (intellect) or physical behavior, while women communicate with feelings and discussion. Subsequently, everything men naturally show us is what they feel. It's not some profound conspiracy that they would want to discuss. It's simply what you see is what you get. When a woman expects a mate to recite poems and give her flowers, she is asking her lover to insincerely express *his* feelings the way *she* would. If a man were to express his feelings sincerely, his testosterone would encourage barbaric behavior. Perhaps he would drag a woman into his bear cave, by the hair. Evidently, men have learned to seduce or manipulate women by doing what a woman *wants* and would respond to. Ironically, woman's pheromones actually respond best to the lover's awkward, crude, and sincere methods (cave man), not the "flowery way." Intellectually, we may think we want a sensitive man who reacts much like a gentleman. Not so. We actually are chemically attracted to the "raw" male. You will always hear the complaint that women are attracted to jerks or that nice guys are attracted to high-maintenance or demanding divas. It's because our hormones instinctively respond best to the sincerity of the chase. None of us, are actually attracted to jerks. Subconsciously, we are attracted to lovers who behave naturally and have confidence without needing to manipulate us. The gentleman might get a marriage proposal, but the "raw" man will get your attention and attraction.

Let's talk about the two types of gentlemen. First, there is the manipulating, manmade *pseudo* gentleman. Ladies, we've trained them to be this way. Then there's the one who naturally evolves into a gentleman, without a motive. Young girls confuse *masculinity* (strength) with being macho. Crude or macho men (a.k.a. boys) are immature. These "macho" men might be able to change themselves into temporary gentlemen to manipulate women insincerely. However, true strength comes from a man who has learned to withhold his primitive behaviors, eventually evolving into a true gentleman. I notice men from the Midwest and South (or from families with good values) naturally manifest chivalry.

Sex and love interrelate to evolutionary and scientific research in the same way that food does. Initially, the experience of love gives us the impression of being fulfilled. Hormones, such as oxytocin, better known as the "cuddling hormone," make us *feel* we are filling our void. The main purpose of oxytocin, which is secreted after childbirth, is to enhance the bonding experience between mother and child. Oxytocin makes monogamy easier for women. Endorphins and other feel-good hormones are released when you fall in love, in the same way certain foods or drugs work. For instance, when you eat chocolate, it releases endorphins, hormones that give us a feeling like we are in love. This feeling chocolate gives us can be compared to the "high" we experience when we are in love. Love and chocolate have the same withdrawal symptoms and both create cravings for more. For example, the neurotransmitter, dopamine (high feeling) actually secretes during the mere memory of your love or treat. This explains why we "can't shake" someone we fell for. Sometimes we insist on "marrying" these *feelings* (we can't live without the person responsible for this feeling), fearing we will lose the feeling this person gives us. Feeling a lack of love sometimes causes women to duplicate these feelings by eating certain foods. Have you ever felt like raiding the fridge when your lover doesn't call? When a man and woman are basically in love, the man's testosterone levels falls and the woman's testosterone levels rises. This enables women to maintain a healthy libido, while men may be prone to straying or fantasizing so they can recapture their testosterone level. Have you ever noticed that female athletes have a healthy sex drive? When a woman is pregnant (or suffers from certain female problems), her estrogen levels usually dominate. This can decrease the sex drive, increase appetite and weight gain (edema), and sometimes cause depression. During this time, the female's progesterone levels are also unbalanced. Progesterone balance is necessary for mental well-being and responsible for bouncing back. It also helps maintain the muscle-building/fat-burning process.

Estrogen, the female hormone, also has a role in filling our void. Estrogen is stored in fat. This could be one reason women subconsciously crave fat or fattening foods, thus connecting the inner woman with their *curves.* Presently, it seems women usually prefer the contradiction of fighting this natural biological urge by starving away their curves. Subsequently, today's men have been involuntarily trained by women to prefer this androgynous image. Modern men subconsciously think this curve-less image represents better health and is therefore better for procreating offspring. Marilyn Monroe would be considered overweight by today's standards. Men and the media are not putting this pressure on women. We, as women, are. Men have always been programmed to be attracted to good health. Early history proves that men were always biologically attracted to youthful and symmetrical women because they were the best for childbearing. Men are physically attracted to women, while women are emotionally seduced by security. At one time, men who were muscular and strong provided security for the family. These days women seem to interpret security in terms of men's wallets and career status, not their muscles. A man who is superficial or a woman who is a gold-digger is responding to *extreme* basic instincts, not society. Society reflects our shameless desires.

Throughout the years, women have transferred their survival mechanisms from one escape to the other, trying to avoid an empty feeling. Perhaps binging is someone's survival mechanism and they want to escape from binging into other areas, such as sex and love. Shopping, modeling, and other escapes can be disguised as necessary events or goals. And of course, relationships can also be disguised fulfillment, replacing *.food* to fill the void. Developing a relationship can medicate a "feeling of lack", the same way food does. A feeling of lack is when you want to fill your "void" with something to make you feel whole. It can be excess food, a man or even an inappropriate behavior. When you *transfer* a craving or survival mechanism, such as binge eating, to a relationship, it is *sex and control*—not love—that then dictates the relationship and defines the person. The "feeling of lack" is replaced by a "controlled substance" or a controlling relationship, out of fear rather than a developing a healthy and honest partnership. Control issues are (manifested in sex) which usually stem from the fear of feeling a void.or incomplete. These new feelings are so powerful they diminish the possibilities for developing lasting love or inner fulfillment. It's simple: Real love does not coexist with fear. Fear is synonymous with any negative characteristic, such a jealousy.

A healthy relationship has the same qualities as a good career: connection and contribution. Control entails neediness, which makes it difficult to share or give to the relationship. Healthy relationships involve support rather than competition, empathy rather than pity, acceptance rather than control, inspiration rather than jealousy, gratitude rather than expectations, and surrender rather than giving up or denial. Obsession eventually overwhelms unhealthy relationships. Unhealthy relationships regress back to the original escape: the obsession of food. However, don't become your lover's friend. Some therapists claim intimacy is lost when there is a feeling of extreme safety in a relationship. It is normal to have *some* level of jealously. Healthy, intimate relationships evolve when the *lover* remains the *lover*; that's it.

This takes us to another level. Some experts claim that women who have a need to constantly dress in a sexy way have a difficult time being satisfied (biologically speaking) with just one partner. One theory claims immodesty is a lack of oxytocin. (For example, adult children of alcoholics are shown to be born with less oxytocin.) Evidentially, these "sexy" women are unable to secrete appropriate lubrication consistently, unless they change partners. This can be perceived as a masculine trait, especially when observing the animal kingdom. It is the male species that reflects the ostentatious showmanship in both their appearance and attitude. Women who act out sexually or insist on an overt appearance usually come from families that had inappropriate boundaries. It's almost a cry for help or a possible need for appropriate closure of unresolved issues with their childhood guardian, usually the guardian of the opposite sex. (A professional can help closure.) These women can easily mistake feeling needy for feeling sexy. With this in mind, it's unfortunate that modeling has been celebrated as the ultimate career for a woman. Models are paid extraordinary amounts of money, are revered as role models, and don't feel any shame about walking into any door without a resume. On the other hand, modeling can be a healthy choice for female athletes or actresses when they want to celebrate their bodies or enhance their careers. This type of modeling seems to compliment their main goal rather than become a validating competition. When modeling is used as the primary goal, it's usually the result of a feeling of lack. Nude modeling, centerfolds, or pin-ups take us to another level. What type of woman would choose that image to define herself. (A desperate woman, from what I've experienced). It has been hypothesized these women had unavailable fathers or unhealthy paternal guidance and obsessively need the approval of a vast amount of men to replace their father. Some objectively compare this career choice to the oldest profession: prostitution, being paid to please a man. Nevertheless, society seems to shamelessly revere these lost souls. This influences our youth's desire, as well, to seek such easy infamy. It saddens me to see young people on talk shows express desire to attain this goal.

On the contrary, women sometimes act out in the opposite way. When there has been some sort of abuse (sexual, physical, or emotional), women sometimes shut themselves off sexually by overeating and subconsciously shielding themselves with a layer of fat. This shield can also manifest itself as anorexia or drug abuse. Although food/weight abuse can be the opposite side of promiscuity, it usually is derived from the same bad experience. For instance, one may be frigid due to a bad experience. Being frigid could be interpreted as using a survival mechanism to control or *discourage* sexuality in the same way anorexics control their food intake. Either of these mental disorders may stem from some sort of abuse. Healthy sex does have its physical and mental benefits as well. During sex, enhancing hormones and chemicals are secreted throughout the brain and body and raise the metabolism's set point. For example, epinephrine (helps blood sugar and muscle activity) is released during sex. This was evident when I had heard about a study about a group of nuns were compared with a group of sexually active married couples. The results noted that the nuns, surprisingly, had lower metabolisms and immune systems on the whole compared to the sexually active married women. (Bummer, I'm getting none!)

Here's the controversy: When is sex or sex appeal inappropriate or unhealthy? In my opinion, when it comes from a feeling of lack. It could be lack of control, lack of feeling love, lack of self-worth, or lack of family security. These feelings of lack subsequently turn into shame. When people are shame-based, as opposed to guilty, they mistakenly see themselves *as*_the problem rather than *having* a problem. Those people's identities are smothered by unrealistic desires that can never be fulfilled. They compensate by placing extreme standards on themselves. Their desperate attempts at gaining control and escaping the shame swing one of two ways: They may inwardly seek self-punishment, triggering over-sensitivity that transforms into some addictive behavior. Or they may outwardly act out and overtly display insensitivity to what others think. Both are signs of depression, which is a form of self-absorption. Self-pity creates self-obsession and a need to escape. Eventually, the obsession loses its potency, which takes the behavior to new extremes. The addictive or radical and destructive behavior is born.

I have heard recently that it's been claimed that, when televisions were introduced into countries that normally don't have TVs, there was a rise in eating disorders. It seems silly to solely blame the media or outside circumstances for our behaviors. This creates a feeling of being helpless or a victim mentality, which prevents us from taking responsibility. We are in charge of our TVs and what is placed on ads. It's supply and demand. Women are the primary consumers. Television experts claim that during ratings sweeps months, *more than 3/4* of the audiences are woman. Women participate by viewing the sensationalized sex on TV! We do have a say by our actions as consumers and viewers. Women complain about the media pushing youth and unrealistic standards rather than boycotting these shows, sponsors, and advertisements. As women, we are giving mixed messages of what we want in the media, because our actions don't match our complaints. Any show, commercial, and magazine that displays average women have been shown to not sell, time after time. Women idolize Marilyn Monroe more than men do. Her image is idolized on postage stamps. How has she contributed to women? Her story was pathetic, not enlightening or empowering. Her image is prehistorically cliché, not inspiring. People mistake Marilyn Monroe's weakness as being *vulnerable*. Being vulnerable actually means being without choice or power. Today, women think it's feminine to imitate and role-play this dated behavior. How discouraging that the world, particularly America, embraces and idolizes women's outsides rather than their insides. We do this by falling into the pit of making the billion-dollar campaign of sex and body image one of our main interests (in magazines, merchandise, on TV, etc.). Don't blame the messenger (or models). Stop buying magazines or watching programs that primarily sensationalize sex. Rather than demanding average looking role models, direct your financial support and ratings. Put your money where your mouth is. America is supposed to have the most liberated women with more rights than in most countries. We abuse that right by prioritizing beauty. In India, they are known for their caste system. Whatever caste you are born into dictates everything you do. There isn't any circumstance that would allow you to break in or out of that certain caste you were born into. In America, if a woman is born beautiful, she is automatically in the top of "America's caste system"—the system we have placed ourselves in. If you are an unattractive or older woman, your chances and choices are not available or easy compared to what the very attractive female can achieve with just her *appearance!* Yet we, as women, continuously choose role models (with what we purchase and view) by the way they look rather than what they've contributed. There are third world countries that revere women as top scientists or prime ministers. These women are not judged by their age or appearance. We've taken our woman's rights and thrown them back into the stone age by glorifying attractive women rather than women who contribute.

My sister and I are always asked the question, "What is sexy?" I think the most feminine quality a woman can embody is *virtue*. Virtue simply means "saving yourself"or waiting for the appropriate time and place. That is sexy to me. This correlates to the theory that women overexposing themselves or constantly dressing provocatively is a masculine trait. That is not sexy; it is a cry for help. I also think that a woman who simply chooses to be a wife and a mother carries that feminine virtue to the highest regard. As basic and outdated as it seems to some, I can't help but respect women who dedicate themselves to their families rather than seeking power, fame, and attention. To me, a sexy man is a man who seeks a woman with virtue and wants to share the desire to dedicate himself to his family above his ambition to succeed. How unfortunate that I came to this conclusion walking down the wrong path.

Where did my sis and I go wrong, if we knew better? While growing up, my sister and I wanted to be veterinarians and horse trainers. We loved sports and animals and only used modeling to support our love of these things. We started modeling at seven years old. It was all we knew. Eventually our dysfunctional eating disorder turned a simple modeling job into a superficial career. Ironically, the image we portrayed on calendars and magazines is the complete opposite of what we really are. Initially it was sort of fun to be in disguise for a while. Then we became what we made fun of. Obviously we had underlying issues that caused our deadly disease (an eating disorder) to dictate and leak into our life-changing decisions. Using food to medicate our feelings of worthlessness was a learned behavior derived from an alcoholic family environment. When our eating disorder was out of control, we transmitted it into weight control, making modeling our *scapegoat*. We negotiated our career with our disease. Our career choices always stemmed from our disease talking. For example, we thought if we were documented as slim on the cover of a magazine no one would judge our eating disorder. We were like walking dry drunks. The "ism" was still there. Our unhealthy childhood environment had left us feeling neglected and unworthy. We associated our self-worth with success (at any cost), so we would be worthy. We turned to society for support and love rather than our unavailable family. It appeared to us that society respected *any* type of notoriety, even pin-up modeling. Being talent-less: That was the perfect career that could help us control and hide our problems with weight. We obtained leverage by placing extreme standards on ourselves, and by doing so we pushed ourselves into a nightmare of extreme diet abuse. This is where we unknowingly crossed the line from victim to perpetrator, or started swimming with the sharks. We were so intoxicated with our insecurities and self-absorbed eating disorder that we became completely unaware of the negative impact we had on women. We didn't think much of ourselves, so we couldn't imagine having any impact on anyone else. That was the turning point when we came out of the closet and admitted to our eating disorder. Our career choice to model was originally transmitted from our food addiction). Modeling or food addictions come from a feeling of lack. Obviously modeling never fulfilled us; it only pushed us back to food. Our solution to weight gain was extreme dieting, which developed the next problem, bulimia, and eventually leaked into our modeling. We were more or less in a symptom-chasing cycle. Rather than dealing with the original problem (which were deep issues that transmitted into compulsive overeating), we solved it with continuous cycles of outside fixes. Our misguided interpretation of approval spun us into a superficial career to cover up the issues we were eating over. In addition, our addiction seemed to replace any relationship, because our only love affair was with food.

Despite everything, it now seems all worth it because we finally touched women who identify with us. Best of all, we finally have a huge female fan following that insists on purchasing our products and pictures, which they say helps inspire them to be healthy and recovered. We are grateful that we can finally utilize our "dysfunctional podium" and turn it into a source of motivation and *solutions* for others through sharing our downfalls and recovery.

Regardless of whether you are escaping or filling a void (unhealthy fulfillment), by using your survival mechanism (food, sex, and so forth), eventually it stops working and backfires , The very reason why you want to escape or fill your void is magnified when you find out your void can't be filled with escaping methods. This is denial. Unfortunately, I can admit we know this from experience. This holds true for any time you try to fulfill yourself with an "outside fix".. If you seek a relationship for sex or money, then it is sex or money that will cause its demise. It is the same for food. If you use diet food to shed your weight, then the diet will bring you back to the reason for dieting: food indulgence or bingeing. The weight struggles begin their cycle, (dieting, binging, escaping, etc.). Of course it's natural for women to have the desire to feel attractive; that's normal. However, sex or concern about your appearance should never be a goal. Simply put, they should be the byproduct or a part of a healthy lifestyle and choices. And simple biology proves this true when you put it in that order.

RELATIONSHIPS:

My sister Shane and her eight-year marriage to actor Ken Wahl: I honestly feel my sister's marriage works for a few simple reasons. Both my sister and I have always been drawn to alcoholics. We had a lot in common with them, especially low self-esteem. We thought that, as long as we rescued our guys, we would be needed. Instead, we fed each other's diseases rather than sharing love. NEVER would I have imagined that my sis, who put the "L" in loser, would end up marrying someone who loved her as she was—without needing anything from her. Along came Ken Wahl. He was athletic, intelligent, and compassionate. He also happened to be a good-looking, popular, and successful actor. Star of the critical acclaimed series "Wiseguy" and about twelve major movies, he also won a few acting and writing awards and was named "sexiest man" on several major magazine covers. Despite all her insecurities, Ken loved my sister's virtue. It was a compliment. They take their relationship one day at a time. They both admit that, if it ended tomorrow, each would be grateful for what the other has given TODAY. Although they both love animals, sports, and shying away from the Hollywood scene, Ken is more like me than Shane. However, they respect each other's independence. Shane NEVER tells Ken what to do or tries to "fix" him. They make compromises respecting each others differences. They realize they don't owe or own each other, so everyday is exciting and new. They also realize nothing is forever and people have the right change their minds, which gives them freedom without feeling obligated. This actually keeps their romance alive. I think romance is killed when there are expectations. That's why most marriages or relationships don't work or last. While people's similarities might bring them together, it is their differences that allow them to grow. "You like because.... you love although!" P.S. My sis thinks it's pretty ridiculous that I am writing about relationships when I haven't been hitched! Oh, well. At least I know what doesn't work!

Who do you think cheats more: men or women? Surprisingly, because women have entered the work field at about the same rate as men, they have also entered the cheating field on somewhat equal ground. I've heard it's about two to one (men to women), or approximately 17 percent of married women. The seven-year itch is a myth that was exaggerated by the movies. Some claim this straying theory has possibly originated from the poison ivy theory. It takes seven years to thoroughly be relieved of the poison ivy itch, without it returning. It's more accurate to call the straying syndrome the "four-year itch." This, again, goes back to biology. Supposedly, every four years seems to be the perfect biological time to bear the next child. The four year space, biologically speaking, gives enough time to find a new mate if necessary. This four-year theory seems to correlate with most relationship breakups. If your mate suddenly has a change in behavior, dress, healthcare, and schedule, then your instincts are usually right. Ironically, the cheater is usually the one who is overly consumed by jealousy and accusations. This is because he or she is projecting his or her own guilt. If your mate was the type to stray when you met him or her, then it will probably happen again. Straying, particularly with men, has nothing to do with with their lack of love for their mate. It usually stems from a personal feeling of lack. Many times, men learn this from their parents or role models. If they outgrow straying, it's because of inner growth, not ultimatums. People change when they have suffered. Unfortunately, the suffering may happen when you leave them for good, without bluffing.

Setting yourself up and putting yourself in precarious situations will also inevitably lead to cheating. "Innocent" computer chats, a need to dress in a sexy way, and partying with friends of the opposite sex is putting the fawn in front of the lion. Trust is important, but denial is condoning disrespectful behavior. There are ways of setting boundaries without being controlling, in order to maintain self-respect. A mid-life crisis is a cry for help and is used as an excuse for cheating. It's a fear of responsibility and the need to recapture youth. Successful relationships are continuous compromises that entail different levels of mutual growth, other than sex. It is really important to treat your mate the way you want to be treated. Though a man may initially fall in love with a woman physically, he *stays in love* with the woman who makes him feel better about himself. Lasting couples learn to agree to disagree. This makes an argument a statement of boundaries, rather than a threat to control. If you are in a relationship to help heal the past, it won't work if you are trying to change and control your mate. Rather than having to be right, respecting and accepting each other's differences and boundaries is more productive.

The divorce rate is more than 50 percent and rising. What does this tell us? People are jumping into relationships on an adrenalin rush, without any thought. In this state they use magical thinking and denial rather than communication and acceptance. Everyone is on a honeymoon high and put their best foot forward, initially. With this in mind, in the beginning of the relationship you won't be thinking straight and the other person won't be showing his or her true colors. Usually what people divorce over was *always* there to begin with. The honeymoon high creates selective denial. There's a saying that "once committed, women want to *change* their man, and men pray that their woman *doesn't* change." It's a mystery that arranged marriages seem to have a lower divorce rate. Perhaps, when there seems to be *no* choice, they work it out. People on their second and third marriage have a higher likelihood of divorcing again. Those divorcees seem to continually attract the same type of mate, who they continue to blame and complain about. I do notice that men or women who swear off the opposite sex are the ones who are *addicted* to relationships. They seem to get "high" during every crisis of the relationship. Their crisis usually brings them a great make-up session, which seems to be the only time they are decent to one another.

There are always the usual complaints when it comes to relationships. Men will complain, "the sex stopped; she nags me about everything; I had to pay for all her past debts" or "she gained too much weight." Women will complain, "I don't trust him and his wondering eye; he doesn't make me feel pretty or sexy; he'd rather be with his buddies than with me," or "he doesn't want to commit and discuss our future." Just because a jeep and a limo are both vehicles does not mean they perform the same way. They are built differently. So are we. Men are physical (visual) and women are connected with their emotions (feelings and romance). Because of our differences, it is important that you choose a mate who grew up with a *healthy* role model of the *opposite* sex. Naturally there is a special bond between mothers and sons and fathers and daughters. That is why we see most people attracted to characteristics of their parent in the opposite sex. If there is an unhealthy relationship between the child and parent of the opposite sex, that child, when grown, may need to heal that unhealthy relationship. A person may do this by being attracted to the same bad characteristics of the parent of the opposite sex. For instance, if a son hated his alcoholic mother, he might have a tendency to be attracted to alcoholic women. This will happen when there isn't proper closure or appropriate therapy before feelings turn resentful. Unfortunately, if your lover has unfinished business from an unhealthy relationship with a parent or guardian of the opposite sex, this will greatly influence your lover's perspective and rapport with you.

Sometimes children of alcoholics confuse rescuing or neediness for love. When lovers pretend to be their mates' therapists, it never works.

Currently, it seems more people are getting involved with addicts of some kind, whether it's a food addict, sex addict, shopping addict, drug addict, alcoholic, or another type of addict. The clues are always there. You either chose not to see them or you unconsciously participate. Just because someone complains about something doesn't mean there isn't a pay off for continually making the same poor choices. If you stay with an addict or continually attract addicts in your life and relationships, you have to reevaluate *yourself*, not them. What is your motive? Addicts are always living in a state of crisis. They are always trying to prevent, cause, or recover from a crisis. You will be manipulated into participating in their continual crisis if you choose to be a part of their lives. You will be forced to rescue them (temporarily) or enable them, but you will never be able to prevent their crisis cycle.

Sometimes people are attracted to bad boys/girls because it gives them a sense of power and it's easier to role-play (masculine/feminine). Some women feel feminine or virtuous when involved with a bad boy. Some men find the chase more challenging when they seek a hard-to-get diva. Continuously being involved with addicts or married spouses shows the need to have an "unavailable" lover. That makes it easier to blame the addict or the adulterer. However, these addicts or adulterers can't survive without enablers: you! Rather than focusing on their problems, ask yourself why you are attracted to or stay with "unavailable" lovers.

When people are in a relationship with an addict or are addicts themselves (whether it's a food addict or drug addict), it's not a relationship. It's what I call a **"hostage ship."** In the past, I seemed to confuse relationships with hostage ships. A hostage ship is when one or both partners are holding the other one hostage. All the unhealthy characteristics of the addict dictate the hostage ship. It's all about control, power, and mistrust. Neither lover is taking responsibility for his or her own actions. Healthy couples learn to agree to disagree. Unhealthy partners end up playing the blame game, diminishing any development of a true relationship.

Because eating disorders and other addictions are so prevalent (and rising), a relationship involving an addict seems to be more acceptable. If there are no serious commitments or children involved, then it would be highly recommended not to be involved in a relationship with an addict. If you are an addict, wait for at least one year of recovery before entering into a relationship. Reputable therapists and recovery institutions agree with this recommendation. This is because the addict in his first year of recovery has not yet evolved enough to make rational decisions. Incidentally, having a relationship with any addict is having a relationship with that person's unrealistic feelings. What I mean is that the addict is usually in love with the "high" feeling, not with you. You are along for the ride. The feelings that that person gets from you are replaceable, and so are you. Their magical thinking is dangerous because addicts refrain from anything that ruins their "buzz," including honesty. If an addict has a hard time getting in touch with his or her own feelings, he or she will hardly be able to be in touch with yours. Moreover, there is no room for any reality, because the addict is busy with "intoxication" rather than introspection.

When the food or drug addict is suffering from his or her disease, he or she lives in denial, numbing all true feelings. A lot of partners of addicts may be threatened by the addict's recovery. They think they will no longer be needed or loved when the addict gets well. This may be true if you were an enabler. For addicts to get well, they need to clean up their environment, including people, places, and things that encourage their addiction. This may be you! Addicts are "unavailable" to give any real love because their priority and focus is on their drug of choice. Simply put, having an addict as a lover is having a relationship with the *"ism,"* not them. However, if you are a part of the recovery without being codependent, then you will continue to be a part of an addict's life. The destructive part about having an intimate relationship with an addict, is that *you* become the problem, instead of that person working on his or her own self-made problems. When someone is detoxing from an addiction and lifestyle, feelings that are usually uncomfortably new will surface. The addict must learn to discover new and healthy ways to deal with those feelings, without having you to blame or enable.

Many times addicts transform their food or drug addiction straight into sex addiction, glossing over any love. Sex addiction, incidentally, is not the love of sex. It's the "need" for sex at any cost. Sex addicts jeopardize their job, health, reputation, family, relationships, and integrity, just to obtain their drug of choice. I laugh when I hear porn stars or strippers claim that they are nymphomaniacs. More like *money-maniacs.* If they were sex addicts, they wouldn't have a sense of priority or the patience to make business decisions. Sex addicts lack good taste or any taste at all. Their only "taste" is the taste of their addiction. Everything revolves around their addiction. Sex addicts have to give sex away for free or pay for it, because addictions don't wait around for responsible, appropriate, or healthy decisions.

Love addiction sounded like a good idea for me. I thought, if I could lose my appetite over a guy, then I could cure my food addiction. Wrong! It's just the opposite. My eating disorder waited patiently beneath my love addiction, eventually smoldering into a volcano. That volcano erupted any time my relationship fell apart or reality set in. Depressingly, I resorted back to my eating disorder, which silently accelerated on its own. That's why I emphasize that all diseases are not about the drug of choice (food, sex, diets, etc.). It's about denial, control, and escape, no matter what survival mechanism is used. It's also trying to use outside fixes for an inside job in order to deal with issues and feelings. In any relationship with an addict, there's usually an enmeshed situation. Your problem becomes theirs; theirs becomes yours. Rather than love, which should be unconditional (ability to let go), there is possessiveness, jealousy, mistrust, fear, obsession, and control. True love and obsession *do not* coexist. Love stems from security. Obsession stems from fear. With obsession, the relationship becomes more about obligation and manipulation. Not only do the partners in an addictive relationship take each other for granted, they feel the other owes them or that they own the other partner.

The dynamics of a relationship with an addict fluctuate between *reward and punishment*. The only time there seems to be peace or love in the relationship is after a huge argument. This honeymoon period is another high. The addict can't seem to live with or without you, but it is impossible to have consistency, commitment, or communication with them. The addict's partner is used to validate of the addict's insecurities. The addict will continuously test the partner's love. Remember, addicts are trying to fill their *void* with love. If they seek it through you or a sexual relationship, then you also become the target for all their blame. They will also blame you for their addiction. You are not filling their void. You become their excuse. Subsequently, the addict's partner takes things personally and guilt may perpetuate enabling. Although the addict will take things personally as well, that person's perception is unrealistic and he or she will take everything out of context. This creates a no-win situation. That is why you should place yourself outside of an addict's crisis until he or she has achieved long-term recovery. You need to remember it's not about you. It's about the addiction; that's all. There was no real relationship to begin with because the addict was suffering from a disease. Perhaps the addict was initially discrete and appeared to be in control. Nevertheless, you were never that person's problem or reason for being an addict, though you may be perpetuating the addiction.

If there seems to be no other choice but to stay in a relationship with an addict, because of major commitments like children, then family counseling is a priority. I would also suggest emotionally detaching yourself totally from that person. You, too, need your own therapy to deal with your feelings about the situation. You can't take these feelings to the addict. There is a fine line between a marriage that survives an addict's abuse and a relationship that thrives on codependency and enabling, or a sick need for each other. The few occasions when a relationship with an addict does survive happens when one or both partners seek extreme recovery. It works if each partner independently focuses on his or her own recovery—not the other person's. The relationship grows when each partner takes his or her own inventory rather than controlling and blaming the other. However, if the addict's destructive behavior is life-threatening or violent, or if repeated rehab attempts have failed, it would be wise to separate with the help of a therapist. If an addict is determined to destroy himself and refuses all help or recovery, then you don't want to let yourself be pulled down with him. The addict will see more clearly when you aren't there to be blamed or enable. When they are alone the effect is like a mirror. This will help them introspect. However, if they continually isolate their sickness will be louder than healthy introspection.

In relationships with addicts, the sober partner becomes the caretaker. This person's role varies between rescuer, referee, the paternal figure, the food or drug cop, and the punching bag. Sex becomes a tool for validation or making up after an argument. Sex is the greatest form of intimacy to share with your loved one, but it becomes a dangerous tool of manipulation when used by an addict. The addict's perception is unrealistic, which makes him or her mistake sex for love. Sex cannot fill the void. This empty feeling causes the addict to resort to the *familiar* drug of choice.

Partners of addicts usually have the same complaints. They feel they are the bull's-eye of the addict's target practice. However, these partners don't want to "abandon" their loved one, especially because they are desperate to help and are afraid to leave them alone. The mistake of the addict's partner is thinking he or she can change, control, or help the addict. Only in rare instances has that ever happened, and it has only happened when the addict was willing to change and surrender to a healthy recovery on the addict's own time. But in most cases, this is not so. It is more important to be the addict's friend, who is better equipped to help, rather than the lover, who becomes the target. The lover should never be a parent, parole officer, or counselor.

I am speaking from the experience of being a food addict myself and trying to transmit my eating disorder into a relationship. The reason I am addressing the addict's partner is because that person will be more objective than the addict living with their disease. The addict usually chooses denial. You can't help someone that doesn't want help. You must allow your partner to hit his own bottom by himself. Unfortunately, only through suffering do we ever change. If you prevent your partner from finding his own bottom and constantly feel the need to bail him out, you are only creating a deeper life-threatening bottom for that person. Addicts must be willing to surrender and humbly accept the help they need to get well. Both the addict and the partner should keep this in mind: To open the door of *opportunity* in front of you, you've got to first close the door of *past actions and habits* behind you. Hope is the essence of positive affirmation. To love is to let go.

(Further details on addicts, enablers, codependency, etc. are in Chapter Nine.)

Brief answers to the relationship questions in the beginning

Rate your Date!

1.   Women usually complain that the subject of long-term commitment is avoided. Every relationship should be lived day by day rather than immediately planning the future. Future expectations can kill any current romance. People who live in the future are magical thinkers, romanticizing the image of love rather than their mate. The mate becomes replaceable. A healthy relationship naturally evolves into mutual commitment. It's frightening for men to hear women speak about future commitments too early in the relationship, because they appear to be shoppers rather than daters.

2.   It's ridiculous to discourage men from fantasizing, because it's natural for them and for some women. You can't train a man. They are biologically programmed that way. Women, on the other hand, have a destructive habit of thinking men should behave as their fantasy hunk from their romantic movies, soap operas, or sappy novels. These imaginary lovers are unrealistic and effeminate because these movies and novels are usually written by women, exclusively for women. Women actually think, if their lovers watch these chick flicks, they might see what a woman needs. It's just the opposite. Men hope women will get over romancing the romance. Most women don't realize their fantasizes are not what they are actually attracted to.

3.   For men, physical attraction is their natural, instinctive nature. It's the same as a woman who is attracted to a man's financial status. If he were to lose all his money, would she leave him? Her instinctive nature is to be attracted to security. If a relationship was based on appearance and money, then that will be that reason for leaving. A man will leave a woman if she gains weight, if the relationship was primarily based on appearance. Furthermore, a woman would leave a man if he could no longer be a good provider, if that was the initial attraction for her.

4.   If you feel insecure when your mate receives compliments, remind yourself that it is flattering that person is with *you*. You don't want to be with a charity case that no one will compliment. Feel good that you are with someone who is admired by others.

5.   If you need constant attention or compliments, then you are not secure enough in yourself or the relationship. A relationship is not about competition. You don't always have to be the best or the first. This can also be a ploy to make the other mate jealous.

6.   Jealousy makes you appear a "hoarder" who has to have *everyone* desire only you. It becomes a competition, not a relationship. You will not be able to truly love the person you are with, if you divert your focus from them to any past lovers. You should not judge your lover for past mistakes; nor should you care about your ex's lover. Instead, support your lover's growth. It's claimed that a woman lacks oxytocin if she feels the need to dress immodestly.

7.   People are naturally attracted to strength. Patience and not overreacting is strength. If you call your lover continuously or always wait for their calls, you are probably obsessed. Don't have expectations. Obsession is the opposite of healthy attraction.

8.   Be careful, constant need for control ruins intimacy. Obsessive control can develop into a "mother-son" relationship or an abusive relationship. Too much control turns a relationship into a hostage-ship. In a healthy relationship, there can only be one person who is in charge. Usually, in a healthy relationship, the man is respected and the woman is cherished. This way, the role playing is a not competition and does not get confusing. That is not to say you can't both make a decision together. On the contrary, women make the mistake of needing both: respect and being cherished. Demanding respect is a masculine trait. Respect is naturally earned. A woman should refrain from telling a man what to do but instead tell him what she *feels* she needs.

9.   I think it's healthy to have your own life independent from your lover's. You should both have friends of your own. If your lover continually carouses without you, that is a clue there is a problem with the relationship. If this was your lover's behavior initially, you should know that people don't change for others—even you.

10.   Usually having "friends" of the opposite sex doesn't work out well. It puts a strain on any relationship because the friend will always appear better than you or your lover. (The grass in greener on the other side.) Women can befriend men without sexual feelings. Men, on the contrary, rarely can separate sex and a friendship with a woman. Men normally have male friends. I would be suspicious about someone who insists on having "friends" of the opposite sex, unless they are gay. Hidden agenda!

11.   When you continuously choose to be with "unavailable" lovers, then you also choose to be a victim. This usually stems from childhood abuse or a poor relationship with the parent of the opposite sex. When you choose to have an imperfect lover, it's easier to blame that person than take responsibility.

12.   Blowing off the plans you made with your friends because your lover has called last minute is not only very rude but is obsessive behavior. Your friends can be a good support system. Your lover will have more respect for you if you state that you need advance notice. Perhaps your lover may join you and your friends.

13.   If you had a poor relationship with your parent of the opposite sex, this will make it hard for you to trust or bond with your lover. Your image of the opposite sex is reflected in your rapport with your parent of the opposite sex. Don't make your lover pay for past wounds or unfinished business. Healing starts when you separate your lover from your negative image of your parent.

14.   Revenge always backfires. Any type of revenge makes it appear as if you can't let go and you care too much. It could appear obsessive or like "fatal attraction." Revenge also gives away your power. The best revenge is no revenge, because it appears as if you've just moved on. ACT. Don't REACT.

15. If you constantly are attracted to the chase rather than the relationship, you mistake need for love. Chasers don't want to join a club that would have them as a member. Chasers would rather have things that are not meant for them and get high on the initial challenge rather than develop longevity. Chasers live and thrive when constantly in crisis mode. Stability and security is boring for chasers.

16. Expecting to be "rescued" is being codependent. You take care of your own responsibilities, and your lover should take care of his or hers. This will define and maintain a healthy relationship. The lover who rescues becomes a parent rather than a lover, therefore ruining any intimacy. When you need someone, it becomes an addiction rather than a relationship. Chivalry is attractive, but you become less attractive if you become a bank withdrawal slip or therapist.

17. It is healthy to give and receive mutually. However, if there are expectations, then it becomes about keeping score.

18. Generalizing about the opposite sex is a sign of possible bigotry. This behavior is a clue to future problems. It can either be used as an excuse to blame or it can escalate into an abusive relationship. The person who generalizes about the opposite sex will speak to you condescendingly. There will be a lack of trust and respect. Look at your lover independently from his or her gender.

19. If your lover has become your best friend, then there is a lack of chemistry. When there is too much safety in your relationship, you will sacrifice intimacy.

20. Losing your appetite when you are with your lover is reacting to the initial adrenalin rush that *isn't real.* This means your appetite will eventually return. If there is no obsession, then there are never any appetite variations. Whenever there is a high, a low will follow.

21. If you are female and you always complain that men just want to have sex, be grateful you are still on the market. Men, regardless of their class, race, age, religion, and so forth, are first attracted to women, sexually. They are wired that way. Perhaps common interests, experience, maturity, spirituality, and other bonus qualities will complete a mutual bond, but sex appeal is the first on a man's list. If there is no sexual attraction, the relationship will not go further than friendship, if that. Men usually prefer male companionship. If your relationship remains purely sexual, then perhaps that was the only common dominator between the two of you and the only thing offered. Rather than complaining about men being "pigs," reevaluate your own dress, attitude, and the type of man you are honestly attracted to.

Answers to:

Is your lover into you? (a "hot fudge sundae or a rotten egg?")

1. Men rarely want to be friends with women, unless they are gay. A man is a "friend" with a women (or a hopeful candidate) because he is hoping for sex. If either a man or a women states to the opposite sex, "Let's just be friends," it's saying "You're not attractive enough to take it to the next level but are safe enough to hang out with, particularly if no one else is asking."

2. Men premeditate their dates just like women do. If a man is interested in a woman, he will call her at least three days before the weekend. If he calls her last minute, then she was the last number on his list and his mind. If a woman calls a man last minute for a date, she is sick of being stood up or waiting for men to call her. She wants control.

3. If you are involved with someone who is heavily into drugs or alcohol, that person will use that as an excuse for infidelity and poor choices. It's also an insult if someone has to get drunk or high in order to be intimate. Having a relationship with an alcoholic or drug addict, on any level, is having a relationship with the substance, or "ism," not the person.

4. When someone is into you, regardless of that person's excuses, he or she will always find a way to call or see you. The person won't be able to get you out of his or her mind. Waiting is torture for the person who is interested, whether he or she is the one making or receiving the call. If someone makes you wait for a call, then that person is testing you while figuring out if he or she is into you.

5. If someone gets nervous when speaking about future commitments or a serious relationship, they simply are using *you* to fill that gap until they find the person that they *know* is their future! However, if the woman asks about careers, family, etc., on the first few dates, the man will feel the woman is profiling for providers rather than asking about the man as a person.

6. If someone speaks like a poem in a fairy tale, then that's what he or she is doing: story telling. Talking about future dreams and making "dreamy" promises without hardcore, immediate commitments is just buying time, or leading you on. They are acting on their "high" and pulling you along for the ride. The person may not want to lose you or their "high" but also doesn't want to seriously commit *right now!* The person seems to know what words to use to keep you hanging. Big stories are BS and whispering sweet nothings is just that: nothing but sweet manipulations!

7. You are in denial if you choose to only accept your lover when he's in a good mood. In the beginning of the relationship, that's as good as it gets. If your lover is a miserable person or cruel to others, you may just be in love with your lover's initial high. Although everyone experiences moodiness, your lover may be using you to escape from misery. This is a problem because you will be replaceable, particularly when your lover's moodiness evolves. Incidentally, you may eventually be the cause of

his or her moodiness. Judge a person by the way he or she acts around everyone, not just you. Is the person kind, generous, and a trustworthy person with everyone else?

8. I've known the busiest people with absolutely *no* time to spare. They will make the time for the right love interest. If someone is into you, that person will want to make you a part of his or her busy life. That person will stop the world for YOU! If they are too busy for a simple phone call, then you are NOT a priority worth pursuing and are last on their mind and schedule.

9. If your love interest complains that he or she needs space or time to figure things out, that person is still looking for better prospects than you! Perhaps it's moving too fast? That's another way of saying the person is attracted to *other* people and may feel bad about going too far with YOU! If they are still hanging onto you, they are just waiting with one foot in your relationship, ready to put the other foot in a relationship they are willing to be *serious* about.

10. Everyone enjoys the challenge of being chased and pursued. Even losers want to be chased (my sis)! Old fashioned or not, men's testosterone increases when they chase. It's the natural innate hunter in them. They sometimes may lose interest once they have caught you. Nonetheless, 99 percent of the time, when the woman makes the first move, it seems to never work out. In this case, the pursued gentleman may be susceptible to any other woman's dominant proposal and will be more vulnerable to straying. Perhaps he will yearn to gain back his manhood by chasing other females. Relationships seem to work when the man chases and cherishes and the woman respects without expectations. Women often complain that men get disinterested once the chase is gone. Though part of that is true, many times women don't seem to realize their own demeanor has changed as well and that they are expecting rather than accepting.

CHAPTER 9:
IDENTIFYING TRIGGERS AND ISSUES

(Definitions and Helpful Organizations)

Are you, a family member, or a loved one a food addict? What are the symptoms of an eating disorder?

SEE HOW MUCH DIETS, FOOD, AND BODY IMAGE AFFECT YOU!

Simply circle "Yes" or "No" next to the question.

1. Are you or someone you know constantly obsessing about diets?	Yes	No
2. Do you or someone you know get anxious around a lot of food?	Yes	No
3. If you or someone you know skip a meal, is it a big deal?	Yes	No
4. Are you or someone you know constantly obsessing about food?	Yes	No
5. Do you or someone you know feel a lack of control or a need for control?	Yes	No
6. Are you or someone you know secretive and isolated a lot?	Yes	No
7. Are you or someone you know constantly worried and unhappy about your body image or worried about your appearance?	Yes	No

8. Do you or someone you know feel worthless, hopeless, and depressed because of eating habits?　　Yes　No

9. Do you or someone you know feel defined by body image (appearance) and weight?　　Yes　No

10. Are you or someone you know always looking for the magic bullet?　　Yes　No

11. Do you or someone you know have ritualistic patterns or rigid rules of discipline (like needing austere schedules)?　　Yes　No

12. Are you or someone you know in denial, dishonest, or defensive about weight, body, and diet issues?　　Yes　No

13. Do you or someone you know, weigh or measure yourself and/or meal portions a lot?　　Yes　No

14. Do you or someone you know blame everyone and everything but yourself for bad situations? (Being a victim and not taking responsibility.)　　Yes　No

15. If you or someone you know blow your diet, is the day "ruined"?　　Yes　No

16. Do you or someone your know have a family history of addiction (alcohol, drugs, food, sex, etc.)?　　Yes　No

If you answered **Yes** to two or more of these questions...feel like bingeing? Instead, continue reading this chapter for answers, solutions, and helpful organizations.

While modeling in Paris, Milan, and other European cities, we had tantrums watching the stick-thin models eat whatever they wanted. To keep up with the models, we would eat just one apple a day (to keep the doctor away). From our five-star hotel, we'd request this single, humble fruit be elegantly placed on a silver platter. It helped that the apple appear important rather than so lonely. Following the fashion shows, my sis and I would neurotically call room service and request everything in the kitchen. Of course, we'd claim we were giving a "fashion party" for many friends. This "Roman feast" (in Paris) extended beyond our hotel suite into the fine dining of several Paris restaurants. Ignoring famous art museums and landmarks, we insisted the only fine art was those French pastries. Disaster soon followed. Shane, "Miss Drama Queen," demanded to be taken to a hospital in Paris. Of course, headline news stated "Barbis' near-death experience." Actually, it was only an acute case of constipation. To put it lightly, Shane never did get to experience those fancy bidet toilets. How do you spell relief? LAXATIVES! Destiny, thereafter, opened up new diet doors in more than one way. I'm sure the South American drug cartel would have been impressed with our stash of laxatives. Our first laxative overdose started with, "Excuse me, I have to use the ladies room," to "Move it lady; this unloading won't be pretty!" We'd drop to the ground so many times from those overdoses you could almost see a chalk outline of our bodies on the floor. Definitely not a calendar shot!

Rarely do people connect dieting and weight problems with having a disease and needing recovery. Because obesity is an epidemic, people assume it is the norm to have a problem with weight and deal with it by using the popular diet or diet aids. If someone has been on continuous diets unsuccessfully, this could be *one* sign of some type of mental ailment that accompanies the physical struggle. Furthermore, if someone is preoccupied with food and/or his or her body, then food is not the problem and diets are not the answer. Weight gain or loss at that point is also not the problem but is the *symptom* of a subliminal issue. The media enables the compulsive overeater, making him or her think that the right diet will fix the problem. The media also perpetuates the anorexic's delusional thinking that they are ahead of the game by using extreme dieting as a way to feel they have control.

These are the key signs of obsessive-compulsive disorders: control, denial, shame-based, self-absorbtion, secrecy, a victim mentality, and repeating one or more destructive patterns. As with any disorder, whether it is alcoholism or bulimia, control is the always an issue. There is either a feeling of lack of control or a need to gain all control. Sometimes it's a combination of switching from one to the other, as with the compulsive overeater who turns to bulimia to compensate for the binges. People without food disorders manage their weight struggles differently than people who have a disease.

Let's go over some of the terms I use in this book.

A *Symptom* is a manifestation (clue or sign) of a destructive or disruptive disorder, usually a disease. When speaking about eating disorders, the symptom is usually weight (physical) or the food abuse (mental).

Symptom-Chasing is addressing the symptom and not the reason for it. Symptom-chasing is dealing with the weight (by dieting) but not addressing the reason for overeating (deep issues).

A *Survival Mechanism* is a defensive or destructive behavior used to control, deny, or deal with honesty and problems. The survival mechanism is the act of binging, dieting, purging, or exercising excessively. This act is used to solve other problems in other areas. For instance someone may starve from food because they feel a lack of control in a relationship or depressed over failure in their career.

A **_Survival Tool_** is a tool or a drug of choice used to enable a survival mechanism and achieve a certain result. The survival tool could be the food, diet, exercise routine, or laxatives. For example, someone may symptom-chase his or her weight gain by dieting.

When people diet to escape, control, or comfort themselves, then it becomes their survival mechanism. Dieting becomes more important for those issues, not just weight. It literally takes a life of its own! _Survival mechanism_ is another term for a problem-solving defense method used for _all_ issues. Denial is also a survival mechanism because it is a destructive behavior used to deal with and deny honesty and problems. If the survival tool or mechanism worked previously, a person will try the behavior again until it becomes a habit or learned behavior. The mere memory of their survival tool working previously keeps the sufferer continually using this method, even when it fails. This is addiction.

As with any addiction, there are chemicals and hormones released with any memory of a high. For example, dopamine creates a euphoric high of its own. Your learned behavior, memory of your own high, and your body's euphoric embellishment makes it nearly impossible to break a survival mechanism or an addiction. People with food disorders actually symptom-chase their weight problems by continually using their survival tools. In addition, they use their survival mechanism for dealing with all problems, including the ones that came from the symptom-chasing. At some point, the survival mechanism becomes a bigger problem than the one they used it for originally. Under normal circumstances, a change in diet and exercise helps someone lose extra pounds. Then you have someone who uses food and diets as survival tools to invent a behavior to cope with problems: a survival mechanism. This is when someone may use food to comfort themselves or escape. The food eventually stops working, which makes the person lose "control" of their weight. The person may turn to extreme methods to get rid of the extra pounds. Perhaps the compulsive overeater will eat because of their weight gain, while bulimics will purge. It doesn't matter which extreme someone resorts to; it's all about control. The compulsive overeater started eating over issues long before the weight became a problem. Turning to a diet or starving is another way to escape real problems. Compulsive overeating or any extreme diet abuse will continue until the real issues are addressed. You have to find out what's eating you or what you are eating over. Simply put, when food and diets are used as survival tools to practice their survival mechanisms or methods of control, there is no longer any problem with weight. The weight is only a symptom. Denial perpetuates this symptom-chasing.

The first signal of any mental disorder having to do with addiction is denial. Denial is also a survival mechanism because it is a behavior used to wipe out honesty or any responsibility. For most, being truly open and honest, and being able to confront people (or problems), is extremely uncomfortable. People often would rather settle for a more convenient way out. Skirting and minimizing problems and issues, or outright denial, allows us to feel safe in our comfort zone so we can escape pain. There are three ways in which we are viewed. First, there is the way we see ourselves. Next, there is the way others see us. And finally, there is the way we really are. Denial keeps us from seeing the way we really are.

One of the key factors in body dysmorphia is misperception. Misperception is our mind learning to lie. Our intuition is not guided by our egos. We always know the truth because intuition is the truth. However, years of learned behavior has taught most of us to live and speak in denial. Most sitcoms on TV are based on some form of dishonest denial. Children are naturally honest. Then they are taught that it is impolite to hurt someone's feelings, even if it's the truth. As grownups, we learned that it is politically incorrect to say how we actually feel; it isn't acceptable. Subsequently, if a child is growing up in a household where denial is the *norm*, that child will grow up thinking communication is about avoiding what is real or uncomfortable. That is why recovery is based on rigorous honesty. Without honesty, there can be *no* recovery whatsoever! The saying "in secrets lies sickness" holds true. It isn't important to overanalyze the reasons for the different survival mechanisms used to deny these feelings. What is important is simply the ability to be honest. Rather than asking *why* we are sick, we should ask *how* to get well. Only then is healthy change possible. I notice that individuals who clench their denial and refuse to be honest are the ones who want to continue their behavior. In order to change, you have to first admit denial doesn't work. Denial is simply a set-up to continue the same mistakes. Next, you need to break the chain of patterns by applying honesty as the first remedy. Willingness is a precursor to honesty and the opposite of denial. It is only at that moment of willingness to be honest and open that we are ready to begin to solve our problems or heal our emotional wounds.

Once you have broken the pattern of solving inside problems with outside fixes, you have begun the recovery process. The key word here is *process*. There is no such thing as being recovered or cured; it's a lifelong process, one day at a time. There is also no such thing as a quick fix, which most try time after time. Insanity is repeating the same mistake over and over and expecting different results. (Try having a twin who also repeats your own mistakes.) Process enables growth. There's no such thing as staying the same. You either regress or progress. When you make a mistake, rather than using an outside fix to change it, learn to face the issue that provoked the destructive behavior. That is growth, and thus progress.

A distinctive characteristic of an addict is instinctive behavior. When a "normal" individual matures, that person outgrows self-indulgences, or instinctive behavior, and uses *intuition*. Through introspection, mature or recovering addicts learn to guide their choices through intuition rather than spontaneous self-indulgence like an animal. Instinct is based in *fear* as opposed to faith and trust. Impulsively making decisions destroys any development of a consciousness of future consequences. Evidently, the addict survives *for that moment only*, constantly trying to find an easier, softer way and relinquishing any thought of repercussions. Acting on impulse also diminishes any development of delayed gratification (waiting or planning for something). Delayed gratification is part of mature behavior, as opposed to immature behavior, which only focuses on fulfilling any spontaneous self-indulgence. Impulsive behavior leaves no time for introspection (intuition) and no room for appropriate choices. Practicing delayed gratification paves the road to commitment.

In order to confront uncomfortable issues, we need to be able to *introspect* from a healthy viewpoint. When we act based on fear, guilt, and shame, it perpetuates and condones self-destructive behavior. Realistically, we should realize that when we make mistakes our normal response is guilt. However, someone who is shame-based rather than guilty thinks he or she *is* the problem, rather than *has* a problem. This can create a paranoid feeling or a victim mentality. A *victim mentality* is when a person thinks he or she is a victim of circumstance rather than thinking there is a *reason* for circumstances and choices. In other words, it is a lack of responsibility, or *giving power away!* This person also thinks that no one can relate to or understand them. This makes it impossible for any healthy action to be taken when thinking this way. Diseases such as alcoholism or eating disorders aren't licenses to condone irresponsible behavior. In other words, giving your behavior a name and calling it a disease isn't an *excuse*. Identifying the disease is giving us the *reason* why we are self-destructive and continue unhealthy behavioral patterns, no matter how much willpower we use to try to stop it. However, as addicts, we *do* have the responsibility to recover so we don't continue these destructive behaviors. Actually, recovery is taking the word *blame* out of the process altogether. If we refrain from being victims, we can't blame others *or ourselves*. Taking responsibility is the opposite of being a victim. Victims wait to be rescued, while they blame themselves and the world. They are *reacting* rather than *acting*. Poor choices are the reason for poor circumstances, which can easily be reversed and remedied by action: healthy choices. Taking responsibility is taking action toward a solution.

I think one of the most important factors in getting well is knowing that you are not alone. Your suffering is not unique. As a twin, I still felt alone. I thought God made a cruel joke by supplying me with a twenty-four-hour mirror to reflect all my problems. Self-absorption is a strong characteristic of someone who is not well. Addicts are preoccupied with their feelings, appearances, and remedies. This really keeps the addict in the disease and it usually manifests into other areas, like body dysmorphia. That's why I prefer group therapy for lasting recovery. This shifts the focus from yourself and disrupts the isolation. Isolation encourages one to ruminate over the problems, not solutions.

Just as important as identifying with the emotional issues is identifying the physical triggers, both of which perpetrate the disease. Don't put yourself in a situation that embellishes your compulsive behavior. Triggers are unhealthy people, places, or things that bring you back to unhealthy behavior (more in Chapter Five). People feed their emotional and physical triggers because they don't connect weight problems with mental diseases. You need to connect the mental with the physical issues in order to get recovery. For example, let's say I feel very uncomfortable with my coworkers in social environments. During my company's functions, I deal with my uncomfortable feelings by compulsively overeating at the scene of the crime. I deal with my guilt by practicing bulimia at home. Neither of these methods fixed my uncomfortable feelings. In addition, my overeating and purging just added two more problems on top of my uncomfortable feelings. As important as my career may be, my physical and mental health are more important. FACE AND REPLACE! This is how I face my feelings: I attend group therapy prior to the company function and "vomit" my feelings at the meeting. I also pre-plan meals of food replacements— enjoyable meals I can look forward to. If I pre-plan my situation and meal plan, I won't set myself up for compulsive, out-of-control behavior.

This is where allowed/disallowed eating comes into play (further details in Chapter Four). Rather than saying "never," allow yourself certain foods at special times. This will also be a good way to wean yourself off of sugar or animal meat. It's normal to enjoy comfortable eating, as long as you aren't eating for comfort. The foods that put your mind into an insatiable cycle of desire are foods to avoid altogether, one day at a time. Certain foods are loaded with tryptophan, which triggers serotonin, a brain chemical that makes us full and satisfied. We think chocolate and other goodies are the exclusive foods that will satisfy us, though they actually can encourage a hypoglycemic reaction, causing repeated cravings. That is why we must educate ourselves about trigger foods, brain chemicals, and hormones that either make us satisfied or make us act compulsively (further details in Chapter Five). There are healthy "non-diet" foods that can replace certain cravings without triggering the "insanity" chemicals. You should educate and experiment yourself so you can learn which enjoyable foods are best for your health and mental state. So you don't feel deprived, you can plan for allowed/disallowed eating. There might be a time when you want to *treat* yourself to something you normally don't eat (not a trigger food). This is done by planning the time and amount of a meal. This prevents the compulsive eating behavior. Compulsive eating is eating unplanned food without any boundaries. For the food addict who is new to recovery, I usually advise staying away from extreme dieting. Use a food plan that is simply *better* than yesterday, one day at a time. Gradually, the food addict will evolve intuitively and learn the difference between enjoying the food guilt-free and bingeing.

Is overeating or starving a choice or a disease?

In the beginning, poor choices can develop into a habit. Depending on other circumstances (genetic predisposition and mental state), the bad habits may develop into an eating disorder (or any disease), which is NOT a choice. However, **RECOVERY** is a choice! That doesn't mean that all overweight or skinny individuals have eating disorders. Genes, learned behavior, and personal choices are basically the reasons for someone's weight appearance. Sometimes simple education can change someone's lifestyle and, therefore, their own body weight. Education and developing good habits are the basics of all recovery.

What makes an eating disorder develop into a disease or an addiction?

1. When it stems from depression, anxiety, obsessive-compulsive disorder (OCD), or any other mental disorder—not the love of food.
2. Low levels of imbalanced hormones and brain chemicals.
3. When it becomes a destructive behavioral pattern, eventually becoming life-threatening.
4. When your WILL has nothing to do with it.
5. When you use FOOD or STARVING as a drug of choice or survival tool.
6. When you use a destructive behavior (survival mechanism) to: DEAL, ESCAPE, or CONTROL.
6. When you lie, cheat, and steal to hide or fulfill your destructive behavior.
7. When you are dictated by fear and shame.
8. When you live instinctively rather than intuitively. This means you live without introspecting about consequences).
- Major weight fluctuation is NOT about the food or appearance. Weight fluctuation is only a symptom of something major going on inside..

How does an eating disorder begin and escalate into a mental illness?

An eating disorder is both a genetic disposition and learned behavior. A *disease* is a condition of abnormal functioning or impaired health. Eating disorders are a disease of mental health. When sufferers chooses to use their survival mechanism (binging or starving) repeatedly, they are entering the addiction phase. Possibly at one time the survival mechanism had worked to help release anxiety or escape from pain. Eventually it no longer matters, because the need to practice the survival mechanism becomes stronger than the reason for doing it. No one chooses to be anorexic or have a compulsive overeater. When speaking about eating disorders, a disease is an addiction that becomes so self-destructive it's beyond willpower. The addiction takes over, like any other disease. There is no rationalization with diseases. Physically, the addict's body chemicals and hormones are radically imbalanced, making the person mentally ill. When someone experiences pleasure he or she excretes chemicals and hormones like endorphins (hormone-love), serotonin (neurotransmitter-satisfied), and others. A food addict will actually over-secrete or experience early secretion (dopamine) with just the *memory* of their drug of choice. Mentally, the addict is constantly in the state of intoxication, craving., or crashing. The addict's perception and self-preservation is not functioning like a person who is well. There are basically two types of mental illnesses: psychosis and neurosis. Most diseases begin with neurosis and gradually transcend into psychosis. Neurosis is a mental condition with symptoms of hypochondria, obsessive behavior, and depression. Depression is a form of self-pity that turns into self-punishment or a self-destructive behavior. Psychosis is a mental disorder that causes people to lose contact with reality, and their perception is highly distorted. Neurosis is thinking YOU are the problem (shame-based), not that you have a problem. People that are affected with neurosis's, act like martyrs. Psychosis happens when people think the world is to blame, not themselves. This is a *victim mentality*. Neurotic conditions have a better possibility for recovery. People suffering from neuroses are capable of being aware that their recovery is their own responsibility. People suffering from psychosis think their recovery is dependent on outside circumstances. They usually don't take *any* responsibility for their situation. I have seen every type of addict get well when *they* initiate the responsibility to get help and apply an *honest* recovery program. This cannot happen when addicts have a *victim mentality* and blame the world for all their problems or wait to be bailed out.

What do you do?

First of all, make *yourself accountable* by admitting to your addition and then become willing to accept help. You are half well when you admit to your addiction, because this is the first step of taking responsibility. Rather than focusing on outside fixes, focus on your *feelings*. Weight, diets, food, etc., should be treated as *symptoms*. Therefore, don't symptom-chase. When dealing with eating disorders, sobriety is called *abstinence*. Abstinence is abstaining from compulsive behaviors such as compulsive overeating or purging. An *abstinence program* may include a certain food plan (with scheduled meal times) and avoiding certain trigger foods and situations. A food plan prevents the insanity of having to negotiate with your food. Compulsive behavior is like an avalanche. Once you start to spin out of control, it's almost impossible to *come back* while in the middle of the insanity. *Compulsive* means unplanned and out of control, which is the opposite of abstaining. *Abstinence* teaches you about a life without obsession and the insanity of compulsive behavior.

Most eating disorders stem from obsessive-compulsive disorder. OCD is a ritualistic behavioral pattern that makes dysfunctional individuals feel safe and in control. Perhaps the ritual simply began as a rigid rule or a strict schedule. Regardless, this behavior eventually manifests as some form of addictive behavior. Then this individual discovers their own survival tool or survival mechanism such as food or dieting, that works for them at the time. This tool is used to escape, to *numb* feelings, or to deal with stress and personal issues. This addictive behavior eventually erupts into a negative mental state or disease. No amount of willpower can cure this disease. You can't cure an addiction, but you can replace it with a healthy behavior pattern. A part of recovery is educating and informing yourself about a behavior so you can take responsibility and work toward healthy solutions (choices and actions). A nutritionist and therapy or group rehabilitation will not only help teach the sufferer how to eat but will also teach him or her how to deal with feelings without using destructive eating patterns.

Do you share these feelings of an addictive personality?

1. Obsessive feelings, an almost a trance-like focus on one thing.
2. A feeling of lack, or emptiness. This feeling is coming from nowhere.
3. Fighting for control when you feel a total lack of control.
4. Feelings of constant contradiction: one moment feeling like a prisoner, the next needing boundaries.
5. Fluctuating between the need to fight or flight all the time
6. Finding safety in ritualistic patterns, strict schedules, or rigid rules.

7. The "pseudo" solution, (unhealthy tool), used to fix other problems becomes a bigger problem.
8. Unable to stop destructive behavior with willpower.
9. Lying, cheating, and stealing to repeat destructive behavioral pattern, though you had not done this previously.
10. Unable to live with or without your drug of choice.
11. Constantly looking for outside fixes or using magical thinking (a new high).
12. Continuously attracting, causing, or running from a crisis situation.
13. Shame-based thinking: Thinking you *are* the problem rather than *have* a problem.
14. The craving for any drug of choice is unbearable: No longer seeking the high; instead refraining from the crash or fearing the *withdrawal* from the absence of the drug of choice.

If you realize that you have a disease or eating disorder then you are half well (no longer in denial). Recovery is threefold: physical, mental, and spiritual.

☞ *Physically, balance your body with a researched food plan. This food plan should be a fail-proof plan that won't allow for setting yourself up. Once in a while, allow yourself allowed/disallowed planned treats to refrain from bingeing or purging. This relieves body/food obsession and focuses on feelings to achieve sanity and peace.*

☞ *Mentally, address the issues that you are eating over. Therapy, group sessions, and journals are helpful. If you focus on the diet and not the issues, you are like a dry drunk setting yourself up for a slip. A dry drunk still carries the "ism" without the symptoms.*

☞ *Spirituality is personal but is the main ingredient that relieves you from relying on your willpower. Willpower eventually sabotages your goal. Spirituality helps you release the results to a higher power (whatever it may be). This makes it easy to concentrate on the responsibility of a recovery. Spirituality is a form of surrender that breaks the misconception that your own will (willpower) can do everything. Charity is form of spiritual surrender. When you reach out, it helps release self-absorption, which furthers the recovery process.*

✓ Bottom line: Live in the SOLUTION!
✓ Rather than symptom-chase, replace with healthy recovery alternatives.
✓ Break denial with honesty.

- ✓ Work both sides of recovery: non-diet food plans and addressing issues and feelings through some type of therapy.
- ✓ Live in gratitude and surrender the results (leave out your self-will and worry)
- ✓ "Connect and Contribute." (Reach out to others.)
- ✓ If you make physical and mental health your goal, then beauty, fitness, and freedom from obsession will be the by product.

What do you do if someone you know or love is afflicted with an eating disorder?

Giving advice when it's not asked for never helps the situation. Incidentally, giving advice can be a "disease" in itself. It actually causes the person receiving the advice to retreat and be more secretive and defensive. You can't make someone get well. That person must be willing. Usually when someone is still "practicing" their disease, it is impossible to talk to them rationally. The most effective method to help another addict is to have someone *share* their own experiences of hitting bottom (sick and tired of being sick and tired) and how they attained recovery (hope). This way it never sounds as if it's a condescending lecture.

In extreme cases, intervention works well. This is when a pre-planned gathering of family members, loved ones, friends, co-workers, etc., all gather to share their concerns about the addict's behavior and how it has impacted everyone. It is advised that a therapist or professional arbitrator guide the intervention. You don't want the addict to feel everyone is against him or her. When carefully planned, an intervention usually works very well. Sometimes an outpatient program or rehab is needed immediately following the intervention. Rehabs are safe environments where therapists and other addicts share their experience, strength, and hope. This makes addicts feel they are not alone. Their focus is on recovery 24/7 in order to break old patterns that trigger the addictive behaviors. Interventions show addicts they have lost their "control" over their secret, which makes them more willing to surrender to help. Sometimes, giving no options is best because addicts are unable to rationally negotiate. Tough love can be misconstrued. A carefully planned intervention should include everyone's *mutual* concern. The <u>solution</u> should dominate the intervention, so the shame doesn't overwhelm the addict.

Most of all, the addict's loved ones should also attend group therapy, such as Al-Anon. You may be unknowingly perpetuating the disease, as a codependent or enabler. You can't work someone else's recovery program. You can give the suffering addict the thirst to get well by setting the example of independent self-help. *Interventions should be conducted with a specialist and family members in a loving, safe environment.*

What do you do if you are in a relationship with someone with an eating disorder or someone who is an addict?

First, ask yourself if you are an addict or are contributing to their addiction in any way. A lot of couples don't realize they are giving mixed messages by participating with the addict. When you don't participate with the addict, they are able to see their addiction as being their own problem. This is also a good silent disapproval. Outsiders sometimes make it about control rather than concern. Next, decide the level of the relationship. If you don't have any commitments or children DO NOT GET INVOLVED WITH AN ADDICT (further details in Chapter Eight). Addicts need an objective friend rather than a mate, which is more helpful. This way you won't make it about you. The addict is "unavailable" for any type of relationship. Addicts are sick and not really responsible for what they do or say. In a relationship, you will take things personally when it's not about you! Addicts claim their true feelings come out when they intoxicated. This only seems true because a dry drunk is in denial. A dry drunk still carries the "ism" (all the characteristics of an alcoholic or food addict) without the alcohol or food. Then, when addicts are "drunk" (with junk food or alcohol), it aggravates the brain, which causes them to spew hateful words and feelings. Their perception is off because they feel they are victims. They will blame you.

If you are married to an addict or committed with children, there are also solutions. There were early clues to this disorder, initially. Perhaps you enjoy role-playing and the need to rescue. In this case, I would suggest emotionally divorcing from the relationship and attending group therapy that specializes with the families of addicts. You should neither condone nor condemn the spouse. It is not your job to fix the addict. However, you can place boundaries and make compromises that directly affect you. If you give an ultimatum, you MUST stand by it. *Bluffing* does not work with sick loved ones. That's not tough love; it's negotiating love. Addicts may die if they don't reach out for help. You, as well, will be pulled down if you try to control an out-of-control addict. An addict needs leverage to move towards sobriety. You can help give him or her the "thirst" for sobriety. Something worth giving up, in order to save, is something worth keeping.

What are the signs or clues of an addiction to look out for?

Any addiction begins with mild obsessive-compulsive behavior. It is said the disease (the "ism") is able to sneak up on you and blow up, out of nowhere. Actually, small **CLUES** are always present:

☞ *depression, mood swings, or fluctuations between deep depression and a "honeymoon high"*

☞ *isolation and not eating with others*

☞ *control issues*

☞ *secretive behavior*

☞ *denial*

☞ *perfectionism or a defeatist attitude*

☞ *self-absorption or people-pleasing*

☞ *obsessive behavior*

☞ *paranoia*

☞ *"committed victim" never take responsibility; blame the world*

☞ *shame-based feelings or grandiosity*

☞ *frigidity and extreme modesty or hyper-sexuality*

☞ *destructive discipline (rituals, schedules, rules) or self-indulgence*

☞ *hopelessness*

☞ *magical thinking*

☞ *always being in a crisis, fixing a crisis. or causing a crisis*

☞ *extreme cautiousness or recklessness*

☞ *inability to live in the present time (NOW) or be self indulgent in the moment without thought of consequences*

All addicts live in the moment, spontaneously indulging without any thought of the reckless destruction. However, their minds are either in the past or the future, never living responsibly in the NOW. All of these things and more can be signs of deeper issues.

What is the best recovery for eating disorders?

You need to treat the disease three ways: mentally, physically, and spiritually. Mentally, the sufferer must join or be active in some type of recovery program and/or therapy. Group therapy, such any twelve-step program, is best because of the sharing experience. It's not about the food or the numbers on the scale; those are just symptoms. It's about the *issues* addicts escape from. The food, body, and mental obsession need to be "released" together. The addict's focus is on control. The addict should learn to deal with issues without trying to control food and the body. It's a LONG-term recovery, usually taking about four to seven years, one day at a time, one meal at a time. In some instances, medication such as anti-depressants, work well with victims of eating disorders. Physically, it is best to have a nutritionist or doctor figure out a healthy food plan and monitor the addict's weight, NOT the addict. If the food plan is *planned* (no obsession involved), the addict is free to work on commitment and his or her inner issues. Addicts need to look at their food as something that will help their health, not as their enemy, drug, or something to fear.

Definitions:

Note: My sister and I are codependent adult children of alcoholics who enabled each other as co-addicts, while suffering from anorexia, bulimia, and compulsive overeating. We also experienced codependent body dysmorphia (I thought my sister's butt was too big.), slips, interventions, and relapses.....you are not alone!

Anorexia nervosa is an obsessive-compulsive personality disorder that focuses on the fear of causing weight gain. Losing weight becomes an anorexic's obsession. Usually anorexia, like other disorders, stems from a psychiatric problem with underlining issues of depression or obsessive-compulsive disorders. Most experts claim there is a genetic predisposition to anorexia. Girls as young as seven years old are showing signs of anorexia and patients have been as young as five. Evidently, learned behavior is also a contributor. Adult anorexia and bulimia is on the rise. There is a growing number of women age forty and up who are suffering from anorexia. There are two types of adult anorexia; one stems from childhood and the other is "born" in later years, usually triggered by stress or some crisis. It was once thought to be exclusive to upper-class female Caucasians. Not any more. Experts claim there is an increasing amount of Asians, Hispanics, and others who suffer from anorexia. Although 90-95 percent of anorexics are women, an increasing number of men have also been shown to suffer from this disorder, particularly members of the gay population. It's estimated that one out of two or three sufferers are men who are too embarrassed to get help. Over 3/4 of female athletes show some signs of an eating/body disorder. Unfortunately there is a 15 percent chance of death from anorexia or bulimia. Eating disorders cause more deaths than any other mental illness. Eating disorders affect 10 million women and 1 million men.

Anorexics live in a constant state of fear, stress, and anxiety. This is partly due to high levels of serotonin, which is caused by overactive neurotransmitters in the hypothalamus. Serotonin usually has a calming effect, but this reverses when it is overabundant. The anorexic feels a loss of control and the need to take control by eating less or not at all (usually less than 1000 calories). Two of the signs are obsession with food content and refusing to eat with others. The anorexic would rather be isolated. Some sufferers combine their anorexia with bulimia. These sufferers will exercise for hours and/or purge along with their starving. Unlike the bulimic, the anorexic never *binges* on large amounts of food.

Anorexics also suffer from loss of body heat. This is due to two things. They lack normal body fat that insulates and protects our organs and body. Also, their bodies' thermogenesis is dormant or interrupted because they lack essential fatty acids. This will increase complications, which include missing periods, easy bruising, and becoming ill often (with the flu and colds). They also will experience non-healing wounds or continuous infections. Many times, anorexics will accumulate unusual body hair, sometimes facial hair, to compensate for immense loss of body heat. Anorexic's reserves are usually depleted of glycogen, causing the body to leech from their bones, teeth, and hair (emergency reserves). They usually have hair loss, dental problems, and frail nails.

Tryptophan is found in a lot of foods, particularly most carbohydrates, and is a precursor to serotonin. This is why an anorexic instinctively feels the need to avoid food in order to keep the serotonin levels down. This constant fight-or-flight state (norepinephrine) signals excess adrenalin (epinephrine) to be manufactured. This interrupts the anorexic's APV, a hormone responsible for appetite. This lack of APV distinguishes anorexics from bulimics. Recovery is not about gaining weight. If the anorexic's only concern is about weight, she is no different than a "dry drunk". A dry drunk still carries the "ism" (sick behavior), of the disease, without having to use their drug of choice. The "dry drunk" anorexic, for example, is when the anorexic doesn't starve but they continue their obsession, (their sickness).. The weight loss or weight gain is only the _symptom._ The anorexic's tool, for instance, might be *starving*, which they use to deal with their personal issues. Anorexics need to learn to deal with issues without using any tool as a reward or punishment. This way anorexics can focus on their feelings rather than their bodies. Everything from the media to magazines *uphold* ultra thin models and actresses. The Internet is also a way for the practicing anorexic to "bond" with other anorexics and to learn new tricks. This "bonding" can be replaced by group therapy with other anorexics, who together share the rewards of the freedom from this obsession. Eventually, in the right environment, the anorexic loses the urge to "disappear" and learns to fight all the unnatural struggles to starve. Although anorexics can also be bulimics, there are the common signs. They are both obsessed with weight and food and try to hide their behavior, bodies, and feelings. Usually they are extremely thin with circles under their eyes. Anorexics will find whatever trick they can use to refrain from eating. Some resort eating paper or cotton to fill their stomachs. Regardless of their methods, they fear fat in their food and imagine it on their body. It isn't any one's fault, but it is suggested that kids often pick up their parents' behavior. If the mother is constantly obsessing about her weight and diet, that will be reflected in her child's behavior. Anorexia and bulimia is accompanied by depression, anxiety, and feeling overwhelmed and out of control. Because it's not about the food or weight, don't make it about that. Anorexics must realize that, without help, they could die. Anorexia is truly a slow suicide. However, anorexics must be willing to get well and desire freedom from the obsession. This will give them peace from the war they have with their bodies and food.

Bulimics have the same obsessive-compulsive personality disorder and control issues as anorexics. The focus is on food, weight, and perfectionism. They also share many traits and habits with the compulsive overeater. The bulimic, unlike the anorexic, eats large amounts of food compulsively (out of control). Like with the anorexic, the bulimic's fear and guilt are extremely overwhelming. This drives the bulimic to extreme behavior to get rid of the food or "make up" for the binge. Bulimia can manifest as purging, laxative abuse, enema or colon cleanse abuse, stimulant or supplement abuse, over-exercising (for hours), or starving (fasting) after a binge. It's a feast-or-famine mentality—never a normal eating pattern. Bulimics might endure other destructive behaviors of their weight control. For instance, bulimics sometimes tolerate or encourage parasites, such as worms, that their systems. They suffer from numerous health problems, such as damaged intestines (stripping their friendly bacteria), esophagus ulcers, liver malfunctions, and tooth decay from constant and unnatural exposure to stomach acid. A bulimic's body is usually full of toxins because she exclusively relies on unnatural evacuations.

Unlike the anorexic, the APV in bulimics is not destroyed. In fact, bulimics' appetites are above average because their abuse leaves them weak and depleted. This cycle is destructive because getting rid of large amounts of food without normal digestion, in a short amount of time, is very harsh and draining on the body. It leaches vital minerals from the body, which can lead to hair loss, dental problems, skin eruptions, crippling bone diseases, candidiasis, and dangerous digestive malfunctions. During vomiting, the hydrochloric acid meant to digest the food in your stomach moves into your throat and mouth, which cause severe problems and can also lead to the formation of fistulas. Fistulas are open wounds that appear in the mouth where the flesh has started to literally dissolve due to exposure to digestive juice.

The excessive diet stress releases a large amount of cortisol. Excess cortisol actually makes it impossible to lose weight. Weight gain or loss is trauma on the body that causes the body to be enervated. An enervated body (drained from nerves) stops working. This means it's difficult to lose weight, and the bulimic will become fat efficient. An exhausted body will experience edema (bloating), usually from adrenal exhaustion (depletion of cortisol). Laxatives, purging, diet aids, and over-exercising create imbalances in the levels of insulin and may cause hypoglycemic reactions. That is why many bulimics are usually bloated, particularly in the face, or don't appear as gaunt as anorexics, no matter how extreme their purging may be.

Bulimics, as well as anorexics, have suffered and sometimes died from heart failure and strokes. Their nutrients and electrolytes are dangerously depleted and this causes fatal consequences. Because bulimics' focus is on weight loss *at any cost,* they rarely consider the damage they are doing to their bodies.

Simply put, every gimmick stops working and eventually backfires. The body learns every trick you have taught it and tries to compensate. Bulimia actually teaches the body to gain weight without digesting food. With this in mind, you can also teach the body to utilize food properly. Slowly introduce small meals throughout the day, which will help the metabolism and digestive system find their own healthy balance. Gradually incorporate more calories into each meal until you are eating normal meals without trying to get rid of it (further details in Chapter Seven). In addition, bulimics should try some sort of therapy, one day at a time, which will relieve the vicious cycles.

The compulsive overeater simply overeats compulsively. Unlike most addicts, compulsive overeaters wear their disease publicly, making them more vulnerable to criticism and judgment. It is the hardest addiction to hide and is the most politically incorrect disease to endure. When people disregard all boundaries concerning what they eat (when they eat and how much they eat), they are eating compulsively. It's only a matter of time until health problems manifest. The more the compulsive overeater eats, the more food he or she wants . It's an unending cycle both physically and mentally. Instead of finishing after a meal, compulsive overeaters continue to eat until they are sick or intoxicated. This may continue until they pass out. Usually, the binges are late at night. When they wake up, they swear to start a new diet. The guilt, shame, and physical detoxification leads them back to their survival tool and mechanism: food and overeating to comfort their self-loathing. Food is their lover, their therapy, their friend, their relief, and the high that won't abandon them. It has also becomes a *sugar-coated poison* that will kill them. Compulsive overeaters usually are closet bingers. They isolate and use nighttime as a safe environment to hide their disease. Finding dark places, such as sitting in movie theaters or in front of the TV, is a familiar routine for the compulsive overeater. Socializing is usually done on the phone or the computer. Many times, their weight becomes so debilitating that they have to resort to medical assistance.

Ironically, a lot of overweight people have more willpower than most normal eaters. The deprivation diets that they usually endure make their bodies extremely fat efficient. This makes weight gain easier and faster than it is for a "normal person," The hormone leptin (in fat cells) isn't present or properly functioning in overweight individuals. This hormone normally decreases appetite and helps boost energy levels. Moreover, the hormone ghrenlin is overabundant in the compulsive overeater's body. This hormone, located in the stomach, is the body's hunger mechanism. It also gives the brain signals to store fat or make it without any food at all. An overabundance of ghrenlin creates an insatiable appetite and weight loss difficulties. Another hormone, PYY336, gives signals that we are full when we have eaten. This is deficient in the compulsive overeater, as well. There is a strong link between sleep deprivation and obesity. Without eight hours of sleep, hormones like leptin do not work properly. Ghrenlin, the hunger hormone, over-secretes right before midnight. Cravings for salty and sugary foods become overwhelming without eight hours of sleep. In some cases, the hormone ghrenlin decreases and the PYY336 increases when overweight individuals choose to have radical weight loss surgery.

Individuals who gain weight in the midsection are more likely to develop medical problems relating to their vital organs. This is particularly true of men. They seem to have a poor insulin response or balance. Women usually gain weight on the outside of their bodies (hips, thighs), while men usually gain around the gut. Although men's weight gain is not as apparent as women's, theirs can be more dangerous for the heart. Muscle weighs more than fat, which give men a little more leeway with their weight gain. Men also have a better metabolism because they are more muscle-bound, which raises the metabolism. When you continually diet, your body learns to sacrifice vital tissue rather than fat. This is because our ancestors helped train our bodies to survive long winters without food. This means that, every time you lose weight, you are telling your body (which has a memory) to save fat while sacrificing muscle and vital tissue. This is the very reason DIETERS end up gaining MORE weight after their diet; they are training the body to live with fewer calories.

We should never look at overweight individuals as weak-willed. On the contrary, they are fighting hormonal imbalances that most could never deal with. One out of three obese adults is born with an unusual drive to overeat. On the other hand, most overweight individuals do NOT have bad metabolisms. In actuality, their metabolisms are ruined when they start restricting their diets. Compulsive overeaters are also more discriminated against than any other weight addict. This is troubling because obesity is one of the fastest growing epidemics in America. Our eating habits have made us the fattest nation on earth. Children's obesity is up to 50 percent. We are also a nation with many diseases that are only related to our overindulgence and are unheard of in third world countries. I have noticed from my own studies that one out of two women in the U.S. die from some sort of diet/weight related disease. Even with this in mind, the world views overweight people as lazy, unsuccessful and not trustworthy, not to mention the fact that the medical field barely recognizes compulsive overeating as a disease, unlike the anorexia and bulimia. The media will go as far as to quote doctors advising compulsive overeaters to diet, but it is NOT about the food or the weight. It is about the issues that compulsive overeaters are eating over. A food plan can only work with a good recovery program.

An eating sponsor can guide the compulsive overeater with a daily food plan, which may change according to different situations. Sponsors are different than nutritionists because they, too, are addicts who will help lead you to concentrate on your issues rather than food. Therapy should always supplement the scheduled non-diet meal plan. Keeping a journal to record the foods eaten and the feelings involved is helpful. Compulsive overeating is as deadly as the other eating disorders. Incidentally, any type of health risk is heightened if someone is overweight. It has been proven that just 10 pounds of extra weight causes stress on every vital organ, not just the heart. Furthermore, every fat cell secretes excess insulin, causing vulnerability to more diseases. When an overweight patient has surgery, the surgeon warns the patient about the risks due to the high weight stress on the body. Drugs are administered or monitored more cautiously because of the unpredictability of the fat cell intrusion. Incidentally, overweight women using birth control pills have a higher risk of getting pregnant because of the complications caused by the excess fat that inhibits proper drug functioning. Overweight mothers have more complications during pregnancy. Our kids are growing up in a sedentary world, condoning a lifestyle of computer games and too much TV (with constant promotion of junk food and fast food). The result is that our kids have adult diseases never seen in earlier generations. It is predicted that our kids won't outlive their parents, unlike generations before us. We are giving our kids mixed messages. We allow them this lifestyle and then we tell them to diet so they don't die of some weight-related disease. No wonder the cycle continues and worsens!

Binge eating disorder is now surfacing in mostly women in mid life. These women usually never had any eating disorder until they reached mid life, their forties and up. Many times this eating disorder is one of many multiple impulsive disorders or was transferred from one disorder to another. Perhaps some crisis or tragedy triggered this behavior, but it is usually accompanied with depression, anxiety, stress, and sometimes hormonal changes. Usually women in their forties and younger face perimenopause, which changes every aspect of a woman's behavior and body. During perimenopause, it is common to experience depression, weight gain, cravings, feeling overwhelmed, and so forth. However, when someone uses binge eating as a survival mechanism to deal with stress or to escape feelings, this eating disorder escalates into an addiction. The common signs of binge eating disorder are eating large amounts of food in secrecy, usually in the middle of the night. Subsequently, binge eaters feel out of control, alone, and ashamed. The binge eaters' usual remedy is diets; they think their weight is the problem. This only makes it worse, because diets and weight are symptom-chasing. These women are fighting both the chemicals changes their bodies are enduring and the compulsion born from the habit of using food to numb and control their feelings. They gain pleasure by turning to food, which stimulates their dopamine, serotonin, and other brain chemicals. Some have used medication, like anti-anxiety medication, which helps compulsions. Others have tried alternative methods such as acupuncture to help break the compulsion that accompanies binge eating disorder. Proper diet with therapy helps target the body's changing chemicals and *wrangle* the feelings of loss of control, shame, and stress.

Balanced, wholesome food plans can restore missing chemicals and help balance the hormones of food addicts. Exercise restores a weak metabolism and releases important chemicals, such as endorphins and HGH. Exercise also balances the blood sugar, estrogen, and other hormones. Therapy and recording everything in a journal can help the food addict deal with the feelings that trigger the food disorders.

Body dysmorphic disorder, better known as BDD, has also become an epidemic. It may accompany other eating disorders. However, you don't need to be suffering from one of the eating disorders mentioned above to be suffering with this disease. The primary symptom is body-obsession with a distorted perception of any physical imperfection that may not be there to begin with. This disease, like others, usually stem from an imbalance of certain brain chemicals or depleted hormones. For example, the BDD sufferer will usually have very low levels of serotonin, which leaves the individual feeling not good enough. The body develops chemical imbalances and hormone depletions as noradrenaline (from adrenal glands), which leaves the sufferer feeling down. BDD sufferers feel the need to compensate for their flaws through extreme discipline or overcorrecting the flaw (or what they perceive as a flaw). It is their only focus in life. They may diet, exercise, become isolated, or even resort to continuous plastic surgery to attain perfection in the areas they see as imperfect. Or BDD sufferers may obsess by complaining, worrying, and hiding their flaw. You can detect hints of BDD in most of the stars in Hollywood or the younger generations who grew up on TV.

BDD becomes a disease when the obsession carries the victim into extreme means of compensation. At this point the sufferer becomes willing to use destructive and risky means to compensate for this "flaw." I honestly think that BDD victims are spiritually bankrupt. They place too much energy on their superficial characteristics rather than their inner development. BDD victims have "dead-man's eyes," appearing vacant, with seemingly nothing inside. They lose touch with what is really important and live in fear of losing what little happiness they have or could have. There lives are a constant "if only."

People of this nature are wise to surround themselves with real victims, people who are dying of a fatal disease and don't worry about their appearance. This disease is not exclusive to women. Men are entering into the BDD disease. The pressure of seeing perfectly sculpted male models gives men a glimpse of what women have been going through for centuries. Charity is the best therapy for this disorder. Refrain from any activity that promotes self-absorption or a superficial focus. Something as simple as shopping for clothes or working out at a gym with mirrors can trigger BDD behavior. We should, as a society, feel somewhat responsible for condoning self-obsession as a nation. Any selfless contribution can help remedy self-obsessed disorders. Severe BDD cases do well with medication, sometimes.

Codependency is when someone is addicted to an addict or someone with an addictive personality. Twins are automatically codependents (like my sister and I). Codependents are usually people who lose themselves in someone else or other people. They are people pleasers. They are usually the caretakers who want to run your life. Codependents want to control, rescue, and fix you and all your problems without your permission. They think they know what's best for you, in spite of your opinion. It may appear that they are generous and concerned, or even martyrs, but really they are addicted to their unhealthy connection, at any cost. Their need is to be needed. "Normal" people who are kind, giving, and generous won't lose themselves in their efforts for others. They want to give what is asked of them. Codependents act based on their own will and need. Part of their disease is that they enjoy complaining. They constantly whine about how much they do for others without receiving any reciprocation or gratitude. However, they can't stop giving of themselves to others. Stage mothers are a perfect example of codependency. They live vicariously through their kids. In my opinion, individuals with stalker mentalities also have a codependent nature. Codependents put their needs and desires onto the person they are "stalking" without permission or consideration of that person. "Stalkers" will go to extreme means when they feel a lack of control. Codependents are obsessed with putting themselves in your life and all of your affairs at the expense of letting their own lives slip away. Codependents also have a need to brag about what they've done so they can be appreciated. I see a lot of codependent mothers dealing with daughters who have serious eating disorders. This unhealthy behavior increases the daughter's need to find her own boundaries and use control through the daughter's eating disorder. All disorders are called family diseases because they influence the whole family. No one can receive or respond to any recovery unless the addict is willing to seek help. You can support, encourage, inspire, and motivate someone toward recovery, but you can't do it for them or tell them what to do. Otherwise, you are just adding to the problem and developing your own disease. When people are alone, without someone else enabling them or coaxing them, they learn to introspect (turn within) and develop inner spirituality. Then the addict has no one else to blame and becomes willing to surrender to help.

Codependent relationships happen when codependents use their codependent "magical" thinking on their relationship. Have you ever heard someone say, "I wish he was the way he was before" or "if only I could find a man who would send me poems and bring me flowers"? This type of thinking is in the clouds and far from realistic. When you are looking for a prototype, you will not love and accept the person you are with. You will place your expectation onto them, needing them to fit into your mold, life, and expectations. When someone says they want a relationship, that doesn't mean they want you. If you happen to fit their description, they will try you out. That leaves absolutely no room to grow together or compromise, which is what a relationship is all about. A person who is *not* codependent is someone who doesn't need a relationship. When that person falls in love, the relationship develops naturally, without any requirements. True love breaks all rules. Codependents demand rules. Love is learning to accept. "You like because, you love although." A non-codependent individual either accepts you or leaves you. They don't stick around to complain, control or to be revengeful. Codependents who thrive on relationships won't leave once they take you "hostage," and the relationship is then called a hostage ship. They feel you owe them. Codependent relationships, without help, rarely end up amicable (further details in Chapter Eight).

Co-addicts are addicts that are addicted to addicts, usually addicts with the same drug of choice. This is a bit different than codependency, because each addict usually shares the same disorder or practices it in the same manner. One is not directing, controlling, or condescending to the other. More or less they are partners in crime, sharing the same secret. If there is any hope for either of these addicts, they both need to have separate recovery paths with different sponsors, etc. Environment is stronger than willpower, and it is too easy to slip back into old ways, living in the same environment, particularly with the same binge buddy. Recovery is letting go of old ways and old partners in crime.

Enablers can also be codependent. The enabler actually knows the addict is suffering and causing self-destruction. Enablers make it easier for addicts to practice their addiction. Enablers are in what I call "selective denial." They realize the addict is in denial and help perpetuate it by pretending they are in denial as well. This way they can condone what they are doing. The enabler's only desire is to be needed at any cost. The fear of losing the person (for themselves) is more than the fear of losing them altogether from the addiction, which could end up being death!. Enablers justify the situation, in the disguise of concern. "I'd rather them to do *their addiction* around me, at home, because I know they are safe" or "I allow them to do their addiction, because they are going to do it anyway." This is the most selfish "love" someone can have for an addict. Enablers lack faith and spirituality, twelve-step programs and rehabs, which are proven to help. The enabler thinks he or she is the addict's only hope. The enabler is as sick as the addict and needs recovery as well. Again, meetings like Al-Anon are good programs where you can learn to detach from the addict and his or her choices.

Adult children of alcoholics should also include adult children of dysfunctional families or families who endure highly unusual circumstances. The symptoms of all of these titles are very similar. Families that experience death, messy divorces, scandal, or severe discipline (military or religious families) can also have issues similar to the adult child of alcoholics. This is particularly true when "extreme discipline" is the disguise for denial. Any family under extreme or highly unusual pressure can experience the same signs (shame, discrimination, denial, and pressure), that an adult child of an alcoholic faces. This may include a "high profile" (famous) family or being the child of a homosexual (like my sister and I). Most of these children who grow up in a dysfunctional family (or highly unusual situation) learn how balance their extreme differences at home with what the world will accept. Their need is to fit in or be accepted as *normal*. This doesn't leave any room for dealing with their own true feelings. It also teaches them at an early age to live in denial or secrecy. Subsequently, this greatly increases the likelihood of them becoming addicts themselves to deal with their own issues smoldering inside. The cycle continues. But it doesn't need to. Without blame and shame, an ACA can take responsibility by turning from a victim to a survivor.

Unlike any other addict, ACA's were victims when they were born to their alcoholic parents (or unusual circumstances). They had no choice. They were taught dysfunctional behavior and survival mechanisms to deal with uncomfortable situations, making denial their first language. They have three strikes against them: genetic inheritance of the disease, learned behavior, and shame (feeling responsible). The ACA's learn to lie, cheat, hide, and steal. Their perception of themselves and life is off because they have learned to look at everything with rose-colored glasses. Dishonesty is justified because, without it, the truth would be unbearable. For instance, let's say a child was about to be placed in a foster home because of their unhealthy environment. The ACA would rather lie about the situation (learned behavior) rather than making a healthier environment. ACA's usually grow into successful people because they learned to compensate, or they bitterly become what they hate: their parents. The caretakers of any household have a big influence on everyone's life. Actually, the ACA becomes the caretaker at an early age. However, rigorous honesty can combat myths, traditions, and superstitions that escalate unhealthy behavioral. An ACA is just like an addict without any drug of choice. ACA's actions are risky and reckless, like the addict's. This type of personality is more susceptible to addictions, if the ACA doesn't turn to a healthy outlet for their feelings.

No matter what disease or disorder is involved, there is hope for recovery. You may have to explore several different types of recovery, particularly in the case of the eating disorders. There are free group therapies, reach out programs, counseling, and twelve-step programs for all of the above disorders.

Relapse is defined as returning to a former state of illness. It usually occurs unexplainably and unexpectedly. This is different from what is known as a slip. A slip is an unintentional behavior that ruined your sobriety. A slip is something usually seen as an accident. Some twelve-step sponsors don't see the difference between a relapse and a slip. This is because they believe that if you work your program you will see the clues of breaking sobriety. They believe you are able to prevent a set-up. The clues to a relapse are in behavior, choices, or environment. Unfortunately, when you relapse, your addiction patiently waited for you to return and give it fuel. Recovery is like remission. Relapse brings you out of remission and right back to the heart of the disease. Perhaps, you might get an immediate high in the beginning. However, in no time, you are at the exact place you were before you became sober. Beware: You actually take off where you left off, as if you were never abstinent or sober. Denial is the biggest clue to relapse. Addiction patiently waits for an excuse. Overindulgence depletes the brain chemicals that are supposed to signal your brain to stop. Most people are able to dry out on their own. All bodies have that capability. This is not so with the addict. Cravings and withdrawals are overwhelming because of imbalanced chemicals. This makes willpower useless. Remember, addiction is not just a physical disease but also a mental disease. Ceasing the symptoms, such as over-eating, purging, etc., is important but not enough. You need to change the brain patterns that control your lifestyle and attitude. Those are the mental and spiritual ingredients of disease and recovery. Cultivate healthy replacement behaviors. Start by developing healthy routines and patterns before being confronted with a bad situation. It's like "putting deposits in the bank" as an *investment*, to be prepared for times you need a "withdrawal." Perhaps you could pack your lunch everyday instead of dealing with uncomfortable food dilemmas. Dry drunks who white knuckle it are usually the ones who wind up slipping or relapsing. It's not the end of the world if you do. On the contrary, it can be extremely humbling, which is exactly what it takes: humility. Begin with admitting that you made a mistake. Then work on preventing a "slippery" situation.

Getting well is not about being good or bad. How many times have I heard someone say "I was good on my diet today" or "I've been very bad about my sobriety." It's about being unhealthy or healthy, sick or well. We don't need to beat ourselves or the addict into recovery. That will only make the addict drown in their survival tool and mechanism more to deal with the shame and hopelessness.

Sometimes, it's a blessing in disguise to have a disease. It develops characteristics like humility, empathy, selflessness, and other honorable traits. You learn gratitude without being a victim. Recovery is taken one day at a time. You do the footwork and give the results (expectations) to your "higher power." The most amazing people I've ever known are recovered addicts, because it takes rigorous honesty and a life-changing attitude to receive the gift of sobriety.

As an addict, you sometimes feel like a soldier who has gone to battle with yourself for years. Hopefully, in time, you learn to surrender to a peaceful way of freedom. It might not be easy, but it is simple.

Brief Answers to Diet, Food, and Body Image Questionnaire

1.   Constantly obsessing about diets seems to be the nation's number-one pastime. Our media actually condones this behavior by calling it normal and encourages it as a solution. Obsession never creates a solution. It creates an addiction in the disguise of a solution. It will only add one more problem to your life. It may become your survival tool and mechanism to escape from dealing with your real problems.

2.   If you get anxious around a lot of food, then you are reacting to the drug-like chemicals your body manufactures in anticipation of your desires. Past actions have rewired your brain patterns to fit your *learned*, compulsive behavior. Certain hormones and neurotransmitters work synergistically with these brain impulses, creating a misperception of your feelings. Like a in drug addict, brain chemicals like dopamine secrete during the mere thought of your past desirable experiences. For anorexics, an overload of serotonin is secreted when they are around a lot of food, making them feel uncontrollably anxious.

3.   Everyone skips a meal at some time. If your missed meal is important enough to ruin your day, then you are living to eat rather than eating to live. When people complain of upset stomachs, a lack of energy, or headaches because of a meal they have skipped, ironically they are in need of a cleansing fast, not their meal. These are signs of detoxing poisons of poor food choices. Healthy people have good reserves and are able to fast for days without any symptoms or lack of energy. Don't use your meals as your itinerary platform (to plan your day).

4.   I have noticed that anorexics, bulimics, and compulsive overeaters constantly obsess about food. Food is and should be delightful and enjoyable. However, if you find yourself constantly entranced by food advertisements or constantly counting calories around you, then that is a symptom of an eating disorder. In recovery I've learned that the world has things to offer other than food. That was a relief and made life enjoyable.

5.   As with any addiction, the food, alcohol, diet, or laxatives is only the survival tool used to enable a survival mechanism (the behavior). The weight, or sign of the abuse (or disease), is the symptom. Don't make the tool (diets) or the symptom (weight) your focus. Control is the root of all addictions and is the method used to practice the survival mechanism. You might constantly feeling a lack of control or a need to gain control. The need to *control* is also a sign of a lack of faith in yourself or a higher power.

6.   The saying "in secrets lies sickness" holds true. I used to call an addict a "secret-aholic" because the sneaking and dishonest lifestyle fuels addiction. The main ingredient in recovery is rigorous honesty. Without honesty there is no sobriety or abstinence.

7.   It seems most females these days are chronically complaining about their appearance. Men are now joining this insecure club. Because society puts too much emphasis on our appearance, we all think it's a priority to look good. Combine

the obsession of looking good with another mental disorder, like depression, and you have an addiction. Particularly when there are brain chemicals missing, such as serotonin, the body misperception exaggerates an obsession about any "flaws." This is body dysmorphia. All addictions, particularly body dysmorphia, are a form of self-absorption. One of the best remedies for that is charity. It forces you to look and reach outward.

8.   If you are depressed about your weight, then you are depressed about the symptom. If you are disappointed with your eating habits, then you are finally sick and tired of being sick and tired. This can go one of two ways. You can regress into another disease to escape or find the root of the problem without *symptom-chasing*. Rather than obcessing about your poor eating choices you can look at this as an opportunity to do research about yourself and your disease. Don't ignore your own cry for help!

9.   If you feel defined by your body image, then you are dictated by impressions. People who are defined by their appearance cultivate or cater to a superficial environment. Women many times blame their husbands for losing interest when they gain weight. They should first take responsibility and realize that they were the ones who chose this superficial mate. Weight gain is not the definition of someone anymore than weight loss is. However, weight management is a clue to taking responsibility. Rather than blaming outside circumstances, it's best to target this problem as a symptom. Weight appearance is the symptom of health management. A healthy lifestyle will manifest as a healthy body. Let the body be a byproduct or manifestation of your inside work, mentally and physically.

10.   Advanced modern technology has made all of us lazy. It seems all we do is look for shortcuts. There is no such thing as a magic bullet. That's giving too much power to something that shouldn't have control over you. Constantly looking for a magic bullet stifles the desire to *earn* things in life. People who always seek the magic bullet are unable to practice delayed gratification. They want it now, no matter what. They feel like they are getting something for nothing. Actually, they are getting nothing for some damage. The damage is making you believe that you are unable to do or get something on your own, without their help.

11.   All eating disorders and other addictions stem from OCD (obsessive compulsive disorder). All OCD behaviors stem from imbalanced chemicals, which creates the need for ritualistic patterns or rigid rules. Rituals and rigid rules gives imbalanced people the feeling of control and safety. It almost becomes a religion or tradition of superstition for them. It's also a form of *magical thinking*. They feel that, if they wash their hands excessively, step over lines, or stick to a strict routine, they've beaten the system and conquered their fears. On the contrary, this behavior heightens the fear and escalates into an obsessive cycle.

12.   Denial is abstaining from truth and escaping change. Denial seems to help someone's comfort level by allowing secrets and destructive behavior to continue. Another phrase for denial is *premeditated ignorance*. What you don't

know doesn't hurt you, right? Wrong. Our intuition always knows and our denial is a tool used to buy time while treading water. Denial is refusing the lifesaver offered. Unfortunately, denial doesn't work for long, if at all. All weight, diet, and body issues worsen without honesty. Then denial become the predominate characteristic.). Being defensive or dishonest nurtures denial, and denial nurtures disorders.

13. Constantly weighing or measuring yourself or your food creates self-obsession. That type of stress actually secretes harmful or inappropriate hormones and chemicals, which eventually sabotages your goal. For example, cortisol is released during any type of stress, which creates weight loss difficulties. Self-obsession creates self-absorbed addiction. It will never feel good enough. You will constantly define yourself as bad or good rather than someone who makes unhealthy or healthy choices. Don't use outside fixes for inside jobs.

14. Constantly blaming outside circumstances rather than taking responsibility is refraining from change. When someone complains "if only," that is a sign the person wants to live as a victim. Being a victim makes it easy to blame everything else rather than make the effort to change. When you blame, you are giving away your power. People who blame are always searching for magic bullets as well. They think that certain people, places, and things will fix their lives just as other things destroyed their lives. Usually these people are psychotic and they can rarely be helped. They would rather remain victims then to choose to be survivors.

15. If your mental stability relies on perfecting a diet, then you are setting yourself up to fail and feeling *shame-based*. Shame based is when you think you are the problem not that you have a problem. People confuse guilt with shame. Guilt is a natural reaction when you do something wrong. Shame is feeling you are the problem. Making your diet rule your day is believing you are defined by whether or not your actions are perfect. If you fail, you feel you *are* the mistake rather than *made* a mistake. Diets are made to fail. As soon as people realize that diets are the pathway to obsession through shame, then they won't buy into the diet conspiracy.

16. Unfortunately addictions are genetic predispositions as well as learned behaviors. This means, if you come from an alcoholic parent, you will be prone to alcoholism as well as learning to medicate yourself with your own drug of choice. I have heard that there is approximately 40 percent chance of inheriting your parent's addiction. However, identifying this preventable "handicap" can curtail behaviors that cater to addiction.

RECOVERY ORGANIZATIONS:

Academy of the Sierras
42675 Road 44
Reedley, CA. 93654
(866) 364-0808

American Anorexia/Bulimia Association,
Inc.
133 Cedar Lane
Teaneck, New Jersey
(201) 836-1800

ANAD–National Association of
Anorexia Nervosa & Associated
Disorders
Box 7
Highland Park, IL 60035
(847) 831-3438

ANRED–Anorexia Nervosa & Related
Eating Disorders, Inc.
P.O. Box 5102
Eugene, OR 97405
(503) 344-1144

Canopy Cove
Tallahassee, FL
(800) 236-7524

Center for Change
1790 N. State Street
Orem, UT 84057
(801) 224-8255

Green Mountain at Fox Run
Fox Lane, Box 164
Ludlow, VT 05149
(802) 228-8885

Institute Of Living
400 Washington Street
Hartford, CT 06106
(800) 673-2411

Hazelden
Incorporates twelve-step program and
rehab for patients eighteen years and
older with food disorders and drug
dependency as the primary addiction, as
well as other programs.
(300) 257-7800

Laureate Psychiatric
Tulsa, OK
(800) 822-5173

Medical Center at Princeton
Princeton, NJ
(609) 497-4490

Medical University of South Carolina
Charleston, SC
(843) 792-1414
(800) 424-MUSC

The Menninger Clinic
P.O. Box 829
Topeka, KS 66601-0829
(800) 351-9058

Monte Nido
Malibu, CA 90265
(310) 457-9958

The National Anorexia Aid Society
5796 Karl Road
Columbus, Ohio 43029
(614) 436-1112

Overeaters Anonymous, World Service
Rio Rancho, New Mexico
(505) 891-2664

Rader Programs (inpatient facilities)
Corporate Headquarters
Los Angeles, CA
(800) 841-1515

Remuda Ranch
One East Apache
Wickenburg, AZ 85390
(800) 445-1900

Rogers Memorial Hospital
4700 Valley Road
Oconomowoc, WI 53066
(800) 767-4411

The Renfrew Center
Philadelphia, South Florida, New York
and New Jersey
(800) RENFREW

Rosewood
Wickenburg, AZ
(800) 280-1212
(877) 74-WOMEN

St. Joseph's Hospital
7629 York Road
Baltimore, MD 21204
(410) 427-2100

Shades of Hope
P.O. Box 639
Buffalo Gap, TX 79508
(800) 588-HOPE

Sierra Tucson
165 N. Lago del Oro Parkway
Tucson, Arizona 85739
(800) 842-4487

Swedish Medical Center
Seattle, WA
(206) 781-6345

Tulane Behavioral Health Center
1040 Calhoun St.
New Orleans, LA 70018
(800) 548-4183

The Willough at Naples
9001 Tamiami Trail East
Naples, FL
(300) 722-0100
(941) 774-4500

Write for a free catalog for books on
eating disorders.
For the "Eating Disorders Bookshelf
Catalog" MPF to:
Gurze Books
P.O. Box 2238
Carlsbad, CA 92008
(800) 657-7533

Also write to:
Health Communications, Inc.\
Enterprise Center
3201 S.W. 15th St.
Deerfield Beach, Florida 33442
(800) 851-9100

CHAPTER 10:
BARBICISE FOR DUMB BLONDES

The "high" benefit of movement
Twenty-minute Barbicise Target-Rotate Workout

More exhausting than bingeing was having to work off the binge. I would exercise up to ten hours a day. My sister and I never worried about weirdoes because we'd outrun them...and then eventually look like one, running all night. Avoiding lectures, judgments, or sight-seeing tours of the "blimpo Barbis" was tough. One gentleman actually tried to stop me during my exercise-athon to hand me his business card. I thought he was "hitting" on me. How embarrassing. It simply stated: "psychiatrist."

Exercise is any type of physical activity for the sake of health and fitness. It's usually recommended to exercise 30 minutes a day. It takes approximately 45 minutes of continual exercise to enter the fat-burning/muscle-building process. I do believe, however, consistency and intensity are more important.

The common question or debate is "which is better: exercise or diet?" Most suggest that diet achieves 60 percent of your goal, while exercise achieves 40 percent. Others suggest that active overweight individuals are healthier than skinny sedentary individuals. The best answer to whether exercise or diet is better is *both!* You can't make one work without the other. Your exercise, however, does not need to be extensive if you eat right. Raw dieters look lean and fit with very little need for activity. Healthy foods actually encourage movement! Poor food choices make us feel lethargic, depressed, bloated, and stiff. Lactic acids build up in the muscles, causing cramping and possible hypoglycemic reactions from the wrong carbs. This further causes edema and lack of energy. Exercise itself releases powerful brain chemicals such as endorphins, which help combat depression and pain. Anaerobic exercises release serotonin (brain chemical that helps satisfy), endorphins (hormone that relieves pain like morphine), CCK (hormone that makes you feel fulfilled), and HGH (human growth hormone responsible for rejuvenation and the fat-burning/muscle-building process). Exercise combats blood sugar imbalances. Smokers get their nicotine replacement from exercise, which helps fight their cravings, depression, and anxiety.

Muscle weighs more than fat, and muscle tissue pumps up the metabolism, meaning the more muscle you have, the more your metabolism stays boosted without any movement. Exercise is obviously good for the heart and lungs, but it is also good for numerous other things we don't think about. For instance, exercise has been reported to boost the immune systems of patients suffering from fatal diseases. It helps fatigue, water retention, anxiety, stress, pain, posture, confidence, diabetes, asthma, and high blood pressure. The testosterone released during exercise benefits women with female tumors, endometriosis, and even cancer. The testosterone helps balance the excess estrogen, which cause female problems.

Sports are a good way to meet and connect with others. My favorite dates were at the batting cage. Exercise heightens good feelings. Forget drugs; exercise helps enhance the libido as well. Furthermore, exercise is good for body and brain circulation. It helps level your brain chemicals and hormones. Exercise triggers norepinephrine and epinephrine. Norepinephrine (neurotransmitter) helps memory, sleep, and emotions. Epinephrine (adrenalin) helps your blood sugar, heart, and muscles. When I need to think about something, it's best if I exercise. It seems to make me level-headed and able to think straight. My best ideas come when I'm exercising. Exercise helps relieve individuals who suffer from rage outbreaks. Excitotoxins, body residue that is linked to diseases such as Alzheimer and Parkinson's disease, are the result of an accumulation of toxins and the wrong carbs. Exercise has been the only known hope for improvement in these areas. There are so many benefits; the list just goes on.

From a very early age, my sister and I have been sports fanatics. We wanted to play, not just watch them. Our parents were into sports, too. Our mother loved to play tennis and our father taught skiing. Our eating disorder never manifested in weight gain, because my sister and I were always extremely active. We loved baseball, track, roller blading, basketball, swimming, surfing, and dance. Playing sports was the few times we had confidence in ourselves.

There was a Surgeon General's Report says that the minimal exercise requirement to maintain general health is 20-30 minutes of exercise three days per week. That doesn't seem like very much until you consider how sedentary our nation has become. Kids, in particular, are more prone to sit in front of computers and video games rather than to exert physical activity. For the best benefits, you should exercise aerobically about 45 minutes 5 times a week, or 3 times a week with 3 extra days of anaerobic exercise. It is better to be fit rather than thin.

EXCUSE LIST: These are basically the excuses people use to refrain from exercise. Check the excuse that keeps you from exercising. Following the excuse list are the ways you can overcome your excuse.

Check next to your excuse(s)
1. Not enough time ☐
2. Too tired ☐
3. Don't have money for a gym ☐
4. Feel too "fat" to be in public places ☐
5. Feel insecure when around a lot of people ☐
6. Lack of desire and motivation ☐
7. Have an injury or discomfort ☐
8. Don't want to get injured ☐
9. Don't know how to work out ☐
10. Feel too old (or too young) to work out ☐
11. Don't want to gain "bulky" muscle mass ☐
12. Doesn't seem to help weight loss ☐
13. Don't need to lose weight ☐
14. Can't stay committed ☐
15. Never had to, so why now? ☐

Excuse Remedies:

1. Just imagine the time you waste watching TV, gossiping on the phone, playing on the internet, etc. All it takes is 20 minutes at home, 5-7 days a week. There is a saying that holds true: Give the busy man something to do and he will find the time. I bought exercise equipment so I could do my phone work and gossiping while exercising! Time management is the key to success in all areas.

2. Exercise energizes a body with poor circulation. Rest is important, but a dormant body eventually slows down the metabolism and other necessary bodily functions to adapt to your "low and slow" mood. Exercise helps you get energized and makes sound sleep possible. I use exercise as my "cup of coffee" in the morning, to get me started mentally and physically.

3. You don't need money to join a gym. There are many community centers, such as the YMCA, public pools, school gyms, and other activity centers that accommodate low budgets. Some thrift stores carry used gym equipment and the newspaper includes specials, like used bicycle sales. Simple dumbbells, jump-ropes, rubber bands, and exercise balls are affordable at your nearby discount

stores. Exercise videos are always on sale at your nearby grocery, drug, and convenient store. I enjoy exercising outdoors, which is free! Best of all, you don't need a gym or equipment for a quick workout. Exercises, as my simple twenty-minute Barbicise, can be done at home, without any equipment whatsoever.

4. If you are overweight, you are *not* alone. Haven't you heard that weight gain is an epidemic? In fact, there are special gyms, classes, and sporting events for the self-conscious person who may be overweight.

5. Most people are self-conscious, overweight or not. All you have to do is explain to the trainer at the gym that you would prefer privacy or a time when it is not crowded. There are gyms that are open twenty-four hours. There are also gyms that are exclusively for women or men. Because I was insecure, I made my gym at home. I eventually noticed that people respect endurance more than appearance. Once you start sweating, you lose insecurities. Exercise helps build confidence.

6. Lack of desire and motivation are the most common excuses. Exercise is known to combat depression. It releases brain chemicals like serotonin, which makes you feel good! I had a friend who was an athlete and trainer that used to say, "You have to get ugly before you look good!" Everything in life has to be earned, including health. Mother Nature may have blessed you with superb genes, but Father Time will take it away if you don't keep up what you were given. It's all a "mind trip." You can train you mind to enjoy exercise. Try music to help motivate you. Explore different sports that you enjoy. Find a buddy who will exercise with you. Exercise also releases endorphins, which make you feel high. Most of our daily routines in life aren't things we want to do, but should do. We were better for it and we should be glad we do them because it's better for us on the long run. Think about the benefits exercise gives you rather than the work it entails.

7. Many injuries are caused from being overweight or out of shape. It's a cycle. Muscles hold your skeletal structure together, which can help prevent or lessen pain and injuries. Movement helps circulation, which speeds up any healing process. Scar tissue, which causes more pain and problems, builds faster on sedentary individuals. Many women complain of menstrual cramps. This is usually due to excess estrogen. Exercise actually releases testosterone that helps the estrogen imbalance, and therefore the pain. Exercise helps bloating

and edema. During activity, the endorphins being released help relieve pain. There are low-impact exercises, such as swimming, that allow movement without impact. Check with your doctor; he or she may have good suggestions for your specific injury.

8. Unless you are going to be a marathon trainer or pump tons of iron, severe injury is not common. It takes simple logic. People who injure themselves with simple exercises are the type to injure themselves crossing the street. Possibly it's a "block" in their heads. However, most gyms have certified trainers that instruct beginners properly. All videos come with explicit instructions. Libraries have easy instructional books about exercise with appropriate injury warnings. Use common sense and start out with light and low-impact exercises, building gradually to reduce injury possibilities. Proper clothing, shoes, stretching, diet, and breathing techniques all help the novice feel safe and secure. You don't need to get all kinds of medical equipment to check your condition if you start out slow and use common sense. If you are on medication or continue to injure yourself, it would be wise to work out a routine with a licensed trainer and healthcare provider. I've known people who were restricted to wheelchairs but continued their exercise routines, which helped their health physically and mentally.

9. There are trainers at most gyms who will instruct any member. Health books, fitness magazines, videos, and fitness shows on TV instruct people at every level. I wanted to learn by myself. I exercised according to the way my muscles felt. I'd experiment until I got the results I wanted. However, to prevent injury, start out with simple exercises and an easy instructional manual that will help guide you. It doesn't take a rocket scientist to learn to exercise properly.

10. I have noticed that families that start their kids out with early activity have a healthier family than most. It's never too early for movement and activity. For those who think they are too old, there are numerous examples of super fit people who are well above seventy years old. There are famous elderly trainers, marathon runners, and swimmers who attribute their avid exercise to their well-being. If you are the oldest at your gym, you will be an inspiration to others!

11. There are two types of exercises: aerobic and anaerobic. Aerobic has nothing to do with "bulky" muscle tissue. It concentrates on your lean, red muscle tissue and burns fat. On the other hand, while

exercising anaerobically, you can use less weight and more reps, which will burn rather than build. People who complain about being bulky are usually people who overeat and build muscle under their fat. Their bulk will lessen if they choose the proper foods rather than give up their exercise.

12. It is proven that movement helps burn fat. In fact, exercise releases hormones, such as CCK, which creates a feeling of satiation. Moreover, when you retain muscle mass, your metabolism naturally raises, without needing movement. If you diet without exercise, the body learns to sacrifice muscle or vital tissue rather than fat. That means when you regain any weight, you will gain fat, which replaces your muscle tissue. When someone is thin but flabby, that person is the type to gain weight very easily. Exercise helps metabolism, circulation, and all the bodily functions necessary for weight loss. Exercise with plenty of water helps food move through your system, which also helps weight loss. Exercise helps balance numerous hormones, such as estrogen, which helps weight loss as well. Exercise also helps motivate someone to eat properly.

13. Perhaps you don't need to lose weight. You might possibly need to gain weight. Weight loss is not *total fitness*. A well-sculpted body is usually derived from exercise. Exercise is not just about looking good. It makes you feel good for good reasons. Everything works synergistically in your body. Good circulation makes breathing, thinking, and functioning easier. Most thin people eventually complain about a tire rim around their mid section. Poor eating habits usually accompany poor exercise habits, which results in poor tissue quality. Poor tissue quality is responsible for cellulite and flabby tissue, which has nothing to do with weight.

14. Commitment and maturity go hand in hand. When people learn to commit and follow through, it builds their self-confidence and it inspires them to take on healthy risks that help them *climb* to higher levels. The trick to commitment is to start out small and easy. Just like a muscle, the brain has memory patterns that thrive on consistency. Once you have established a good habit (daily commitment), you can start trusting yourself to take bigger steps. People who don't exercise because they are unwilling to commit are training themselves to be irresponsible. There are clues to people's success and failures. Success at anything stems from small commitments like exercise. If you have to start out with 20 jumping jacks a day, do that just for the commitment. Learn to trust yourself and follow through so you can depend on YOURSELF!

15. If someone has poor health habits, it will not go unseen. Poor health habits smolder in the body, eventually manifesting when it's too late. Movement is critical for all life. It helps you physically and mentally. Athletes rarely encounter serious diseases. Have you heard of preventive medicine? Well, exercise is just that. When healthy individuals over the normal old age (above ninety years old) were asked what their secret was, all of them had one common denominator: movement! You don't need much; you just need consistent, daily movement. A brisk walk every day can be easy and relaxing. Many people do their best thinking or meditation when they are exercising. Exercise is a guarantee to improve anyone's life!

Exercising aerobically means to work out "with oxygen," indicating any sustained, moderate activity that keeps heart rate raised and steady over an extended period of time. Aerobic exercise focuses on the red, lean muscle tissue. Examples of aerobic activities include, walking, hiking, and swimming. Aerobic (or cardio) exercises can last anywhere from 10 minutes to several hours, depending on your fitness level. They create a demand on the heart and lungs to deliver oxygen to the bloodstream, where food is metabolized as energy (fuel). A good indicator of aerobic exercise is to be able to have a breathy conversation while exercising continuously. If you struggle to have a conversation, you are entering anaerobic exercise. This stage doesn't put you into the fat-burning/muscle-building stage until your body has used up its reserves (glycogen).

The anaerobic workout (without oxygen) typically refers to stop-and-start activities that require quick bursts of energy followed by a lull—weight lifting, tennis, and wind sprints for instance. As in aerobic exercise, the fuel that makes an anaerobic activity possible comes from glycogen (calories stored as byproducts of the food we eat), which is provided mainly by carbohydrates and fat. Proteins are used very sparingly as available energy. They are too busy repairing and building muscle cells. The fuel for high-intensity anaerobic activity typically runs out after a few seconds or minutes, whereas aerobic fuel can last much longer. Anaerobic exercise focuses on the white, bulky muscle tissue. Isometrics are another example of anaerobic exercise.

You actually need both aerobic and anaerobic exercise for balanced fitness and weight loss. Aerobic is good for the heart, lungs, and fat burning. Anaerobic is good for stronger muscles and bones and for speeding up the metabolism. Anaerobic releases CCK hormone (satiates) and the HGH (human growth hormone for muscle-building/fat-burning process and rejuvenation). There are conflicting opinions about the most effective exercise mode and workout intensity. Most experts claim that extended periods of continuous (but not bone-breaking) moderate cardio exercise burns more fat. In fact, training at very high aerobic intensities adds the anaerobic element, which may oppose your goal. I have found that varying the exercise and intensity shakes up my routine so my body does not try to compensate for what it already knows. I really believe that sweat is a good indicator of burning calories. I will always "peak" at the end of my run to emphasize the sweat and to add a little anaerobic to my aerobic. Most claim aerobic exercise only burns lactic acid. Anaerobic, which conserves more energy than aerobic, draws straight from the fat for fuel. This claim insists anaerobic is best for individuals that have exhausted themselves with diets and exercise.

Weight lifting (anaerobic) is for your total health, not just for big muscles. It all depends on the type of exercise, the intensity, and the total reps you apply. Strength training is for people who want to build muscle, sculpt their bodies, improve appearance and posture, kick-start their metabolisms, help prevent injuries, improve body composition, and help build stronger bone connections. In fact, one of the most important reasons to lift weights regularly is to build denser bones in order to help prevent osteoporosis. As muscles get stronger, so do bones. Here are some facts about *osteoporosis* that may motivate you to lift your first set of free weights.

- ☞ 80 percent of all osteoporosis patients are women.
- ☞ Half of all women will get the disease at some point in their lives.
- ☞ You achieve peak bone mass by the age of thirty and it dwindles from there.
- ☞ Strict dieters and people with eating disorders are at much higher risk.
- ☞ Caucasians, smokers, and very small-boned people are at a higher risk.

The best strategy for weight lifting is learning how to strength train regularly. To sculpt muscle definition and improve functional strength, the American College of Sports Medicine recommends lifting three sets of 8-15 repetitions per exercise. Most experts suggest choosing three different exercises per body part to get optimal results, as well as lifting weights for different parts of the body at least three days per week. Always skip a day of lifting in between sessions to rest and repair your active muscles.

It is best to ask a trainer about your intensity level and weight amount if you're just starting out. My sister and I worked up to lifting fairly heavy weights three to four times a week, trading off with isometrics (using your own body weight as leverage).

Do not overdo it. When you are ready to increase the weight or try a new exercise, go slowly and raise the intensity in weight little by little, to avoid injury. Stretching after each lifting session is recommended by most, to relieve symptoms of the delayed onset of muscle soreness.

Most avid body builders prefer resistance training with free weights (dumbbells) instead of the resistance machines found in health clubs nationwide. If you just want to tone-up, *any* form of weight (tubing, body bars, or exercise bands) will do the job. However, you have to watch your form. (There are excellent how-to videos on the market today.) For those who fear being bulky, remember it is *impossible* to build muscle and gain weight at the same time. Lighter weight with more reps will help sculpt the body rather than build it.

Exercises like yoga, tai chi, palates and other stretching activities seem to tone, sculpt, and strengthen. These are good low-impact exercises and are great for people who suffer from frequent injuries. These exercises help enhance balance, focus, and endurance. There is no cheating with these exercises. It all works together with your breathing. This is why health experts promote these kinds of exercises; they are safe exercises for *every* part of your body. When one body part or muscle is worked on one side, it can create injuries. Yoga and other stretching exercises work on the body as a whole with the mind. It's like a meditation technique. Most people underrate the importance of breathing. Breathing itself can be considered an exercise, because if done properly, it can give you the same benefits as a moderate workout. I think these exercises are an excellent way to give variety to your routines along with the usual aerobic activities. Many yoga athletes combine the spiritual philosophy with their exercise to help benefit themselves, and their body, mind, and soul.

~ ~ ~ ~ ~ ~

A term we've become fond of is **peaking.** This means going beyond your normal intensity range in either aerobics or weight training sessions. I usually know I'm peaking if I start sweating profusely or I can't catch my breath. I'm at the point that I know my body and I know when I peak. But many exercisers do not, so they use other methods to test themselves.

Many active people depend on measuring their performance by taking their heart rate before and after exercise, particularly during cardio activity. A heart rate monitor is extremely accurate but can be expensive. It also does not allow you to become accustomed to your own body's fluctuations. It's best to spend our time focusing on solutions. Below, we've listed three easy methods to measure your workout intensity. The third method is the most accurate and complete, also allowing you to measure your own recovery rate after the workout. Your recovery heart rate is a significant indicator of your cardiovascular fitness.

1. Talk Test Method: If you can hold a breathy conversation while exercising, you are working at an efficient level. If you cannot hold a conversation, you should lessen the intensity. If, on the other hand, you can converse easily during a workout, then increase intensity to see better results. It should never be too easy to chat with your exercise buddies.

2. Perceived Exertion Test Method: This scale demands that you rate your own exercise intensity depending on how difficult it feels to you intrinsically. This is a great way to get know your own body, incidentally. Consider "0" as no workload and "10" as working so hard you cannot continue for more than a few seconds. Keep self-checking your intensity during each session. Experts say the most effective calorie-burning ranges fall between 6, 7, and 8. But you should fluctuate throughout each session.

3. Heart Rate Test Method: If you have a heart rate monitor, the gadget does these calculations for you. If not, become adept at taking your own neck or wrist pulse.

    a) First thing in the morning, take your morning pulse for one minute and remember the number. The lower the number (50, 60, or 70), the more fit you are. Then subtract your age from the number 220. For instance, if you are 20 years old, subtract 20 from 220 (to get 200).
    b) If you know your most effective training heart rate zone, you can boost cardiovascular health and blast body fat. To determine intensity via heart rate during a cardio workout, take that number (200) and multiply it by 0.70 and 0.85. Now try to keep your workout pulse in that fat-burning zone for most of your exercise sessions. For example, when that twenty-year-old takes a neck or wrist pulse during exercise, she should effectively try to stay between 140 and 170 beats per minute for best body results.
    c) Recovery heart rate is how long it takes for your heartbeat to return to normal. After your workout, keep walking slowly and take a one-minute pulse. Register that recovery number, and see how close it comes to the morning pulse you took above. The more fit you are, the more quickly you will recover. Be sure to take your pulse immediately after each workout to get an accurate baseline.

The different methods of **weighing** or **measuring** yourself are numerous. Just like weighing or measuring food doesn't work because it's about the quality not the quality, it's the same for the body. Muscle weighs more than fat, and when muscle replaces fat there is water retention. So why weigh yourself with these variables? Measuring yourself can be obsessive and deceiving. BMI (body mass index) is one popular method now used to determine if you are overweight. BMI measures the fat compared to your bone structure. It's criticized because it does not take your body *type* into consideration. Determining your fat percentage seems to be the most accurate. It is done by either by the pinch or water test. Another method used to determine if your health is at risk is simply to measure your waistline. Men should be less than 35 inches and women should be less than 33 inches for good health. If you a man and are over 40 inches, there are health risks. If you are a woman and are over 35 inches, there are health risks. Then again, during my days of measuring myself, I thought I was fine to put plastic wrap around my waist and sweat all night without drinking water. I had a great waistline until I ate a piece of celery. It was better when I treated my body holistically instead of obsessing about numbers. Thank God my days of ridiculous weighing and measuring methods are over—the lengths I went through to get to an expensive hospital or sometimes a truck stop scale). I'd always carry a bag full of traveling measuring cups and *stretched out* measuring tapes (to achieve the perfect waistline). No more!

The best time to exercise really depends on the individual. At nighttime you have more energy, and it's a good way to clear your mind and relax. Your metabolism is sluggish in the evening so this can help pump it up. Mornings are best to get you started, like a cup of coffee. Exercise first thing to get your body in shape for the whole day, mentally and physically. I liked mornings because it was my anxiety medicine for the day. My boyfriend would throw me out the door in the mornings because I was not in the mood until I exercised. Afternoons are good for people who feel they are too sluggish in the morning to get into it. Splitting up your routine is the best for the metabolism and preventing injuries. There is a theory that dawn and dusk are the best times because of the positive ions in the air. These are the times that are best for meditation as well.

DO NOT exercise on a totally full or empty stomach. You'll feel crampy and gassy if you've eaten a meal within ninety minutes of a tough workout. You ruin the digestion and you will *not* be working off that meal. An empty stomach cannot fuel you properly for a long routine, either. Although you burn-off the calories you had twenty-four hours ago, a light nutritious snack before a workout is best. This will help prevent a burn-out or the so-called hitting the wall. Otherwise, enervation might develop, which causes the body to sacrifice vital tissue rather than glycogen or fat, because it feels stressed. The stress can eventually lead to adrenal exhaustion as well. Do not eat refined carbs or take caffeine before a workout. This usually causes excess insulin secretion, which hinders the fat-burning/muscle-building process. Drink plenty of water before, during, and after your workout.

Simply put, exercise gives you every benefit there is for your body, physically, mentally, and spiritually. The byproduct is great muscle tissue. The more muscle you build, the more fat you will burn.

BARBICISE: 20-MINUTE TARGET-ROTATE WORKOUT—fast results!

🖐 *Check with your doctor. Use proper shoes and check your exercise area for safety issues to prevent any accidents.*

Regardless of your schedule, everyone can take 20 minutes out of their day. It's amazing what we have time to do if we want to. Knowing that only 20 minutes of the Barbicise Target-Rotate Workout can work as well as hardcore torture, it is easier to incorporate this into your lifestyle. Just like eating a huge salad with nothing but lettuce in it, a long workout without focus and intensity is a waste of time and is mentally draining. It's best to do these exercises 6 days a week; they're easy!

Alternate days between aerobic and the anaerobic target freeze exercises in this way:

First Day:

20 minutes of continuous cardio of any one choice:

1) Jumping rope (My favorite; I can do anywhere, anytime.)
2) Step aerobics (along with a taped routine if you wish)
3) <u>Brisk</u> power walking with 5 lb. weights
4) Stationary bike (or elliptical training, which is better for your joints)

Second Day:

Isometric-type exercises, equal in intensity, using your body as "free weights"

These are all very intense exercises that use only your body as weight, except for some common instruments (like a chair) to attain certain angles and positions.

1. Sit on a wall: This is particularly good for the quadriceps (upper thighs). It also helps your back, bottom (glutes), and knees. You appear as if you are sitting on a wall without a chair or any help. Your upper legs are parallel to the floor while your back and calves are perpendicular to the floor. (You may want to have a pillow under your bottom just in case you slip down, until you build up your leg muscles) You do this for about 2 minutes or until you are shaking. Remain as long as you can with short rest periods. Do this until you have completed at least 2 minutes. Eventually, after practicing daily you will be able to do it for at least 2 minutes straight without a rest period..

2. Push up freeze: This focuses on the shoulders and triceps (underneath upper arm). It also works on the neck and stomach area. On something similar to a kitchen sink, you place yourself in a push-up position with you feet slightly back and your hands on the sink (Don't use the bathroom sink; it may not support your weight.) Lean in as if you doing a push-up, and when your arms are at a 90-degree angle, freeze for 2 minutes. Remain in that position unless you have to rest. Continue until you finish 2 minutes. Every day you should improve until there is no need to rest during your two minute freeze.

3. Leg-lift freeze: This works the lower stomach area and lower back as well. You sit on floor with you legs straight in front of you. Then lean back on your forearms by your side that are bent with your elbows slightly behind you.. You lift your legs straight up together to about a 45-degree angle. If you get tired spread and bend your legs to rest, but don't lay them down. Continue this without laying your legs down for 2 minutes. If you have to rest by bending the legs try to resume immediately back to straight legs after breaking position. This should be done until you can hold your legs still in a 45-degree angle without movement.

4. Sit-up wall freeze: This works your upper stomach area. While sitting on the floor, facing a wall, you place your feet in front of you onto the wall. Lay your torso down to make it easier to place each foot flat against the wall in front of you. Your knees should be bent. This position should look like you are sitting on an invisible chair against the wall. Your legs should make a perfect 90-degree angle. That will mean your calves will be parallel to the floor and your thighs will be horizontal (perpendicular to the floor). Put your hands behind your head as if you are going to do sit-ups. Pull your head up with the help of your hands locked behind your head. As soon as your stomach feels like it is in full crunch position (about a quarter to halfway up), hold it. Stay in this position as close to 2 minutes as possible or resume immediately after resting back into position.

5. Chair push-up freeze: This works the back of your upper arms (triceps). You take a chair with NO WHEELS and arm handles that are normally at your waist when you sit down in it. You sit in the chair, making as close as a 90-degree angle while sitting as possible(sitting very straight). You put your hand on the arms and push up until just before your elbows straighten. Your bent arm will have a slight angle during this freeze. Remain in that position until 2 minutes or resume immediately back into position after brief rest periods.

6. Three-legged lift freeze: This completely concentrates on your rear (glutes) and backs of your thighs. On all fours on the floor, position your back so it is parallel to the floor. Lift one leg at a time (to the side or straight out and back) so you have two arms and only one leg holding you. You bend your leg into a perfect 90 degree angle, with the thigh parallel to the floor

and your back but higher and your calve perpendicular to the floor. Hold that freeze position for 2 minutes. Repeat on other leg for 2 minutes as well.

7. Sway freeze: This focuses on your lower back. Laying on your stomach, lift your head and neck off the floor while you raise your legs and feet as much as possible. Do this with your hands stretched out in front of you or clasp behind your back. Hold and freeze this position for 2 minutes or as long as you can. Try to remain in position for a complete 2 minutes.

8. Chair butt-pinch: This works your stomach area and rear. In any chair, with or without arm handles, put your legs straight out in front of you. With just your heels touching the floor and your knees locked, squeeze your butt cheeks as tightly as you can. Hold and freeze that pinch for 2 minutes. When done properly, you'll feel yourself lift slightly.

9. Power-calves lift. This works on your calve muscles. On the edge of a sturdy stair, with a wall or something to hold onto, stand on the step with only half of your foot so you heels are in the air. With your weight on just your toes, raise yourself up. Feel the muscles in your calf tighten. Freeze this position right before you are completely on your toes, at the highest position. Hold position for 2 minutes. Resume this position immediately if you did not complete 2 minutes. (Raising and lowering your body weight slowly in this position is also a good lower leg workout.) *BE CAREFUL!

With each one of these freeze position exercises, you should be able to work up to a solid 2 minutes. Later, if it begins to get too easy (need to sweat or shake a bit), add leg and wrist weights to add intensity. All of the exercises are 2 minutes, including the three-legged lift (exercise #6), which is done for 2 minutes on each leg. That makes a total of only 20 minutes. The intensity and position of each of these freeze positions targets those specific target areas to the max. You will quickly see results.

Rotate your 20-minute aerobic workout (like jumping rope) with your Barbicise isometric freezes every other day to receive the best benefit. This way, your muscles heal while boosting the metabolism. You will never get bored, which will help your body refrain from getting "sour" if you rotate these extreme opposite exercises every other day. You should be able to do these 7 days a week for best results. These exercises are simple with no hardcore instruments and are convenient enough for people on the go who want FAST results.

CHAPTER 11:
NATURAL Rx REMEDIES FOR THE
BEAUTY WITHIN THE BEAST

"Chemical Warfare"...
    Which Beauty Tips and Home Remedies Are Best?
Weight-loss Aids and Energy Boosters
HGH; "Fountain of Youth"
Everything from Amino Acids to Vitamins

Like Nobel Prize winning scientists, we'd create the perfect diet aid to prevent us from eating. Like dream team lawyers, we'd negotiate delicious meal-like diet aids. Oops. We forgot to make these diet aids calorie free.

This chapter goes through the popular diet aids, energy boosters, healers, enhancers, etc. Beauty tips were included, which is pretty funny to my sister and me. We think we brought the "cheap" look in, because we don't have a clue about make-up and fashion...obviously! However, there are some natural beauty tips included that we found helpful. For the addictive personality, there are remedies to help quit stimulants, such as smoking and coffee. This chapter also has the breakdown of vitamins, minerals, amino acids, antioxidants and herbs.

Many people benefit from supplements and enhancers, but these products can't take the place of a healthy lifestyle and diet, and you must remember that not all products are made the same. So do your own research on any product before you start using it.

Most people look to supplements and aids for a quick fix. A healthy lifestyle does not include any shortcuts, because they always backfire. You need to learn what is best to take for your body's needs and in what amount. You body is better at figuring out what it needs. Rather than being your own pharmacist, learn to listen to your body so you can learn what it really needs . Many times, people will take things for what they believe is a deficiency when in truth they already have too much of that substance in their systems and end up poisoning themselves. We have to be careful about what we put into our bodies. Certain supplements are extremely helpful, but nothing is a magical potion.

The four basic nutrients are water, carbohydrates, proteins, and fats, which are also the basic building blocks of a good diet. Along with the basic four nutrients, there are micro nutrients that are also needed in smaller amounts. These are vitamins and minerals. The amount needed varies according to your health, lifestyle, and circumstances. Supplements are something added to help complete or enhance proper nutrition. Nothing can take the place of a proper diet or food plan.

Your skin is the largest organ of your body. It is can be used by the body as an emergency exit for toxins in the body, so certain health problems will manifest outwardly as skin problems. Covering your skin with creams, oils, lotions, or anything else can restrict the proper function of this exit. Your skin absorbs toxins, too; it doesn't just excrete them. When you put products with chemicals and fragrances on your body, you are absorbing those chemicals into your bloodstream.

A swallowed substance is recognized through digestion as a food or poison. If the body can't digest a substance (drug), then your body "clones" it in order to recognize it. Vitamins, minerals, and certain herbs should only be used as supplements in addition to proper nutrition and under supervision. These non-food substances try to replace your own natural chemicals while building a tolerance to them. Eventually you become immune to then. Nothing is a cure-all. With proper rest, exercise, sunshine, and clean air, our bodies manufacture almost everything we need. At times what appears as a deficiency in our bodies may well be a vitamin overload. *Always check food labels and confer with a nutritionist.*

Supplements can't cure diseases without proper nutrition. They can help you work through your health dilemmas, but at other times they may be harmful. Iron is recommended for anemia. Usually sick people have some level of anemia. Too much iron can actually be harmful and toxic or sometimes won't give you any energy at all because it is symptom-chasing the root problem. All vitamins and minerals work synergistically, needing each other (or their absence) to complete their job. Supplements can actually cancel each other in certain combinations. The lack of vitamin B-12 prevents the absorption of iron (and also vitamin D). Vitamin E is good for the heart and blood (blood thinner) but is not recommended before surgery. Too much vitamin C can mimic estrogen and destroy your B vitamins. Calcium needs iron, magnesium, and vitamin D to work properly. Excess vitamin C cancels the B vitamin's effects. Echinacea hinders zinc, and so on. Vitamin A, D, E and K are fat-soluble, so they need to be taken with a fatty meal. Vitamins B and C, on the other hand, are water-soluble. They should be taken one hour after the meal, with a glass of water. Chelated vitamins include an amino acid molecule to make the vitamin more absorbable. Bioflavonoids are a vitamin C complex that makes vitamin C more absorbable. Coenzymes are vitamins that work with enzymes (catalysts, or activators). Sometimes the additives or fillers combined with the supplement are very unhealthy. Certain herbs act as or include harmful substances, such as ma huang, which contains ephedra. I don't think people are comparable to scientific labs. People are not Petri dishes. Just because a certain substance reacts a certain way in a laboratory Petri dish doesn't mean it will be the same for me. A man reacts differently to substances than a woman (because of the different hormones) and my twin reacts differently than I do. Most credible animal organizations claim experimenting on animals is scientific and medical fraud and used only for the benefits of medical insurance. Laboratories can't take into consideration all of our hormones and brain chemicals (all working synergistically), which respond to any substance ingested. All supplements are fragmented or oxidized, therefore, they are an imperfect nutrient source, unlike nature's food. Nature supplies the pulp and fiber in fruit and vegetables to slow down the insulin spills when the fruit is breaking down. Pectin, present in fruits and vegetables, aids our digestion. Our bodies can take a perfect acidic fruit and break it down to an alkaline residue. Our bodies are more sophisticated and complicated than a laboratory or a lab rat. So it's best to keep it simple and let the body rest so it can do its thing.

Unfortunately, health food stores are not regulated by the Food and Drug Administration (FDA), so there is almost no proof of the safety, efficiency, or content of the products they sell. I researched the reputation of specific brands before purchasing supplements. Some supplements and herbs act like drugs and can cause liver damage. For example, tobacco is a plant and marijuana is an herb. Just because a product is natural does not mean that it's good for you. The labeling is usually for promotion only, with very little truth. *Organic* literally means the substance contains carbon compounds. Today, *organic* has come to mean pesticide free, and it has to be labeled *certified organic.* Eating too much of anything, even if it's a good thing, can cause harm as well. Beta carotene is supposed to be a good cancer fighter, but too much of it can actually cause cancer.

Supplements should only be a temporary aid that compliments a healthy lifestyle; they should not take the place of it. Remember, though, that whatever aid you used for certain results, will eventually be the very thing that will reverse the results. For example, if you use a diet aid to lose weight, that diet aid will stop working or need to be increased to a new, higher level to keep working. Because of this, all of the pounds lost will return and they will bring new friends, too. You will just end up being fatter. Lots of people take mega-doses of vitamins, thinking they are harmless. This causes their bodies to limit or stop their own manufacturing of these supplements. When that person forgets to take the daily mega-dose, he or she gets sick. As with anything, moderation and balance with a lot of research is the way to take supplements, aids, and enhancers.

You can't *buy* your health; you have to *build* it!

☞ *Popular Weight Loss, Energy, and Rejuvenation Boosters*

Ergogenic aids are a source of energy or performance enhancers. That means that these enhancers imply they help metabolism, weight loss, muscle building, etc. Please note that they are all controversial and are still being tested.

<u>DHEA</u>: A.k.a. dehydroepiandrosterone, a steroidal hormone (androgen) produced in the adrenal glands and ovaries that is a precursor to testosterone. Testosterone, in male or females, is responsible for libido, energy, and muscle structure. DHEA helps our immune system, increases bone density, helps lower "bad" cholesterol (LDL), and helps with energy and sleep. It helps rejuvenate. Age, illness, and an overdose of stress depletes our own DHEA. It's important to test regularly for this if you take the synthetic form. Natural forms have very little potency. It is best taken if you are over forty.

<u>Chromium Picolinate</u>: The combination of chromium and picolinate acid, a natural substance secreted by the liver and kidneys. Chromium helps level the body's insulin. Some claim that this helps build lean muscle and decrease body fat percentage.

<u>L-Carnitine</u>: An amino acid that aids fat metabolism. Carnitine in actuality is more like a substance related to the B vitamins, which are responsible for your energy and muscle-building process. Helps lower LDL and raises the HDL ("good" cholesterol). Sometimes our body has a hard time manufacturing this supplement, thus creating difficulty burning body fat.

<u>Creatine</u>: An amino acid that is a constituent of the muscles of vertebrates. It occurs naturally in meat. As a supplement, it increases muscular cell water-retention, allowing increased energy for muscular contraction, thus facilitating muscle gain. One Tbsp. of Creatine is said to have the same benefits as 2½ pounds of beef.

<u>Co-enzymeQ10</u>: Vitamin-like antioxidant compound that helps the immune system and the cardiovascular system. It boosts energy, circulation, and athletic performance. It helps slow the aging process.

<u>Melatonin</u>: Hormone secreted from pineal gland. There are claims that this supplement helps rejuvenate and reset your body clock so you are able to sleep. (It is useful for jet lag.) It helps rest the body and, therefore, rejuvenates.

<u>Lecithin</u>: Fatty acid found in egg yolks and soybean products that helps lower "bad" cholesterol and boosts energy and memory. It is also known to help fight disease and aging. Lecithin is loaded with the B vitamins, and is thus an energy booster.

Ginseng: A tonic herb that provides energy, helps stress and fatigue, and builds endurance. It stimulates brain activity, aids memory, and enhances male reproductive and circulatory systems. Ginseng is used for athletic performance and decreases the level of cortisol and also insulin.

Green drinks or sea greens: Includes all sea vegetables like chlorella, seaweed, spirulina, kelp, etc. Most contain large amounts of chlorophyll, carbohydrates and all of the B vitamins, vitamin C and E, amino acids, and rare trace minerals. This is why they are considered a complete food, better known as the "super-food." They are a good source of iodine which helps the thyroid and, therefore, the metabolism. They also help balance the blood sugar. Cancer patients use sea greens as protein because meat is toxic.

Desiccated Liver: Concentrated, dried liver that is put into powdered or tablet form. It contains vitamins A, D, and C; the B-complex vitamins and the minerals calcium; copper; phosphorus; and iron. This is used for anemia to increase energy or relieve stress.

Wheatgrass juice: A concentrated form of chlorophyll, loaded with vitamins, minerals, enzymes, and all important nutrients. This is a good blood cleanser and energy booster. It helps energy return to anemics.

EFA oils: Especially Omega 3, found in fish oils and flaxseed. These oils repair tissue and thus helps slowing the aging process. These essential fats replace the "bad" cholesterol and help balance hormones (insulin and blood sugar), creating better weight loss. They are the building blocks of eicosanoids.

Stevia: An herb "sweetener" to substitute sugar. Synthetic sweeteners have been linked to health problems and disrupting the hormone balance, thus making weight loss difficult. Stevia has no side effects like diarrhea, headaches, or hormone imbalance.

Gotu kola: Widely known as a memory herb that increases circulation to the brain and body (energy). It is a stimulant and should not be taken at bedtime.

Bioidentical hormones: "Natural" hormones made in a lab from hormone precursors found in soybeans and yams. Female problems and synthetic hormones cause weight loss difficulties, unlike these natural hormones which actually fight edema, depression, and PMS.

Acidophilus: A type of "friendly" bacteria that assists in digestion. Acidophilus also helps reduce blood cholesterol levels and helps absorb nutrients. Poor health and problems with weight are connected with digestion problems. Weight loss occurs after digestion and elimination.

Aloe vera: This plant is best known for healing, internally and externally. It has a gentle laxative effect

Citrimax- Extraction from citrus fruit in South America. There are claims this fruit extraction breaks down and dissolves body fat more easily.

Bee pollen: Nutritious tonic and full-spectrum building and rejuvenating substance good for energy.

Royal jelly: Supplies key nutrients for energy, mental alertness, and general well-being. It enhances immunity wellness and is a rich source of pantothenic acid, which fights stress, fatigue, and insomnia.

Noni: Natural fruit extract. It helps eliminate chronic fatigue, detoxifies, cleanses, and helps headaches.

Licorice Root: Herb that fights viruses. It helps with energy and helps balance blood sugar.

Kava: Herb that helps calm the nervous system. It enhances serotonin release and sleep (rest is needed for slowing the aging process).

Green tea: Contains an abundance of antioxidants and anti-allergens. Use it when fasting. It is a good replacement for coffee.

Alpha-lipoic acid: An antioxidant that enhances vitamin C and E and glutathione, neutralizing the effects of free radicals. It promotes two key enzymes that convert food into energy.

Glucosamine: An "amino-sugar" responsible for body tissue structure and digestive system. It is helpful for asthma, candidiasis, allergies, osteoporosis, skin problems. For athletes it's good for joints and cramps.

Garlic: Lowers blood pressure, thins blood, and fights infections. Garlic is good for the heart, circulation, and energy.

Lemon: Liver cleanser that helps with edema or dehydration. The natural sodium in lemon helps the electrolyte balance in your body.

Black strap molasses: good natural source of calcium, magnesium and iron. It is good for energy, bones, cramping, and insomnia.

✦ QUITTING KIT FOR SMOKING, SODAS, CAFFEINE, AND OTHER STIMULANTS

All stimulants are addictive. When you use your stimulant, you will experience a temporary high, releasing such brain chemicals as serotonin (helping you feel calm) and hormones like endorphins (which binds to opiate receptors). Over time, the mere thought of your stimulant can release dopamine (neurotransmitter), giving you a false high. This makes it impossible to attain your goal while using any type of stimulant, regardless of the stimulant. This is especially true if you are using stimulants for weight loss. All stimulants and non-foods react like a drug, eventually creating a hypoglycemic reaction. Your stimulant may enhance the metabolism, but when it detoxifies from your system, it usually turns the hyperglycemic reaction (high blood sugar) to a hypoglycemic reaction (low blood sugar). This triggers excess insulin and cortisol secretion, making weight loss difficult. Dieters use cigarettes, diet sodas, coffee, and other diet aids without realizing they are creating a hormone and brain-chemical imbalance. Cigarettes contain nicotine, which is a stimulant and a muscle relaxant. This dual effect creates an addictive behavior both physically and mentally. At first the nicotine helps block the insulin flow and slows down the blood sugar drop. Coffee and diet drinks work in the same way. However, this reaction is counterbalanced by a lower drop in blood sugar and an insulin difficultly, creating a hypoglycemic reaction. This reaction is the cause of feeling tired, bloated, and hungry. Some athletes use caffeine before their workouts. It may initially cause a false energy, which is enervating (nerve energy). However, caffeine eventually impedes the fat-burning/muscle-building process. The tissues are not as "clean" as those of an athlete who does not use any stimulants. The synthetic sugar substitutes used in sodas have the same negative effect on the insulin as well. All stimulants, especially ones that contain ephedra, eventually cause adrenal exhaustion (cortisol depletion). This is why I stress don't count calories or fat grams. What counts is the way the ingested substance reacts with your own hormones and chemicals. All drugs cause digestive and elimination difficulties in some way as well.

Quit smoking: Use Eco Anti-Diet #2 because the mini-meals help balance the blood sugar and the high carb content helps calm the sugar cravings. Licorice root sticks, eucalyptus, and mint (which comes in gum and lozenges) all help the nicotine craving. Tea tree toothpicks also help. Kava, as well as DLPA (an amino acid), helps with depression, (the feeling of "crashing"). Chromium picolinate helps with the insulin levels.

Sea greens help level your hormones and brain chemicals and give you energy. Alpha-lipoic acid is an antioxidant that helps reduce the effect of free radicals caused by smoking. Aloe vera and acidophilus are good for the constipation side effect of stopping smoking. This can help clean the body of smoke residue: Mix 1/3 cup of apple cider vinegar and 2/3 cup of water with 10 drops of Chinese woodlock. Cook on stove. Drink.

Quit sodas: The caffeine, synthetic sugar substitutes, and carbonation all interfere with your insulin level and blood sugar. Replace the soda with green tea, lemon (or diluted fruit juice), and sparkling water. If you need more sweeteners, add Stevia or fruit juice concentrate.

Quit coffee or caffeine enhancers: Try green tea, gota kola, licorice root extract, ginseng, sea greens, and kava. Try wheatgrass juice instead of caffeine enhancers.

✦ MIRACLES OR MARKETING?

It shouldn't be a surprise that the constant demand for a miracle drug always gives birth to some new discovery or invention. Sophisticated steroids and undetected enhancers have slithered their way through various drug tests. I know many celebrities who use various hormone and steroid combinations just to appear extra fit and rejuvenated. Unfortunately, they will find out that there is no such thing as a shortcut. Somewhere they will pay. Everyone who has used the popular weight loss drugs, has gained back their weight plus more. Women who take HGH or other drugs and steroids usually find themselves with gynecological concerns. Many use the natural herb containing ephedra, which is also very dangerous. Natural or not, we are meant to get our nutrients from food, not pills. I have found that it's what you *don't* eat, rather than what you eat (or supplement), that makes you healthy. Your body is sophisticated enough to figure out how to stay fit and healthy with *simple* fuel and rest.

The new and promising "miracle aid" seems to be the hoodia gordonii, a cactus plant found in the semi-deserts of South Africa, Botswana, Namibia, and Angola. It's said to contain a natural appetite suppressant. It also has the added advantage of being able to stimulate the libido. The hoodia cacti seem to contain a molecule that is about 10,000 times as active as glucose. It stimulates the hypothalamus and actually signals your brain that you are full, without eating. This might be a dangerous discovery with the rise of eating disorders. It still does not teach a compulsive overeater how to choose healthy foods. However, this may be a new way to help study the different responses to satiation.

✧ **ANTIOXIDANTS**: Vitamins, minerals, and enzymes that help protect the body from destructive oxidation reactions at the cellular level (free radicals). Free radicals are atoms (or groups of atoms) that damage cells. Examples are pollution, smoking, and sun damage. This can cause infections that lead to extreme diseases such as cancer and heart disease. Antioxidants are found in sprouted grains, fruits, and vegetables. Common supplements: CoQ10, green tea, grapeseed extract, vitamin A and beta-carotene, vitamin C, vitamin E, zinc, and selenium.

✧ **ENZYMES**: Protein catalysts that interact or speed chemical reactions in the body. They are important chemicals involved in every bodily function. These activators are the chemical reactions responsible for the breakdown of your food and other bodily activities. As we age, we lose our own function of enzymes, especially digestive enzymes. When you eat heavy meals of animal meat, your digestive tract has a difficult time eliminating the partially digested protein. Digestive enzymes can be used to help digest meals. Common enzymes: bromelain (from pineapple) for fat, papain (from papaya) for protein, protease (from aspergillus) for protein, lactase for milk sugar, amylase for starches, and cellulase for vegetable fiber.

✧ **AMINO ACIDS**: These are the building blocks of proteins. The are 29 amino acids from which over 1,600 basic proteins are formed, comprising over 75 percent of the body's solid weight. There are 22 nitrogen-containing organic acids essential for synthesizing proteins in your body. There are 8 essential amino acids. *Essential* means the body does not supply them so you have to. *Non-essential* are those formed by metabolic activity. Vitamins and minerals cannot be effective without amino acids. The body's liver makes about 80 percent of the amino acids, leaving 20 percent that are essential and need to be obtained from your diet. Some of the common or essential amino acids are alanine (helps metabolize glucose), arginine (retards tumors), carnitine (energy for muscles), cysteine (collagen: skin), glutamine (burns fuel), histidine (essential for growth and repair), phenylalanine (essential antioxidant that helps neurotransmitters), methionine (essential antioxidant that breaks down fats) and tryptophan (essential antioxidant that helps boost serotonin).

✦ **VITAMINS, MINERALS, AND HERBS**

VITAMINS

Vitamins are essential but cannot replace a proper diet. They help you maintain your health by contributing to the biochemical processes that are responsible for metabolism, energy, elimination and major body production. A slight vitamin deficiency can make the body very sick because the body's cells will function less efficiently. Therefore, if we can't supply vitamins with the foods we eat, we take supplements. Vitamins are used immediately, excreted in the urine, or stored until needed. There are so many vitamin theories than continually change or contradict one another. This complicates choosing the right supplements. It's best to be advised by a nutritionist or limit supplementation that should be thoroughly researched.

Vitamin A aids in resisting infections and healthy skin, hair, eyes, bones, and teeth. Found in milk, cheese, leafy greens, yams, sweet potatoes, liver, dairy, fish oils, and fruits as melons. Deficiency: dry eyes; night blindness; dry, itchy skin; weak tooth enamel; chronic diarrhea; and bladder infections.

Beta carotene is an antioxidant that is a precursor to vitamin A. It is best for the immune system, allergies, etc. Found in leafy greens, green peppers, carrots, cantaloupes, kale, peaches, mangos, nectarines, papaya, prunes, squash, sweet potatoes, spinach, and sea vegetables. Deficiency: blurred vision, kidney stones, and impaired growth.

Vitamin B1 (thiamine) aids in nervous system and immune function and increases mental capacity. It also aids growth and motion sickness. Individuals taking diuretics and oral contraceptives or those who are pregnant require an increased intake. Smoking, pollutants, stress and alcohol deplete B1. Found in whole grains, asparagus, brewer's yeast, nuts and seeds, wheat germ, oatmeal, red meat, and dairy products. Deficiency: loss of appetite, edema, depression, fatigue, loss of energy, poor mental abilities, insomnia, weight loss, and constipation.

Vitamin B2 (riboflavin) aids in metabolism and energy and promotes healthy skin and eyes. It also reduces the impact of drug toxicity and environmental chemicals. It controls cataract buildup. Extra B2 is needed during pregnancy, oral contraceptive consumption, lactation, depression, when using diuretics, and in times of stress overload. Found in milk, nuts, brewer's yeast, eggs, mushrooms, yogurt, liver, kidney, cheese, and whole grains. Deficiency: hypersensitivity to light, skin irritation, reddening of the cornea.

Vitamin B3 (niacin) aids in proper circulation and healthy skin. It helps the metabolism (of cholesterol and sugars) and enhances digestion and the production of sex hormones. It is good for nerves, acne, diarrhea, and migraine headaches. Found in milk, poultry, almonds, avocados, brewer's yeast, fish, liver, beans, legumes, bananas, whole grains, and green vegetables. Deficiency: cause pellagra, canker sores, dementia, depression, diarrhea, fatigue, headaches, limb pains, low blood sugar and skin eruptions. Too much may cause liver damage.

Vitamin B5 (pantothenic acid) is an antioxidant that aids in immune system function and adrenal activity. It may help prevent arthritis and lower cholesterol. It helps fight infection, strengthen antibodies and decreases stress, adrenal exhaustion, fatigue, and nerve disorders. It enhances healing after surgery. Found in brewer's yeast, brown rice, poultry, yams, whole grains, liver, kidney, broccoli, legumes, peas, bran, and molasses. Deficiency: insomnia, vomiting, and lack of energy and coordination, skin problems, dizzy spells, adrenal exhaustion, digestive malfunctions, and foot pain.

Vitamin B6 (pyridoxine) aids in metabolizing fat and protein and helps make red blood cells. It also eases nausea and skin disorders. Found in meat, fish, fruit, wheat germ, egg yolks, cantaloupes, cabbage, milk, and brewer's yeast. Deficiency: anemia, nervous system disorder, insomnia, edema, skin abnormalities, and loss of muscle function.

Vitamin B12 aids in the production of healthy red blood cells, hinders anemia, and enhances children's growth. Found in meat, shellfish, eggs, and dairy products. Deficiency: anemia, poor appetite, growth retardation, loss of energy, and pale skin.

Biotin (member of B complex) aids in energy metabolism and growth and boosts metabolic function. Found in brewer's yeast and most fruits and vegetables. Deficiency: appetite fluctuations, energy loss, and decreased muscle function.

Choline (B complex) aids in liver function and metabolism and the breakdown of fat. Found in egg yolks, leafy greens, legumes, yeast, liver, and wheat germ. Deficiency: dysfunction of the liver, problems with fat breakdown, and hardening of the arteries.

Inositol (B complex) aids in hair growth, has a calming effect, and helps to reduce cholesterol levels. It also helps prevent hardening of arteries and helps with the metabolism of fat. Found in lecithin, fruits, brewer's yeast, legumes, meats, milk, unrefined molasses, raisins, vegetables, and whole grains. Deficiency: hair loss, high blood cholesterol, constipation, irritability, mood swings, and skin problems.

Folic acid (member of B complex) aids in building new cells and helps protein metabolism and growth. It also helps build red blood cells in bone marrow. Found in dark, leafy vegetables; liver; legumes; kidney; and yeast. Deficiency: anemia, heartburn, constipation, depression, and frequent infection.

PABA is an antioxidant that fights skin cancer and acts a coenzyme in the breakdown of protein. It also helps with red blood cell formation, healthy intestines, and stress. Found in kidney, liver, molasses, mushrooms, spinach, and whole grains. Deficiency: fatigue, depression, intestinal disorders, graying of the hair, irritability, nervousness, and skin problems.

Vitamin C aids in healthy teeth, gums, and bones. It helps fight infections and speeds up wound healing. It also builds connective tissue. Found in citrus fruit, broccoli, Brussels spouts, kale, papaya, mango, cabbage, and red and green peppers. Cooking destroys the efficacy of vitamin C. Deficiency: hair loss, anemia, soft gums, tooth decay, loss of appetite, bruising, muscle degeneration, and bone fragility.

Vitamin D aids in kidney function and boosts healthy teeth and bones. It is vital to children's growth. Found in natural sunshine, fish and liver oils, fat, eggs, milk, and butter. Deficiency: rickets, tooth decay, growth retardation, and loss of muscle tone and energy.

Vitamin E is an antioxidant that builds the immune system and acts as an anticoagulant (eliminates blood clots). It helps fight heart disease and stimulates kidney function. Found in wheat germ, whole wheat, leafy greens, vegetable oils, meat, eggs, nuts, seeds, and whole grain cereals. Deficiency: anemia, leg cramps, weakness, decreased reproductive function, and muscular disorders.

Vitamin F aids in the growth process and healthy skin, hair, and glands. It also lowers blood cholesterol and helps fight heart disease. Found in oils such as soybean, peanut safflower, cottonseed, and corn. Deficiency: skin disorders such as eczema.

Vitamin K aids in blood clotting and liver function. It helps regulate calcium. Found in milk, cabbage, liver, alfalfa sprouts, green vegetables, soybean oil, and egg yolks. Deficiency: hemorrhaging.

Vitamin P aids in protecting vitamin C. It is beneficial for hypertension and can help build up a resistance to colds. Found in the peels and pulp of all citrus fruits. Deficiency: skin spots and weak capillary walls.

Rutin aids in the same way as vitamin P. Found in buckwheat. Deficiency: same as P.

MINERALS

Minerals, like vitamins, are vital to the body's functions, energy, growth, and healing, but they must be obtained through diet. Constituting the very few inorganic compounds in the body, minerals also serve as electrolytes. Electrolytes are vital mineral compounds that maintain the body's fluid balance and are capable of conducting electrical impulses. Electrolytes enable the neural transmission and complement the ionic exchange. The best mineral supplements are ionic; they are absorbed naturally into your body. With age, mineral assimilation reduces. The body's ability to assimilate minerals and sodium affects the body's ability to hold water. Our cells do not appreciate distilled water, only water with a certain electrolyte balance. Babies contain 75 percent water. A grown man contains about 50-70 percent. This affects the way our skin appears as well as our overall internal health. Minerals also help maintain the blood pH at 7.35-7.45. A poor diet causes the body to be too acidic. Raw-food diets make the body more alkaline.

Boron aids in healthy bones and muscle. Found in leafy greens, apples, carrots, nuts, and grains. Deficiency: bone and muscle deterioration.

Calcium is the most abundant mineral in our bodies but our bodies are also the most deficient in calcium. Women with female problems lack in calcium. It aids in creating healthy bones and teeth. It lowers cholesterol and helps with insomnia, muscle cramps, and numbness. Found in kale, greens, broccoli, brewer's yeast, oats, dairy, salmon, clams, soy, bancha tea, and molasses. Deficiency: eczema, heart palpitations, high blood pressure, insomnia, dental problems, and brittle bones. I have heard about some research which indicates the calcium molecules in dairy and meat are too large to absorb and thus leech more calcium, creating calcium deposits.

Chromium aids in energy and metabolizing glucose. It helps cholesterol, blood sugar, and breaking down fat and protein. Found in brewer's yeast, brown rice, cheese, meat, and whole grains. Deficiency: anxiety, fatigue, glucose intolerance, and arterial disease.

Copper aids zinc and vitamin C. It also helps with energy, healing, hair and skin coloring, plus the formation of bones and red blood cells. Found in almonds, avocados, garlic, liver, mushrooms, seafood, and leafy greens. Deficiency: osteoporosis, skin problems, anemia, baldness, lack of energy, and respiratory dysfunction.

Germanium aids in detoxification and blocking free radicals. It also increases cell strength and helps fight pain. Found in garlic, shiitake mushrooms, onions, aloe vera, comfrey, and ginseng. Deficiency: escalating food allergies, elevated cholesterol, arthritis, candidiasis and chronic viral infections, and is especially needed for individuals with cancer, and AIDS.

Iodine is only needed in trace amounts. Iodine helps metabolize fat and maintain thyroid health. Found in fish, sea vegetables, garlic, mushrooms, sea salt, sesame seeds, soybeans, Swiss chard, and spinach. Deficiency: can lead to mental retardation, breast cancer, ,fatigue or weight gain.

Iron is most needed for the production of hemoglobin. It is important for a healthy immune system and energy. Excess iron, however, can be harmful as well. Found in eggs, fish, liver, meat, poultry, leafy greens, whole grains, almonds, black strap molasses, and dried fruit. Deficiency: may include anemia, bone and hair problems, fatigue, nervousness, obesity, and slow mental reactions.

Magnesium aids in calcium and potassium functions. It is important for enzyme activity and the body's pH balance and helps with depression and PMS. Found in dairy, fish, meat, seafood, apples, avocados, bananas, garlic, kelp, nuts, and whole grains. Deficiency: insomnia, confusion, poor digestion, and even diabetes; can lead to cardiac arrest, asthma, and depression.

Manganese aids anemics. It helps control fat metabolism and blood sugar levels. It also contributes to a healthy immune system. Found in avocados, nuts, seaweed, whole grains, egg yolks, and parsley. Deficiency: confusion, eye and hearing problems, memory loss, tremors; can lead to high cholesterol, convulsions, and breast ailments.

Molybdenum, only in small amounts, is need for cell function. It helps gum disorders. Found in beans, grains, and leafy greens. Deficiency: impotency in older men; may cause cancer.

Phosphorus aids in bone and tooth formation as well as cell growth, heart, and kidney function. Phosphorus should be balanced with magnesium and calcium. Found in whole grains, asparagus, bran, corn, brewer's yeast, dairy, eggs, fish, dried fruit, nuts, and seeds. Deficiency: may lead to anxiety, bone pain, weakness, numbness, and problems with weight.

Potassium aids in nervous system and heart rhythm. Also can prevent strokes, muscle problems, and water retention. It helps with acne, constipation, bloating, weakness, and the body's fluid balance. The elderly need potassium most. Found in dairy, fish, legumes, whole grains, chicken, bananas, apricots, dried fruit, peanuts, potatoes, and leafy greens. Deficiency: may include skin problems, confusion, constipation, depression, diarrhea, reflex problems, heart and growth impairment, high cholesterol, insomnia, muscle fatigue, nausea, respiratory distress, and salt retention.

Selenium—like as iron, zinc, iodine, and fluoride—is a trace mineral. Only small amounts are needed for important functions such as boosting the immune system and slowing down the aging process. Selenium is an antioxidant like vitamin A, C, and E. It prevents abnormal oxidation of body fat that can cause cancer. Found in Brazil nuts, brewer's yeast, seafood, whole grains, garlic, and egg yolks. Deficiency: may lead to cancer, heart disease, growth impairment, infections, and sterility.

Silicon aids in formation of bones, tissue, nails, skin, and hair. It also helps prevent Alzheimer's disease and osteoporosis. Found in alfalfa, beets, brown rice, soybeans, whole grains, and leafy greens. Deficiency: may lead to osteoporosis and skin problems.

Sodium aids in the body's pH and water balance. A sodium deficiency is are but can cause problems with weight and depression. Found in almost all foods, especially in pickled foods, canned foods, seafood, and dairy products. Deficiency: may lead to anorexia, cramping, fatigue, depression, heart palpitation, vomiting, confusion, and muscle impairment.

Sulfur is an acid-forming mineral that helps resist bacteria, stimulate bile secretion, protect against toxins, and slow down the aging process. Found in Brussel sprouts, eggs, garlic, dried beans, wheat germ, kale, soybeans, meat, and onions. Deficiency: skin problems.

Vanadium aids in growth and reproduction. It also helps reduce cholesterol levels and aids bone and teeth formation. Found is dill, fish, olives, meat, radishes, and whole grains. Deficiency: has been linked to cardiovascular and kidney diseases, reproductive problems, and infant mortality. Vanadium is not easily absorbed.

Zinc aids in cell reproduction. Zinc is present in all human tissue and is essential for enzymatic activity in the body. Zinc is also vital for reproductive functions, skin care and a healthy immune system, particularly in healing wounds. Zinc also helps fight free radicals. Found in brewer's yeast, dulse, egg yolks, fish, kelp, legumes, liver, mushrooms, pecans, poultry, pumpkin seeds, sardines, soy lecithin, soybeans, sunflower seeds, and whole grains. Deficiency: may result in loss of taste and smell. White spots or peeling nails can indicate a zinc deficiency. It can also cause fatigue, growth impairment, hair loss, high cholesterol, impotence, infections, colds, memory loss, slow wound healing, and a low resistance to the flu.

HERBS

Herbs can be remedies, performance boosters, and energy enhancers. They can even be deadly, if taken in excess. Herbs are plants with leaves, seeds, or flowers that are used for flavoring, food, medicine, or perfume. They lack a permanent, woody stem. Some herbs have medicinal properties, while some are pests or are used in cooking for savory qualities. For hundreds of years, as prescribed by learned alternative healers, herbs have been used to treat a large variety of conditions, such as mild burns and indigestion. They have also been used to supplement cosmetics. Others have been used to help cure serious medical problems. Most bitter-tasting herbs are medicinal herbs. The pleasant-tasting herbs are potentially less toxic and can be used more often. Most plant roots and bark are naturally fungicidal and bactericidal. They can retain their medicinal value for years if thoroughly dried and kept dry. You can find them in natural form (leaves, bark, and roots) or in tablets, capsules, liquid beverages, bark pieces, powders, extracts, tinctures, creams, lotions, salves, and oils. You can use them as compresses, teas, or as an oil or powder.

Alfalfa aids in the function of calcium, magnesium, phosphorus, chlorophyll, vitamin C, and other vitamin and minerals.

Aloe vera in a gel or cream aids in soothing burns or small wounds. It lubricates the skin and improves healing. Aloe vera juice has been known to treat acne, balance the endocrine system, and prevent constipation.

Black cohosh aids in reducing edema. It also eases PMS, menstrual symptoms, and fights nerve dysfunction. It can reduce blood pressure and prevent headache and arthritis pain.

Capsicum aids in thermogenesis for weight loss, especially when combined with caffeine, herbs, or ephedra. It increases circulation.

Cayenne cream aids in eliminating cramping and helps with other injuries.

Dandelion root aids in the purification of the skin, liver, blood, and endocrine system.

Echinacea strengthens the immune system, especially against infection.

Garlic has an antibiotic effect and fights infection. It is a blood thinner as well.

Ginger decreases cramping, indigestion, nausea, coughs, sinusitis, and a sore throat. It's a good warming circulatory stimulant or body-cleansing herb, especially for candidiasis.

Ginkgo bibloba aids in memory and concentration.

Ginseng aids in energy and rejuvenation.

Goldenseal aids in fighting colds. It's a natural antibiotic.

Green tea contains large amounts of antioxidants and anti-allergens. It is used as a fasting tea.

Guarana/Kola nut is a natural stimulant like ma huang (not recommended) but contains caffeine, not ephedrine.

Kava aids in calming nervous system without side effects. It enhances sleep and naturally enhances serotonin release.

Licorice root aids in fighting viruses and symptoms of herpes, and it helps boost energy.

Ma huang is NOT recommended. It stimulates the adrenals and expands bronchial tubes but causes the constriction of blood vessels. It contains ephedrine.

Red clover aids in the alkaline balance. It contains large amounts of minerals.

Rosemary is an antioxidant herb that aids brain and memory stimulation.

Saw palmetto helps with prostate problems.

St. John's Wort helps combat herpes. It is much like anti-depressant that has calming and relaxing effect.

Tea tree oil is an antiseptic and antifungal agent. It helps cure athletes' foot and helps candidiasis.

Valerian root aids with insomnia without the side effects of addiction.

White willow has an aspirin-like effect on arthritis and headaches. It's an analgesic, anti-inflammatory, and astringent.

Yellow doc root high content of iron to prevent energy loss. This herb aids in circulation. It also reduces skin eruptions and pale coloration.

✦ ANTI-AGING SECRETS

The term *fountain of youth* is used often. Cynical shoppers are prone to go to radical extremes to reach this so-called fountain of youth. Expensive creams, injections, and surgeries seem to be the norm to combat anti-aging effects. Young adults are also turning to these extreme measures to "prevent" aging and to receive the other bonus benefits of HGH.

The latest rage with celebrities is the off-label use of HGH (human growth hormone). Human growth hormone naturally occurs in the pituitary gland (the master gland of the endocrine system located in the base of the brain) and is at its optimal level between birth and adolescence. Our natural growth hormone (a polypeptide hormone) is produced by the anterior part of the pituitary gland, which promotes normal growth. It also promotes protein building in all cells, increases use of fatty acids for energy, and reduces the use of carbohydrates. The release of our growth hormone (controlled by nervous system) occurs in bursts. More than half is released during sleep. HGH also helps trigger the muscle-building/fat-burning process. HGH levels usually peak between twenty-one to thirty years old and quickly decline thereafter. Every year from that point on, the HGH levels drop approximately 14 percent and can be nearly 50 percent less than normal by age forty. Growth hormone deficiency in adults is called *somatopause*.

There has been promising evidence that synthetic HGH may help reverse the effects of declining hormones in elderly adults. Young adults (some as early as their twenties) also obtain this hormone for the other promised effects. HGH is reported to reduce wrinkles, increase skin's elasticity, reduce body fat, increase muscle and bone mass, increase libido, and so forth. There is an obvious difference in someone who is taking HGH. Celebrities who experience sudden weight loss and muscle tone are quite possibly using HGH. Normally extreme weight loss and increased muscle tone takes time and a lot of consistent, hard work. It takes approximately six weeks to see a radical change from HGH. I have never achieved such a bionic body, even though I followed a strict diet and exercised up to ten hours a day for months at a time.

There is the bad news, of course. Taking any hormone is dangerous because our bodies are dictated by hormones. HGH should only be given to individuals with pituitary problems by an endocrinologist, not a plastic surgeon or a sports trainer. Under certain circumstances, endocrinologists have been able to help elderly people who are deficient in HGH. They do this by carefully monitoring the declining hormones frequently. However, any type of off-label usage can cause negative side effects such as joint soreness, elevation in blood pressure and blood sugar, liver and kidney difficulties, and possibly diabetes.

Here's how it works. HGH (synthetic) only lasts a short time in the bloodstream. It's usually injected in various places in the body, particularly in the stomach. Sometimes the injections are evenly distributed throughout the body. The HGH stimulates the IGF-1 and 2 (insulin-like growth factors) in the liver. It's the IGF that creates the benefits and shoots the glucose levels up. This causes the body to rush into the muscle-building/fat-burning stage without having to diet or exercise. (Though muscle mass is increased, there isn't any noticeable difference in energy levels.) The skin thickens and wrinkles disappear. Sleep and hair growth is enhanced. As with any drug, no one should use these products without taking scheduled break intervals. Withdrawal symptoms may occur, such as edema, a lack of energy, and sometimes depression. This may cause the user to return to HGH or continually use it. All the benefits of HGH disappear when HGH usage is stopped. Many people also supplement HGH with insulin injections to increase the effects and to help balance the blood glucose levels. This may cause serious liver and endocrine problems. Reported side effects of HGH usage are increased blood pressure, increased blood sugar levels, and joint pain. Some experience kidney pain or difficulties. Your own natural HGH levels usually decrease when using the synthetic form. Taking HGH can also dangerously interfere with other medications. IGF-1 and 2 in excess can also lead to cancer. I know of some female celebrities who complain that HGH mimics testosterone, which causes them unwanted masculine symptoms. All shortcuts have a payback.

Many people have turned to "alternative" HGH supplements in order to bypass the alarming side effects of the synthetic form. HGH is a protein-based hormone. Over-the-counter HGH distributors sell their version, made from safe and simple amino acids, sometimes adding ginseng. I have found these to be worthless. HGH would be destroyed in the stomach if taken orally. The HGH sprays are ridiculous because the molecules of HGH are too large to be absorbed.

The good news is that there are four ways of secreting HGH naturally, without side effects. The first is during sleep. The second is during a fast. The third is during a protein diet or when heavily into ketosis. The fourth is during anaerobic exercise. You can trigger your own HGH secretion and help prevent the levels of it from dropping in your body by eating light, clean mini-meals, resting well, and incorporating a good exercise program. The pituitary gland is the master of your body's hormones and helps regulate sugar metabolism. That is why I stress that our bodies are dictated by hormones and our lifestyle choices dictate our hormones (health). With this in mind, health should be your goal, not weight or beauty; those will come.

Secret foods that rejuvenate you!

Anti-Inflammatory = Anti-Aging

☑ Foods high in antioxidants (antioxidants =anti-inflammatory, which fights free radicals, the cause of disease and aging)
> Blueberries are the best (high in antioxidants).
> Green tea (high in antioxidants)
> Vitamin E

☑ Foods low on the glycemic index (low sugar and low insulin; prevents aging)

☑ EFA oils and fish oils (essential fatty acids that replace bad fats and plump the skin)

☑ Leafy greens and super sea greens (help hydration and are a good source of B vitamins for circulation)

☑ Foods high in beta-carotene (precursor to vitamin A, also an antioxidant which is good for the skin, hair and eyes and brings natural color to skin).

☑ Garlic (antibiotic effect that helps circulation and detoxifies the body, including the liver)

Things to avoid!

(Inflammatory = Aging)

☒ Sugar (causes skin to sag, insulin imbalance, edema, and enhances free radicals)

☒ Coffee (causes insulin imbalance, which escalates aging)

☒ Meat (in excess, dehydrates the skin and clogs up the colon, tiring the body)

☒ Unnatural sugar and fat substitutes (dehydrate the skin and cause digestion and insulin problems)

☒ High-glycemic foods (insulin surge causes bloating)

☒ Excess sodium/table salt (causes edema and aging)

☒ Excess makeup or heavy creams (unnatural substances that clog pores and the weight causes skin to sag)

☒ Excess sun or smoking (dehydrates skin and ruins elasticity. Five to ten minutes of sunshine before 10:00 AM or after 2:00 PM is sufficient and helps bring melanin to the surface, which helps protect skin.)

☒ Stress and negativity (causes excess cortisol secretion, which escalates aging and causes bloating)

✦ NATURAL HOME REMEDIES AND BEAUTY TIPS

Facial scrub: Mixture of cornmeal a few drops of olive oil and sea salt.

Wrinkles away: Mixture of mayonnaise, vitamin E with egg whites, honey, crushed cucumbers, almond oil, lemon, and sea salt. Also try ginger root, borage seed, flaxseed, lemongrass, or parsley.

Exfoliating skin: Mixture of milk, oatmeal, eggs, honey, and cornmeal.

Exfoliating face peel: Mixture of papaya, eggs, and oatmeal.

Skin firmer: Mixture of plain yogurt, wine vinegar, and brewer's yeast.

Acid peel: Mixture of apple cider vinegar, lemon, and tomatoes.

Smooth and brighten skin: Mixture of ester C powder with lemon and white willow.

Night moisturizer: Mixture of butter and buttermilk with avocado.

Acne cure: Mixture of lemon, vinegar, baking soda, honey, and almond meal (or try ingredients separately).

Face astringent: Mixture of lemon, vinegar, tea tree oil, and tomatoes.

Detox facial mask: Mixture of yogurt with bran (or baking soda), oat flakes, vinegar, and eggs. Or try green clay, honey, and lemon.

Eliminate age spots: Mixture vitamin E, castor oil, lemon, and wheat germ paste. Rub with vitamin K cream.

Reduce puffy eyes: Place cold figs and cold cucumbers or iced chamomile tea over eyes.

Reduce large pores: Mixture of almond meal, salt, oatmeal, and buttermilk.

Reduce red skin: Comfrey.

Smoother skin: Mixture of oatmeal, egg, mild rose water, and rosemary tea.

Oily skin: Use witch hazel first. Then make mixture of yogurt, tomato, lemon, wheat germ paste, brewer's yeast paste, and cucumber juice. Also try lavender with lemongrass and rosebuds put into a facial steam.

Dry skin: Mixture of dried apricots with honey, papaya, milk, butter, avocado, and mayonnaise.
Peppermint, calendula, and chamomile is good when you put it into a facial steam.

Hair loss: Apple cider vinegar and sage tea as a rinse. Try taking licorice extract and horsetail.

Cuts and stings: Vitamin E, Aloe vera, or cayenne pepper.

Poison ivy: Aloe vera gel, lime water, white oak bark, black walnut extract, bloodroot, and myrrh.

Itch or rash: Mixture of cornstarch, baking soda, oatmeal, and Epsom salts with aloe vera. Then follow with an iced watermelon to relieve itching.

Fight infection: Black walnut and myrrh.

Swelling: Bloodroot.

Nausea: Black tea when sick, but not on empty stomach. Regular tea and diluted apple juice with a few drops of lemon.

Pain relief: Sitz bath (which is also good for muscular disorder, constipation, blood poisoning, congestion, headaches, and swollen ankles). A sitz bath is a form of hydrotherapy. It is the use of hot and/or cold water, steam, and/or ice to restore and maintain health. The sitz bath helps the blood flow, thus helping edema or circulation. It's best to consult with your health care provider before choosing the type of procedure for your illness.

Sinus problems, congestion, and asthma: Steam inhalation with these herbs: comfrey, elecampane, eucalyptus, and licorice. To relieve irritation of the mucous membranes, use steam inhalation with slippery elm, peach bark, Irish moss, lungwort, chickweed, burdock, and marshmallow.

Surgery preparation: Acidophilus, CoQ10, echinacea, goldenseal, milk thistle, pau d'arco, and rose hips.

Healing from surgery: Echinacea, goldenseal, EFA oils, Aloe vera, vitamin E oil, garlic, and sea vegetables.

Toothaches: Epson salt and warm water rinse with a few drops of tea tree oil. Topically, clove oil is good for pain Peppermint calendula, chamomile, and yarrow are all herbs that are naturally anti-inflammatory..

Headaches: White willow, St. John's Wort, and kava kava.

Candidiasis (yeast infections): Ingested: acidophilus, garlic, ginger, milk thistle, and sea greens. For topical use yogurt (lactose free), tea tree oil, vinegar, and Epson sat.

Toothpaste: Baking soda, tea tree oil, peppermint, and cloves.

Bad breath: Chlorella, tea tree oil, and eucalypts.

Bath oil: Lavender, tea tree oil, and olive oil.

Natural laxative: Epson salt, aloe vera, garlic, senna leaves, cascara sagrada, rhubarb root, and cayenne pepper or fennel seed tea.

☞ Drink about eight glasses of water (with lemon) one half hour before meals and two hours after meals. The natural sodium in lemon helps with the electrolyte balance (dehydration). A squeeze of orange changes the molecular structure of the water, making it a little more "clean." If your diet is raw, you don't have to overwork your kidneys. Distilled water is best.

☞ Ten to twenty minutes of sunshine a day will bring your melanin to the surface, which is a natural sunscreen. The vitamin D you accumulate naturally is a catalyst to other nutrients in the body. The sun penetrates the pineal gland through your eyes, which is good for depression and hormone balance. Use natural sunscreen like PABA, otherwise. All the chemicals in other sunscreens sometimes causes problems because your skin is an "emergency organ," or exit, that picks up chemicals and carries them through the blood. Poisons are sweated out naturally. It's best to use an umbrella or hat and scarf.

Hair and skin sauna: This is a good way of detoxifying your skin. If your hair and skin are prone to dryness, try a "hot-oil treatment" by applying a light oil like sunflower on your hair or skin.

Lips: Use vitamin E and Aloe vera. Take a soft toothbrush and lightly brush away the dead skin.

Hair lightener: Vinegar, lemon, and chamomile tea.

Hair darkener: Sage and/or rosemary.

Hair conditioner: Mayonnaise at night. Rinse hair with vinegar. Turn water from hot to cold.
Over processed, damage hair or spilt ends: Jojoba oil

Body lotion: Avocado, sesame oil, and mayonnaise with beeswax.

Brighten skin: Use a natural loofah dipped in hot water in an upward, circular motion. Then dip loofah in very cold water with lemon. This brings a bright color to the cheeks, closes skin pores, and helps clear away dead skin.

Full hair: Use natural gel on the roots of the hair only. If it makes it oily, put on a bit of body powder, as well. Then blow dry the hair upside down.

Eyelash thickener: Brown powder on top of petroleum jelly.

Nails: Use a natural lemon "polish" to whiten them.

Deodorant: Baking soda, vinegar, and tea tree oil.

Perfume: Use natural oils that you can mix. Clean citrus smells don't usually clash with other smells. Remember to keep it light. Men have a different sense of smell than women do. They like the smell of lavender, vanilla, and cinnamon. As long as your perfume smells like detergent, everyone will enjoy it. My favorite combination is almond oil and honeysuckle.

Meditate: This brings all your atoms and cells towards an upward energy (quantum physics). Positive affirmations and clearing the mind of worries is the best beauty secret. If it is a proven fact that certain chemicals are excreted during certain thoughts, then take control and excrete good chemicals only. You can manifest beauty by thinking beautiful thoughts. Your whole face changes when you are in love. People notice the "brightness" when you smile and think positively.

CHAPTER 12:
DUMB BLONDE MENUS, CHARTS, AND SURVEYS

I was a martyr while dieting. I loved to look at things I could not eat. Then along came the Food Network. That was my "porn" station. The food would seduce and tease me like a 900 number. My only complaint: the time factor. I ate most of my ingredients raw. I thought that made me a raw-food dieter.

✋ *Check with doctor or healthcare provider:*

☞ **Sample Menu Meal for Eco Anti-Diet 1: Curb-Carb Corrector**

<u>Breakfast</u>: Energy smoothie: whey protein powder, low-fat yogurt, berries, almonds, vanilla, and flax seed oil blended together.

<u>Lunch</u>: Mexican egg (or substitute) omelet with mushrooms, bell peppers, scallions, tomatoes, and olives topped with salsa.

<u>Snack</u>: Apple slices with cream cheese (soy) or nut butter, or bean soup.

<u>Dinner</u>: Italian pouch: protein choice (tofu, fish, or poultry substitute) with broccoli, cauliflower, eggplant, and tomato sauce. Fill bell pepper with mixture; sprinkle on top grated cheese and sliced olives. Cook in oven till bell shells are soft.

<u>Dessert</u>: Handful of frozen grapes or blended frozen strawberries with sprinkled nuts on top.

☞ **Sample Menu Meal for Eco Anti-Diet 2: Veg Metabolizer**

<u>Breakfast</u>: Slow-cooked oatmeal with black strap molasses, skim or substitute milk, berries and flaxseed. Green tea.
Or two slices of French toast (sprouted bread grilled in egg batter), topped with strawberries. Hot green tea with lemon.

<u>Snack</u>: Small fruit and avocado salad (papaya, apple, strawberries, and avocado).

<u>Snack</u>: Oven-roasted yam topped with whipped non-fat sour cream or soy cream cheese, scallions, and herbs.

Lunch: Veggie slices, rice patty, or nut burger on sprouted bread with avocado, mixed with pickles, sun-dried tomatoes, cucumber, and sprouts.

Snack: Germinated seed crackers with nut butter, bean dip, salsa, or muffin with soy cream cheese.

Snack: Vegetable soup with rye crackers.

Dinner: Tostada Pocket: lentils (or bean mix) and cooked whole rye (or multigrain) blend together. Lightly sauté cabbage, onions, and garlic; then blend into protein bean/grain mixture. Add a mixture of raw shredded greens and tomato. Stuff mixture into warm pita bread pocket. Top with an avocado dip (yogurt, avocado, olives, garlic, onions, and herbs).

Dessert: Mix low-fat yogurt with vanilla and cinnamon. Layer between mixture of nuts, berries, and raisins. Put in small cups and freeze.

☞ Sample Menu Meal for Eco Anti-Diet 3: The Garden Tonic

Breakfast: 6-8oz. of coconut juice

Snack: ½ melon or 1 cup of berries

Snack:1-2 small fruit (preferably sub-acid such as a pear/peach)

Lunch: apple with ½-1 small avocado

Snack:1-2 small citrus fruit (orange or grapefruit)

Snack: 4-6 oz. of sprouted seeds with carrots or 2 oz. almonds with 2 tomatoes

Snack: green juice mixed with green apple, carrot, and beet juice (with spirulina)

Dinner: In chopper mix cabbage, spinach, red bell pepper, scallions, tomato, avocado, and garlic, or make cold soup by blending tomatoes, cucumber, celery, and corn with garlic until fairly smooth.

☞ Sample Garden Tonic Fast: (Not for hypoglycemics, diabetics or anyone with severe medical problems, unless supervised. Any fast that is four days or more should be supervised.) Always check with your doctor.

Breakfast: coconut juice (straight from the coconut)

Snack: lemon, grapefruit, and lime with warm water

Snack: repeat above

Lunch: green juice with green apple juice

Snack: repeat

Dinner: Carrot and Beet juice

Follow with this natural laxative and liver cleanser: chopped ginger, garlic with cayenne pepper, and aloe vera. Lemon helps your liver and water balance. The natural sodium helps the electrolyte balance or helps combat edema (bloating).

☞ **Mother-to-be diet:** Under doctor's supervision, eat at least 6-8 balanced and nutritious meals per day with supplements, particularly EFA oils and natural calcium sources (like black strap molasses, greens, and tofu).

DIET AND WEIGHT SURVEY

Since our last book, we've surveyed about 500 people about their diets, goals, and perceptions. This survey is from a list of 100 people between the ages of twelve to sixty years old. Eighty percent of the individuals surveyed were women, because men don't care or don't really pay attention to food and diets like women do. Nevertheless, men finally are finally challenging women in the weight and diet battles. The first answer was the most popular.. The answers given are independent, sometimes opposite, of my own opinions. We don't endorse or support this survey and did we advise anyone who takes this survey

1. What is the most popular diet?
    a) The Atkins Diet.
    b) South Beach Diet.

2. Which diet works best?
    a) The protein diet.
    b) None. We are all getting fatter.

3. Which diets last the longest?
    a) Diets without starvation.
    b) Ones that change with your lifestyle.

4. How many people diet?
    a) Almost every woman and some men.
    b) According to advertisements, it appears everyone has tried at least once.

5. What is the most ridiculous diet you've heard of?
    a) The all-you-can-eat diet.
    b) The spiritual diets, that claim weight loss is a "blessing."

6. What diet would you never try and why?
    a) Starvation diets because eventually you sabotage it.
    b) The most popular ones because obviously they don't work.

7. What do you expect to gain from your diet?
   a) Lose couple of pounds to wear new clothes rather than sweatpants.
   b) Lose enough so I can be fit and healthy.

8. How long does the average diet last?
   a) Until the weekend, Monday through Friday afternoon.
   b) When you don't see good results (disappointment).

9. If diets are the number-one obsession for many people, why are there so many contradicting theories (all protein, no-fat, all-you-can-eat, etc.)?
   a) Money.
   b Different strokes for different folks.

10. Which professional body type would you like to look like?
    a) A celebrity.
    b) Professional athletes or dancers.

11. What is your dream body?
    a) Lean and mean; thin and super fit.
    b) Tall with a good metabolism.

12. What is the blame for the obesity epidemic?
    a) Sedentary lifestyle. Everyone is not as active as they used to be.
    b) Easy access to "super-sized" fast foods.

13. What causes weight gain or someone to appear "fat"? (Weak willpower, genes, medical problems, or environment?)
    a) No discipline and cliché excuses.
    b) Poor choices of foods, activities, and environment.

14. If you could take a pill that would guarantee safe weight loss without any side effects, would you?
    a) 95% of women answered: Yes.
    b) 65% of men answered: No, don't trust it!

15. Does economic status have anything to do with weight issues or eating disorders?
    a) Rich people have better access to personal trainers, fat farms, diet chefs, and outrageous rehabs.
    b) High profile people have pressure to be perfect, which is motivating.

16. What is the most popular enhancer used to cheat for body improvement and weight loss?
    a) Steroids (HGH) or over-the-counter diet aids.
    b) Liposuction.

17. What is your reason for dieting?
    a) To look good for a special occasion (party, graduation, shopping, beach, boyfriend).
    b) To be able to fit in with society's image and to be healthy.

18. Would you rather be rich and fat or thin and poor?
    a) Rich, so I could "buy" my way to get thin.
    b) Thin, so I could attract a rich soul-mate.

19. If your lover was to gain a considerable amount of weight, would you consider leaving him or her?
    a) Women: 75% No or depends on other circumstances.
    b   Men: 80% Probably.

20. How do you judge morbidly obese individuals?
    a) Lack in desire and discipline and very insecure.
    b) A slow suicide with deep issues.

21. What food or treat is the hardest to give up?
    a) Women: Chocolate.
    b) Men: Beer.

22. When should people start thinking about dieting?
    a) When they are young, so they don't deal with weight problems their whole lives.
    b) When they can't fit into their old clothes.

23. When is it dangerous to diet?
    a) As a child, because it can give them an eating disorder.
    b) When people are doing it for something other than themselves (boyfriend, parent, job).

24. What is an eating disorder?
    a) When someone starves and purges or eats beyond boundaries.
    b) When all a person thinks about is losing weight at any cost.

25. Are eating disorders considered a real disease?
    a) Although it is dangerous, it's a choice, unlike cancer.
    b) It's a good excuse, particularly for medical insurance or being "politically correct".

26. Do you know of someone who has an eating disorder?
    a) Yes, everyone in Hollywood.
    b) Everyone I know diets and sabotages their diets.

27. Is Marilyn Monroe considered a perfect body type for today's woman?
    a) Women: For her day, but now she might be a little overweight.
    b) Men: Sexy but too "soft."

28. If our pin-ups are getting thinner, why is our nation getting fatter?
    a) We can't compete with the super models.
    b) Pressure to be thin can make you go either way: starve or give up.

29. Is diet or exercise more important for weight goals?
    a) Women: 95% Diet.
    b) Men: 95% Exercise.

30. Which could you give up first: food or love?
    a) Women: 75% Love.
    b) Men: Under forty years old (if love meant sex): 80% Food. Those above forty years: 80% Love.

GLYCEMIC INDEX CHART: Glycemic index is the relative potency of carbohydrates and their propensity to raise and stabilize blood sugar. There can be advantages to consuming lower glycemic foods for use in exercise, athletic function, and weight maintenance.

Note: These are sample of acceptable glycemic foods (low-glycemic index) and unacceptable glycemic foods. Though some charts list ice cream as more acceptable than carrots, I do not endorse poor food choices over what is an acceptable glycemic food. This chart will have foods that are included in my Eco Anti-Diets. Therefore the chart excludes ice cream, fast food, and soda drinks, although these are listed in other charts as acceptable. It is better to compliment high-glycemic index foods with a proper protein/fat rather than eat poorly.

Acceptable Glycemic Index Foods (lower glycemic index)

Fruits
Honeydew melon
Berries
Cherries
Apples (especially green)
Grapefruits
Plums

Starches
Beans like lentils
Slow-cooking oats
Slow-cooking rye
Sprouted bread
Yams or sweet potatoes

Dairy
Eggs
Low-fat cheese
Low-fat yogurt
Whole, raw milk

Oils and Dressings
Apple cider vinegar
Olive oil
Canola oil
EFA or flax seed oil
Avocado dressing
Lemon

Juices
Green juice
Diluted apple juice
Grapefruit juice

Vegetables
All leafy greens
Broccoli
Cauliflower
Mushrooms
Eggplant
Cucumber
Celery
Bell peppers
Zucchini

Snacks
Avocados
Nuts
Seeds
Olives

Drinks
Green tea or any natural tea
Sparkling water with lemon or lime squeeze (Lemon's sodium helps electrolyte balance, which prevents dehydration.)

Unacceptable Glycemic Index Foods (higher glycemic index)

Fruits

Raisins or dried fruit

Watermelon

Bananas

Mangos

Persimmon

Starches

Rice cakes

Fast-cooking grains

Potatoes

Bread, including whole wheat that isn't sprouted

Corn bread

Cereal (except for homemade without sugar and with whole oats and whole grains)

Pasta

Popcorn

Oils and Dressings

Dressings with sugar

Low-fat cheese dressings

Vegetables

Corn

Carrots

Peas

Sweet onions

Dairy

Whipped cream

Nonfat milk

Nonfat cheese

Coffee creamers

Snacks

Chips

Rice cakes

No-fat crackers

Drinks

Fruit drinks

Artificial drinks

Sodas

HEALTHY ALTERNATIVE CHART FROM A-Z

- ✓ Aloe vera: for digestion and soft laxative
- ✓ Acidophilus: enhances "friendly bacteria" for candidiasis and digestive problems
- ✓ Barley grass: the best of all the greens for green drinks; easily digestible unlike wheatgrass
- ✓ Bee pollen: good source of energy; complete food; good for allergies
- ✓ Charcoal: antidote for all poisons
- ✓ Chlorella: an algae plant that is a complete food; good for energy
- ✓ Date sugar: healthy sugar alternative
- ✓ Dulse: healthy seasoning that is alkaline or used as a dieting tea
- ✓ EFA oils: healthy alternative to other oils; contains essential Omega 3, 6, and 9
- ✓ Eucalyptus: good for congestion or asthma; used to help quit smoking
- ✓ Flaxseed: healthy alternative to fish oil; contains Omega 3, the essential fatty acid
- ✓ Fennel: used as appetite suppressant or eyewash
- ✓ Garlic: detoxifies body and protects against infection; enhances immune system and circulation
- ✓ Guar gum: an herbal fiber
- ✓ Hyperbaric oxygen therapy: delivers high-pressured pure oxygen, which enhances all healing
- ✓ Horsetail: herb that promotes healthy skin, bones, nails, and hair
- ✓ Juicing: good cleansing, healing, and resting regimen
- ✓ Juniper: acts as diuretic and relieves congestion (asthma and obesity)
- ✓ Kelp: seaweed rich in vitamins and B's; good for therapy
- ✓ Kava kava: herb that helps anxiety, depression, stress, and insomnia
- ✓ Lecithin: lipid having B's; helps immune, fat, and triglycerides control
- ✓ Licorice root: herb cleanses the colon; promotes adrenal function; helps energy
- ✓ Meditation or massage: use to relax instead of turning to food or addictions
- ✓ Melatonin: antioxidant that is used for sleeping problems
- ✓ "No": saying this to unhealthy foods, stimulants, or environments
- ✓ Niacin: vitamin B3 needed for proper circulation and healthy skin
- ✓ Oat bran: good fiber source

✓ Oregon grape: root that purifies blood; liver cleanser; good for skin (acne)
✓ Psyllium husk: good fiber source; also used as a laxative
✓ Primrose: GLA, EFA that aids in weight loss and helps PMS
✓ Quercetin: a bioflavonoid that is therapeutic for allergies and asthma
✓ Quinoa: gluten-free grain filled with nutrients
✓ Rice syrup: healthy sweetener
✓ Royal jelly: from bees; contains B vitamins; excellent for immune system
✓ Shiitake: Japanese mushroom that helps T cells fight diseases
✓ Spirulina: most promising of all micro algae; helps fasters or blood sugar levels
✓ Tea tree oil: good for external itching and cuts
✓ Thyme: herb high in B-complex that lowers cholesterol; good for fever and candidiasis
✓ Utensils: Don't use aluminum or nonstick cooking pans. Use glass, stainless steel or iron.
✓ Uva ursi: herb that acts as a diuretic, helping kidney and bladder problems
✓ Valine: essential amino acid with stimulant effect
✓ Valerian: herb that improves circulation and acts as sedative (stress)
✓ Wheat germ: excellent source of vitamin E
✓ Witch hazel: used as an astringent; has healing properties; good for itching and skin care
✓ Yeast (like brewer's or torula): rich in B's, amino acids, and many minerals
✓ Zinc: antioxidant usually taken to prevent flu and colds

ENZYMES

Amylase	Digests starches in the mouth.
Bromelain	Aids digestion of fat. An anti-inflammatory food enzyme. You can find it in pineapple.
Catalase	Helps fight free radicals. Antioxidant.
Cellulase	Enables cellulose digestion. Found in most vegetable fiber.
Chymotrypsin	Helps neutralize the stomach acid when semi-digested food passes from the stomach into the small intestine.
Diatase	Enables digestion of vegetable starch.
Glutathion	An antioxidant enzyme (peroxidase) that turns free radicals into oxygen and water.
Lactase	Enables digestion of lactose (milk sugar). Very common.
Lipase	Breaks down fat in the stomach.
Mycozyme	Plant enzymes that help digest starches.
Pancreatin	Important for prevention of degenerative diseases. Animal pancreas derivative. Helps digestion.
Papain and chymopapain	Derived from papaya. Helps digest protein (vegetable pepsin).
Pepsin	Breaks down protein. Can help digest 3,500 times its weight in protein.
Protease	Digests protein.
Rennin	Helps digest cow's milk.
Trypsin	Breaks down fat, protein, and starches. Secreted by the pancreas.

BAD BREATH AND BODY ODOR

FOODS THAT HELP	SUPPLEMENTS THAT HELP
Juice fast occasionally. Eat lost of greens and cultured foods, such as yogurt and tofu, to boost intestinal bacteria. Vinegar and lemon juice help digestion and breath. Drink 8-10 glasses of water daily to keep kidneys clear. Avoid red meats, fried foods, sugar, too much dairy, and junk food.	Oat bran, Psyllium husks, Rice bran, Vitamin C, Acidophilus, Garlic caps, Zinc, Vitamin A and beta-carotene, Vitamin B complex, plus extra B3 and B6.

HERBS THAT HELP	ALSO HELPS
Alfalfa, Goldenseal, Myrrh, Peppermint, Rosemary, Parsley.	Exercise to detox: Long, slow sweats will help. Take a mineral salt bath. Baking soda is good for breath and body odor. Use natural toothpaste and rinse! Use tea tree oil mouthwash. Wear loose cotton clothes. Use crystal rocks from a health store instead of commercial deodorants. Eat slowly for digestion. Brush teeth and clear coating off the tongue.

CELLULITE

FOODS THAT HELP	SUPPLEMENTS THAT HELP
Reduce dietary and body fat. Eat small, easily digestible meals. Use unsaturated oils. Avoid junk food. Avoid caffeine, carbonated drinks, and too much dairy. Eliminate saturated fats from your diet. Consume oat or wheat bran to lower cholesterol.	Enzyme supplements, EFA oils (flax seed or fish oils), Kelp, B-complex, Lecithin, Oat or wheat bran.

HERBS THAT HELP	ALSO HELPS
Bilberry, Gotu kola, Kola nut, Butcher broom, Seaweed tea.	Start exercising at a young age. Massages may help circulation. Stimulate lymph glands with loofah. Regular aerobic exercise. Do not smoke.

COLDS

FOODS THAT HELP	SUPPLEMENTS THAT HELP
Liquid fast on juices. Eat fruit and greens. Avoid heavy meals that strain the body during fever. Drink 8-10 glasses of liquids a day. Take 2 Tbsp. of cider vinegar and 2 tsp. of honey twice a day, or 2 Tbsp. of both lemon juice and honey. Limit dairy to decrease phlegm.	Echinacea, Goldenseal, Vitamin A and beta-carotene, Vitamin C, Garlic caps, Acidophilus, Kelp, Multivitamins and minerals, B vitamin complex.

HERBS THAT HELP	ALSO HELPS
Ginger, Slippery elm, Yarrow tea, Eucalyptus oil (in bath or steam), Tea tree oil (to gargle).	Do not smoke or drink alcohol. Apply ginger compresses on the chest. Use eucalyptus steams in steamer or vaporizer. Commercial drugs often mask or make a cold worse later. Get plenty of sleep. Only exercise if you are fever-free; moderate walks are fine.

DEPRESSION

FOODS THAT HELP	SUPPLEMENTS THAT HELP
Need protein, fresh vegetables, and whole grains. Include legumes. Drink carrot or green juices. Drink wheatgrass juice. Eat plenty of brewer's yeast, wheat germ, seeds, and nuts. Include EFA oils in your diet. Avoid alcohol, drugs, caffeine, stimulants, and junk food. Drink lots of water.	L-Tyrosine, Zinc, B-complex (B6 and B12, pantothenic acid, niacin, folic acid), Calcium, Magnesium, Chromium, Black currant oils, Evening primrose, Vitamin C.

HERBS THAT HELP	ALSO HELPS
Balm, Ginger, Ginkgo biloba, Licorice root, Oat straw, Peppermint, Ginseng, St. John's Wort.	Anti-stress therapies including yoga, meditation, self-massage, biofeedback, etc. Get adequate sunshine, which impacts mood and gland function. Stop smoking and drinking alcohol. Exercise is crucial. Stretch in the morning to start the day and in the evening to help sleep. Practice coping and deep breathing skills, and go to group therapy. Get plenty of sleep.

DIABETES

FOODS THAT HELP	SUPPLEMENTS THAT HELP
Cooked fruit and vegetables. Reduce the intake of dietary fat and calories. Increase the intake of fiber and complex carbohydrates. (Fiber binds with cholesterol and eliminates it from the body.) Eat whole grains, brewer's yeast, string beans, eggs, soy foods, cucumbers, onions, dried fruit, wheat germ, mushrooms, and garlic. Eat a salad daily	Chromium picolinate, Brewer's yeast, L–Carnitine plus L–Glutamine and L–Taurine, B–complex plus extra biotin and inositol, B12, Zinc, CoQ10, Magnesium, Manganese, Psyllium husk, Vitamins A, C, E, Calcium, Copper, Garlic capsules.

HERBS THAT HELP	ALSO HELPS
Cedar berries, Ginseng tea, Huckleberry, Goldenseal, Dandelion root, Bilberry.	Exercise reduces the need for insulin. Massage helps reduce sugar cravings. Do not smoke; it may increase the need for sugar. Avoid desserts, sugars, fake sugar or phenylalanine. Lose weight on high-fiber, high-carb diets. Get plenty of rest. No caffeine.

EATING DISORDERS
(Anorexia Nervosa and Bulimia)

FOODS THAT HELP	SUPPLEMENTS THAT HELP
Eat at regular times: small portions, light meals. Eat high-quality, high-fiber foods. Eat balanced, frequent meals (blood sugar). Brewer's yeast, Wheat germ, Black strap molasses, Wheatgrass juice or Chlorophyll.	Multivitamins and minerals, Beta-carotene, Vitamin A, Calcium, Magnesium, Potassium, Selenium, Zinc, Copper, Acidophilus, Amino acids (freeform), B-complex, B-12 shots, Liver extract, Vitamin C.

HERBS THAT HELP	ALSO HELPS
Dandelion, Milk thistle, Red clover, Wild yam, Ginger root, Ginseng, Gotu kola, Peppermint.	Improve self-esteem and be positive. Exercise moderately almost every day. Do not strictly diet. Develop lifestyle changes instead. Do not smoke or use drugs. Read self-help therapy books and get therapy if necessary. Join twelve-step programs and enter group therapy or an institution specializing in eating disorders. Eat slowly and calmly; chew well.

FATIGUE

FOODS THAT HELP	SUPPLEMENTS THAT HELP
Adhere to high-energy diet of mostly complex carbohydrates, fresh fruit (sea and regular vegetables, whole grains, and legumes, including such protein sources (to allow for about 20 - 25% of protein content) as whole grains, legumes, soy, and sea foods. Aim for little dietary fat. Drink high-protein drinks with spirulina or bee pollen granules and brewer's yeast. Consume foods high in vitamins B and C and rich in iron	Bee pollen, Amino acids (free form), Brewer's yeast, Iron, Multivitamins and minerals, Vitamin A, Chromium, Potassium, Selenium, Zinc, Vitamin B complex (plus extra B12, B1, pantothenic acid, and choline), DHEA, Calcium, Magnesium, L-Phenylalanine, Royal jelly.

HERBS THAT HELP	ALSO HELPS
Cayenne Pepper, Gingko biloba, Gotu kola, Ginseng, Guarana, China gold.	Reduce alcohol and caffeine intake. Do not smoke. Regular cardio and strength exercises help circulation, ease stress, and improve energy. Try regular massage. Get regular sunshine. Try acupressure and deep breathing exercises.

HEALTHY HAIR

FOODS THAT HELP	SUPPLEMENTS THAT HELP
Help your hair by incorporating into your diet a lot of vegetables and protein. Wheat germ (oil or flakes), Black strap molasses, Brewer's yeast, Seeds and nuts, Avocados. Foods good for hair are all greens, carrots, green peppers, bananas, strawberries, apples, peas, onions, eggs, cucumbers, sprouts, and unsaturated fats, especially olive oil. Avoid saturated fat and junk food.	EFA oils, B-complex with B6, Biotin and inositol, Vitamin C, Vitamin E, Zinc, CoQ10, Kelp, Copper, Silica, L-Cysteine, L-Methionine.

HERBS THAT HELP	ALSO HELPS
Sage tea rinse, Horsetail.	Brush hair upside down. Massage the scalp every day. Use alcohol-free products. Wash hair in warm, not hot, water. Rinse in cool water. Rinse with cider vinegar or lemons. For added hair shine, try coconut oils. To brighten hair color use chamomile. Avoid tobacco, alcohol, and caffeine. Occasionally use natural home products like mayonnaise and olive oil to condition hair cuticles.

LEG AND MUSCLE CRAMPS

FOODS THAT HELP	SUPPLEMENTS THAT HELP
Eat plenty of leafy greens, citrus fruit, brown rice, sprouts, broccoli, tomatoes, green peppers, bananas, beans and legumes, whole grains, dried fruit, sea vegetables, molasses, nuts, and seafood. Drink green shakes. Avoid sugars and processed foods.	Kelp, Calcium, Magnesium, Vitamin E, Potassium, Silica, B-complex (plus extra B1 and niacin), Vitamin C, Vitamin D, CoQ10, Lecithin granules, Multivitamins and minerals, Zinc, Brewer's yeast.

HERBS THAT HELP	ALSO HELPS
Alfalfa, Dong quai, Elderberry extract, Gingko biloba, Horsetail grass, Valerian root.	Massage legs; elevate feet to stimulate circulation. Take a couple of days of rest from exercise each week. Apply hot and cold alternating compresses to the area to ease pain and promote circulation. Get bi-monthly massages. Always warm-up, cool down, and stretch thoroughly before and after exercise.

MENSTRUAL PROBLEMS

FOODS THAT HELP	SUPPLEMENTS THAT HELP
Eat more lean proteins. Stay away from saturated fats. Consume foods rich in vitamin E, such as wheat germ. Try molasses for an energy boost during your period. A raw vegetarian diet during your menstruation may help. Avoid sugar, caffeine, and junk foods. Eat more things with essential fatty omega oils.	Make sure you take your multivitamin now: Vitamin K is an important supplement for heavy bleeders. Iodine helps the thyroid control the estrogen levels. Essential oils help balance hormones. Iron and antioxidants are important. Brewer's yeast and calcium supplements may ease bloating and insomnia. Try B6 and zinc to combat water retention.

HERBS THAT HELP	ALSO HELPS
Dong quai and chamomile tea for cramping. Licorice root or other herbal teas to battle edema. Black cohosh is excellent for uterine fibroids; burdock root and evening primrose oil are crucial for hormonal balance.	Exercise helps ease tension and balance hormones. Massage helps bring a natural rhythm and improves circulation. Lower salt intake to help bloating. Fiber helps constipation. Soy products are a natural source of estrogen and help boost the body; they also may help regulate hormonal imbalances.

OBESITY

FOODS THAT HELP	SUPPLEMENTS THAT HELP
Cut back on saturated fat but do not cut it out. Fat is not all bad; it's the chief source of energy for normal bodily function. Do not eat "empty calories," like processed and junk foods. Eat fruit and vegetables (raw). Do not go lower than 1000-1200 calories. Eat carbs, protein, and fat at every meal. Choose foods rich in complex carbs (starch), also containing protein such as beans and whole grains.	Multivitamins and minerals, Psyllium husks, Chromium picolinate, EFA oils (esp. flaxseed, primrose and salmon oil), Kelp, Lecithin granules, Spirulina, Vitamin C, Calcium, CoQ10, DHEA, L-Arginine, L-Ornithine, L-Lysine, L-Carnitine, L-Glutamine, L-Methionine, L-Phenylalanine, L-Tyrosine, Potassium, Vitamin B.

HERBS THAT HELP	ALSO HELPS
Alfalfa, Corn-silk, Dandelion, Gravel root, Horsetail, Hydrangea, Hyssop, Juniper berries, Oat straw, Parsley, Thyme, Aloe vera juice, Butcher's broom, Cinnamon, Ginger, Green tea, Mustard seed, Cayenne.	Exercise most of the days of the week (a three-mile walk can burn about 250 calories, depending on your weight). Lift weights to increase lean muscle mass and metabolism. (Muscle tissue uses up calories for energy. The greater the amount of muscle tissue you have, the more calories you can burn.) Try twelve-step programs, group therapy, or individual therapy. Use meditation to reduce stress.

SMOKING AND RELATED PROBLEMS

FOODS THAT HELP	SUPPLEMENTS THAT HELP
Fast on fresh fruit and vegetable juices to neutralize and clear the blood from nicotine. Then eat leafy green salads and lots of citrus fruit to promote body alkalinity. Include lots of vegetable protein. Eat yellow and deep orange vegetables like carrots, pumpkins, squash and yams. Eat smaller meals more frequently to maintain blood sugar levels. Avoid junk foods.	CoQ10, Vitamin C, Vitamin B complex (plus B-12 and folic acid), Vitamin E, Vitamin A and beta carotene, Zinc.

HERBS THAT HELP	ALSO HELPS
Cayenne pepper, Catnip, Hops, Lobelia, Skullcap, Valerian root, Dandelion root, Milk thistle, Ginger, Slippery elm.	Practice yoga and deep breathing exercises that deliver more oxygen to the body and its organs. Try patch treatments, support groups, and therapy. To help curb cravings, chew licorice root sticks, calms root, or cloves. You must exercise to help blood sugar levels (insulin excretion) and to build and regulate your metabolism. Regular workouts also ease food cravings.

VARICOSE VEINS (and spider veins)

FOODS THAT HELP	SUPPLEMENTS THAT HELP
Eat only fresh foods with plenty of green salads and juices. Then follow a predominantly vegetarian, high-fiber diet. Include beans, whole grains, brown rice, and lots of raw fruit. Take lecithin granules, brewer's yeast, and wheat germ daily in nonfat yogurt. Reduce dairy products, fried food, prepared and red meat, and saturated fat. Avoid salty, sugary, and caffeinated foods.	CoQ10, EFA oils, Vitamin C, Vitamin E, Brewer's yeast, Lecithin granules, Multivitamin complex, Vitamin A and beta carotene, Vitamin B complex plus extra B6, Vitamin D plus calcium and magnesium.

HERBS THAT HELP	ALSO HELPS
Butcher broom, Gingko biloba, Gotu kola, Hawthorn berries, Horse chestnut, White oak bark tea (soak legs in it).	Bike, walk, run, stair climb as much as possible to increase circulation and strengthen tissues. Elevate the legs during rest. Massage feet and legs regularly. Go barefoot and wear flat sandals. Take mineral salt baths. Apply Aloe vera gel. Do not use knee-high hosiery. In advanced or painful cases, surgery will help.

WATER RETENTION

FOODS THAT HELP	SUPPLEMENTS THAT HELP
Fasting flushes excess water. Reduce salt intake. Avoid junk foods. Drink at least 6-8 glasses of bottled water daily for free-flowing functions that help appetite suppression and elimination. Eat fresh, raw foods to flush out excess water. Eat green salads every day with cucumbers, parsley, and celery	Free-form amino acids, B-complex, Calcium, Magnesium, Silica, Bromelain, Garlic caps, Kelp, Potassium, Vitamin C, Vitamin E.

HERBS THAT HELP	ALSO HELPS
Alfalfa, Cornsilk, Butcher's broom, Dandelion root, Horsetail, Juniper berries, Parsley, Marshmallow.	Drink at least 8-10 glasses of water each day, and more if you exercise regularly. Try steam baths or saunas but re-hydrate immediately. Exercise regularly.

CHAPTER 13:
"DEAR BARBI," FACT OR FICTION?

(Plus Answering Personal Questions)

"Dear Barbi, is this fact or fiction?"

Protein diets are the best because they are the most popular, right?
FICTION: Protein diets, like others, have been around for years and go in and out of style, like all other gimmick diets. One size does not fit all. Therefore, it is dangerous to say the protein diet is best for everyone. If they are so popular, then why are we getting fatter as a nation? Because protein diets, like all diets, eventually stop working!

A diet of 1,200 calories (or less) per day is best in order to lose weight, right?
FICTION: A calorie is not a calorie! What works in the laboratory doesn't work with us, because we are dictated by hormones, unlike Petri dishes. For instance, carrots can be low in calories and fat but have a high glycemic index (poor blood sugar effect). It is recommended that you are supposed to have ten calories per pound of body weight, but that's relative as well. Muscle weighs more than fat. Low calories only create a sluggish metabolism and a fat efficient body. It's the quality of the calorie, not the amount that counts.

Overweight individuals just need willpower and discipline to get thin, right?
FICTION: Extremely overweight individuals are battling excess or deficient hormones and brain chemicals that "normal" eaters don't usually encounter. For instance, the hormone leptin, which is responsible for making us full, is dormant in overweight people. They also have an excess of ghrenlin, a hormone responsible for making us hungry and making fat, even if you don't eat. Furthermore, they lack in PYY336, the hormone that fulfills us, and serotonin, the brain chemical that helps curb appetite and is triggered by tryptophan, which is abundantly found in carbs and sweets. Compulsive overeating is called a disease because willpower has nothing to do with it. Eating disorders stem from mental disorders, which are illnesses or diseases. There is hope for recovery, however, when overweight

individuals learn certain foods either help or hurt these hormones and brain chemicals plus work on confronting their issues, or what they are eating over.

Overweight people usually have low metabolisms, true?
FICTION: False! On the contrary, eating a lot of calories actually *raises* the metabolism. It is the yo-yo dieting that creates a sluggish metabolism. People are fatter not just because of poor choices but because they DIET! This trains the body to hold onto all food as storage rather than burning it, because it is the body's natural survival instinct.

All fruits, particularly citrus are acidic in the body, true?
FICTION: Organic acids within the fruits stay acid until they hit the bloodstream. They combine with other acids, leaving the mineral salts (alkalis from the fruit) in the blood. The blood's pH is balanced from these alkalis.

Using caffeine supplements before a workout is harmless because it gives a "boost" without any fat or calories, right?
FICTION: Regardless of the stimulant's food content, all drugs (including cigarettes, diet aids, and some herbs) usually cause a hypoglycemic reaction, further causing water retention, lack of energy, eventual hunger, and moodiness. Stimulants usually cause excess cortisol to be released or adrenal exhaustion. This all makes it impossible for the body to achieve the fat-burning/muscle-building process. The temporary lift is followed by the crash. Stimulants also cause a buildup of dirty tissue, making the body flabby (cellulite). We are dictated by hormones, not fat or calories. Empty calorie substances can sometimes cause harm. Though trainers claim stimulants cause thermogenesis (fat burned by body heat), they can also create a plateau (set point) that will backfire.

In order for anorexics to get well they just need to gain weight, right?
FICTION: False; that is their very problem: weight obsession. Weight loss is only the symptom of their disease. Eating disorders stem from depression, OCD, anxiety, etc., and manifest in some self-destructive behavior. These diseases are based on control and fear and can easily be transmitted into body obsession, especially because they are shame-based. (People think they *are* the problem, not that they *have* a problem.) Recovery should include a healthy food plan without focusing on the meal intake or the weight gain. Anorexics use "control" rather than confronting their inside issues. Again, don't use outside appearance for an inside job. Weight gain is the byproduct of a good recovery program.

Rich people are thin because they have access to fat farms, good chefs, and private trainers, right?

FICTION: Most thin people are thin, rich or not, because they make better choices. However, some wealthy celebrities, whom we usually look up to, think that money can buy anything and seek further methods to attain a super-fit body, like through HGH and liposuction. Nevertheless, shortcuts eventually backfire, rich or not.

Genetics override diet and exercise programs for your weight outcome, right?

FICTION: Reportedly, genetic factors account for about 40 percent of the influence. Though some are burdened with a family's poor health history, RADICAL life changes *can* override genetics, for the most part. Most studies are done by comparing very ill individuals on "normal" diets to a healthy person on the same diet. I have witnessed individuals with one foot in the grave completely change their lives 180 degrees. They view everything they eat as a health investment, not a perverted entertainment for the mouth. Though food does not work as quickly as medicine, health gurus claim it's their medicinal investment. Usually these are raw dieters who change their ways mentally, physically, and spiritually. If they had depended on genetics, they would have been victims of drugs and surgery.

Good, healthy weight loss is only about one or two pounds per week, true?

FACT: This is true. Any diet that promises more is depending on water loss through ketosis (an unnatural rapid fat burning without burning glucose).This is temporary and can cause kidney damage. Initially, all diets cause water weight loss, before they burn fat. Fast weight off is fast weight back on...plus more. If you are used to eating a lot of junk, your first week or two may result in extra weight loss. However, true and lasting weight loss should never be more than one or two pounds per week, because that is fat.

Aerobic exercise (cardio) is far superior to anaerobic exercise (weight lifting) for weight loss, true?

FICTION: Both are important. Just as a one-nutrient diet is imbalanced, so is a one-type exercise routine. Although aerobic exercise works on the red, lean muscle tissue to achieve the fat-burning/muscle-building process, anaerobic exercises (that focus on white bulky muscle tissue) release CCK (hormone that creates a satiated feeling) and HGH (human growth hormone that also clicks you into the fat-burning/muscle-building process). Muscle mass burns calories even when sedentary and *boosts* the metabolism. You need to shake up your exercise routine just like a diet so your body doesn't learn to compensate. Your muscles need to recuperate, as well. Therefore, it is best to switch between anaerobic and aerobic exercises, every other day.

There are some overweight people who simply love food without mental issues involved, true?
FICTION: There is no such thing as being extremely overweight because you love food. True, certain out-of-control brain chemicals and hormones will make the addict believe that because of the unbearable cravings. Chocolate actually raises endorphins (hormone that makes you feel high and in love). True hunger does not stem from uncontrollable cravings. Food becomes the food addict's tool to deal with every emotion, including the shame of their disease. The food tool is used as their survival mechanism, which is all they know. True feelings don't manifest until the food addict is detoxified from all sugars (drugs) and other mind-altering foods. Food addicts are in the constant state of intoxication or detoxification, leaving no room for confronting issues. Their "hunger" is for love and acceptance. Filling that void with food only makes them more shame-based, thinking they *are* the problem, not that they *have* one. They don't have any boundaries for hunger or fullness.

An apple keeps the doctor away, right?
FACT: What the actual saying means is that the alkalis (minerals) in the apple neutralize the acids within the body, which stops any leeching of alkalis from the teeth, hair, nails, and bones. Acidity causes hollow bones and cavities. When you eat sugar (acid), it robs the alkalis from your teeth (as well as bones and hair), which causes cavities. This is not the same thing as direct contact of the sugar on the teeth. The high content of pectin in the apple is a natural fiber that helps you evacuate. An apple a day keeps you regular and balanced!

There is no such thing as a cure when speaking about recovery, true?
FACT: Recovery is a process, not an event. Recovery includes changing the brain patterns and life choices that at one time brought you to your drug of choice. There is no logic to their disease; there is an only obsession. You can reason yourself right back into the disease. Obsessions can be confronted or transferred but not controlled. Recovery is contingent on the addict's daily progress, not perfection.

Changing your food plan and attaining recovery is always easier with a buddy or friend, true?
FACT: <u>Discriminate; don't isolate</u>! Environment is stronger than willpower. Having a buddy or a sponsor who is on a recovery path also helps you connect and contribute. You are helping that person as much as he or she is helping you. Solitude is good for introspection, however, in

numbers there is power. Sharing your experience, strength, and hope with a fellow sufferer will allow you to be less self-absorbed, which causes you to ruminate on your disease.

Meat- or nitrogen-based protein diets are far superior to plant protein diets, true?

FICTION: Plant protein has fiber and other nutrients. Meat only has protein. Furthermore, meat is loaded with antibiotics, hormones, and chemicals, making it harder on our kidneys, liver, and digestive tract. Remember, our body has a priority system; first it digests; then it eliminates; and only after that does it heal (rest) and burn fat. Some meat can take up to ten hours to digest, leaving your intestines fermenting with toxins that open your immune system to diseases and parasites. Nature made the best diet for humans: organic plants. When an animal is slaughtered (stressed with fear), it excretes dangerous hormones and chemicals that we ingest. Try this: Compare a person who solely lives on an extreme meat protein diet to someone who lives off of raw food only. Which one is free of illnesses, fatigue, and wrinkles? You make the decision.

It's better to be fit and overweight rather than thin and sedentary, right?

FACT: I've found this to be true. I have heard that when overweight individuals who were physically active were compared to thin people who were sedentary, the active overweight individuals were healthier than the thin people who were inactive. However, some experts claim that people who are ten pounds or more overweight, also put a *strain* on every organ, muscle, and bone. I don't advise using this theory to condone extra weight. Use this theory to inspire your exercise routine, regardless of your size.

Drinking water is important when dieting, true?

FACT: This is true for several reasons. One is that, when you enter into ketosis or weight loss, you lose a lot of water. Your kidneys are already working overtime because many diets, like the protein diet, cause a diuretic effect. Water itself can have a diuretic effect. It's very good to drink lots of water to prevent water retention. Usually, by the time you are thirsty, you're already dehydrated. Use lemon for dehydration. The sodium in lemon retains the water because of the sodium (electrolytes). Water without sodium (or other minerals that can act like electrolytes) can further dehydration. It is said to drink eight eight-ounce glasses of water per day because our bodies are composed of approximately 70 percent water. However, you want to be careful not to get "water logged." Drink two hours after a meal and one half hour before a meal. When your diet is full of fresh fruit and vegetables, you don't need to drink as much water. If you have unusual thirst, there is something wrong. This will happen after a binge (sugar) or too much protein.

Moderate exposure to sunshine or a light tan is very healthy?

FACT: Only in moderation. Deep tans are not healthy. Sunshine is a must, not only for the vitamin D. Sunshine is a catalyst for other vitamins and minerals. It also penetrates the pineal gland through the eyes, helping relieve depression and release serotonin. It also helps with anemia. Though skin cancer is serious, there are more health problems in people who refrain from the sun than people who are always outdoors. Compare surfers to people who sit at computer day in and day out. A slight tan, just about 5-20 minutes a day, actually raises the melanin just enough to act as a natural sunscreen. There are those who claim most skin cancers are the result of toxins *baking* on the skin—poisons within corrupting poisons on the outside. They also believe a toxin-free diet and a *little* sunshine is the answer to superior health, not refraining from Mother Nature's vitamin enhancer. Also, try using natural sunscreens that are chemical free.

A food addict is much like being a drug addict, true?

FACT: The food addict goes through the same issues of control and fear. Whether the tool is food, a drug, or alcohol, the behavior is compulsive—dictated by obsession. The weight is only the symptom. The brain chemicals react in the same way. For instance, dopamine (induces a euphoric feeling) and endorphins (which is a hormone that binds to opiate receptors) are depleted or sometimes over-released when we experience pleasure over and over. In anticipation, the memory of such an experience also causes the release of dopamine, which further causes cravings. Overindulgences in this pleasure deplete dopamine. This process then creates a need to acquire the food (drug of choice) not for the pleasure anymore, but to refrain from crashing. Food addicts can be depleted of other vital hormones as well. Many of them are low in norepinephrine, the flight-or-fight hormone. This makes their crashing worse and creates a need for a pick-up. Food addicts experience the same blackouts, highs, and hangovers of the drug addict. Other brain chemicals are depleted as well, like serotonin which is a neurotransmitter that makes you "feel full"), when we overindulge. The addict's only memory is the habit of recouping these missing feel-good chemicals is by using their drug of choice. The addiction is born when the need supersedes the pleasure. An addict is an addict no matter what survival mechanism he or she chooses for an easier, softer way. Addicts can't live with or without their drug. Their drug is used to escape, cope, and medicate themselves from feeling their feelings. They will lie, cheat, and steal for their addition, food or otherwise.

Just because someone is extremely skinny does not mean they have an eating disorder, right?

FACT: Weight is only a symptom, not a problem. Some individuals are naturally thin or suffer from hyperthyroidism (over-active thyroid).

However, obvious weight loss is a warning sign that some obsessive-compulsive disorder is beginning, even if it is enhanced by drug use. If someone uses drugs for weight-gain fear, that person is possibly treading the path of two disorders.

Fasting and dieting causes acidosis, right?

FICTION: Acidosis is commonly produced by the fermentation of proteins and carbohydrates due to their lack of minerals. Ketosis, on the other hand, cleans the body of excess fat by having an empty or nearly empty stomach. It does this to give energy. Acidosis is abnormally high acids in the blood and fluids. Sometimes the cleansing process of a fast can create temporary acidosis, in the beginning.

An eating disorder is not really a mental illness (disease); it's just an addiction, right?

FICTION: An addiction eventually develops into a disease, meaning the addiction takes over the body and mind much like a disease. No one chooses to be an addict. Eating disorders stem from some type of mental disorder (OCD, anxiety, depression, etc.). Mental illness is a disease. It has nothing to do with food, diets, weight, or starving. Those are symptoms and tools. Once it has become a disease (mental illness), no amount of willpower can stop it. Brain chemicals, like dopamine, are released upon the very memory of the drug of choice, making the addiction stronger. When the addiction becomes self-destructive and self-preservation is absent, it has become a disease. There are basically two types of mental illnesses: neuroses and psychoses. *Neurotic* is thinking YOU are the problem (shame-based), and you become hypochondriac. *Psychotic* is thinking everyone but you has the problem. Psychotic individuals blame the world because they have a victim mentality. Neuroses can transcend into psychoses. Once it has regressed into psychosis, it is hard for addicts to get or seek help, because they don't think it is their responsibility.

Wine, chocolate, and other taboo treats must be good for you because they contain antioxidants and other helpful substances, right?

FICTION: Everything in you ingest is recognized as a food or a poison. You just need to weigh out the food qualities. An orange has traces of arsenic. Tobacco has vitamin content, like vitamin C. Does that make it healthy? No. Wine and chocolate can enhance addiction as well. For normal people without addictions, wine and chocolate in moderation are fine. However, to make these goodies a daily requirement for antioxidants is only condoning an unhealthy pattern that can lead to addiction. There are better ways of receiving antioxidants without side effects.

Some people are just born unlucky, no matter how much discipline they exert, right?

FICTION: There is no such thing as continuous bad luck. People who usually complain about their bad luck are in denial and won't take responsibility. There are clues to people's circumstances. Perhaps someone may have poor genes or a bad circumstance coincidentally. Regardless, it's all about perception. People with severe handicaps or healthy disadvantages are basically more positive about life than people who appear successful . They are known to excrete "happier" brain chemicals, than successful, "lucky" ones. I look at my disease as a blessing in disguise because my recovery was threefold: mental, physical, and spiritual. I had to work on all of those things to attain true fulfillment, not just food abstinence. Luck is being able to see opportunity when it goes by. Individuals who are negative don't notice positive, OBVIOUS signals, because they have a victim mentality. We can choose to be a victim of our circumstances or we can choose be positive in spite of our circumstances. The biggest success stories come from individuals who have had to overcome unusual obstacles and then just kept going up!

If something is labeled organic or natural, you can't believe it, right?

FACT: It needs to be labeled CERTIFIED organic. Natural is relative. Poison can be natural. *Natural* is a term used for packaging. It can be misleading or a downright lie.

It's important to eat a large carb meal for energy prior to a workout, right?

FICTION: First off, the meal should be light and "clean" so it doesn't interfere with digestion and hormones. Going without food can cause excess cortisol release or adrenal exhaustion, causing weight loss difficulties and bloating. Eating high carb contents before a workout can also cause a hypoglycemic reaction (bloating, fatigue, hunger). It's best to have one small carb snack or a small balanced meal with protein or fat to block the insulin. Your food is not actually burned off until twenty-four hours later. True energy actually comes from the process called catabolism, which takes time. All foods at first act as a slight stimulant. Your food is then used for anabolism (building tissue).

Modeling seems to be a good career choice, true?

FICTION: Modeling is body-obsessed and is the worst choice for anyone with an eating disorder or someone comes from a dysfunctional family. Many times I see food addicts, for instance, use shopping as a reward after they have completed their diet. Modeling, shopping, or any "outside," body obsessed escapes or rewards only breeds the self-absorbed disease. When I see, for instance, athletes choose to model in order to celebrate their bodies or actresses who want to further their career, that's fine. But to use modeling as a goal (or as a scare-tactic, as we did to lose weight) is unhealthy. It's never good enough or fulfilling.

I am prone to be an alcoholic if someone in my family is, right?

FACT: There is a 50 percent chance of having a predisposition for two reasons: genetic and learned behavior. Genetically, a child of an alcoholic might have certain brain chemicals that are missing or unbalanced (serotonin, dopamine, and endorphins), which draws them to other chemicals (or foods) that supply them with these feel-good feelings. They might have an inherited hormonal imbalance as well. Learned behavior is both traditional eating habits and self-medicating (survival mechanism). If your family eats poorly, then that will also pass along the same imbalances that trigger an addictive personality. If you are surrounded by role models who live in denial and deal with everything by self-medicating, it will impact you greatly. The good news is that we don't need to be dictated by tradition, bad habits, and denial. We have a choice, though for some it will be harder. Fighting your battle will also improve other parts of your life, that would normally be unnoticed or unimportant.

Sugar (included in most ingredients) is claimed to be a DRUG, true?

FACT: Sugar has all the qualities of a drug. It acts as a temporary stimulant at first, eventually causing a crash when it's excreted. Excess sugar causes the same withdrawal symptoms and cravings as a drug and can cause a hypoglycemic reaction. Manufacturers use corn syrup and other cheap sugars as ingredients. These are actually worse for the blood sugar. However, sugar is used in all products because of its addictive nature. It's in toothpaste, cigarettes, and even athletes' drinks that are supposed to be filled with vitamins and minerals. Sugar actually leeches most of the nutritional value that your food may give you. American companies put sugar in the very products that are supposed to combat sugar-related diseases. For instance, candidiasis is a fungus in the lower intestine that is triggered, caused, or encouraged by sugar. Acidophilus is one of the main combat supplements that fights candidiasis. Yet most acidophilus products contain sugar! All manufacturers agree that we can't live with or without it as a drug, so they include it.

It's hard to communicate with the opposite sex because of our differences, true?

FACT: Yes, biologically and evolutionary we are different in almost every aspect, so why complain or try to change another person? Women think with their whole brains, taking longer to make a decision. They guide their intellect (left side of the brain) with their intuition (right side). Men think simply and logically (left side). Women tend to overanalyze and over-emotionalize, while men minimize their feelings (and others'). Men also want to solve their problems alone in their bear caves and then be done with it. Women may want to openly discuss something without getting to a point. This could be construed as "nagging." Women have the hormone oxytocin (cuddle hormone) that helps maintain loyalty. Unfortunately men have the four-year itch (not seven), which makes it easier for them to stray because of their testosterone (hunter). They are attracted to women physically (young and symmetrical for breeding), while women are attracted to the protector" and provider (security). Men, dominated by testosterone, are stimulated in the brain by sex and alcohol (and protein meals) in the same area of the brain where women are stimulated by food (serotonin). Women would rather eat sweets (bountiful in tryptophan, which triggers serotonin). It is ridiculous to compare or complete with your opposite-sex mate. The best relationships accept the differences and make a team with each of the good attributes.

To prevent dehydration, water is a good source because it helps balance electrolytes, true?

FICTION: Water by itself acts as a diuretic. It contains inorganic materials (minerals) rather than having a source from organic tissues. It's the minerals (like sodium, potassium, phosphorus, etc.) in fresh fruits and vegetables that help prevent dehydration in the body, with the help of electrolytes. The body makes electrolytes (needed for water balance) with the help of the minerals, which are only derived from fresh fruits and vegetables (organic tissues). Electrolytes are of various ions, like potassium, sodium, chloride, etc., required by cells to balance the electric charge and flow of water molecules in the body. Lemon is magical. It can help with edema when you are bloated and with dehydration when you need electrolytes. A squeeze of orange helps the molecular structure of tap water. Sugar and manmade salt, on the other hand, purely dehydrate you and leech minerals. Always stick with nature's nutrients rather than turning to something that contains other additives. Nature's clones usually backfire.

Although both my triglycerides and cholesterol are fairly high, only the cholesterol is life-threatening, right?

FACT: Triglycerides and cholesterol are lipids (fats). Although triglycerides are 95 percent of your body fat and usually your diet (protein), cholesterol is only small percentage. Triglycerides are food fats and represent most of your body's fat, like the fat stored in the muscles and breasts. Cholesterol is vital to the brain and nerve cells and all other cell membranes, nerve fibers, bio salts, and sex hormones. It is found in animal-based foods and can be found in the body. It can harden around the arteries and cause fatal heart problems when in excess. Usually high triglycerides go hand in hand with high cholesterol, but only high cholesterol is fatal. It is a good indicator of a person's chance of suffering from cardiovascular disease and also indicates a diet high in animal protein. Raw dieters never encounter this problem.

Meditation and positive affirmation helps weight loss and recovery, true?

FACT: It's like quantum physics. The body is moving energy and the power of our mind dictates every function in our bodies. Deep breathing, meditation, and positive thinking all enhance our body's hormones and brain chemicals. A mother can actually poison her child while breast feeding if she is extremely upset. During stress, excess cortisol is released, which eventually exhausts your adrenal glands. This makes weight loss difficult. Meditation has been proven to lower blood pressure and help enhance our immune systems.

The color orange helps increase appetite, right?

FACT: Certain colors have subtle connections to our emotions and feelings. Warm colors like orange have been known to induce hunger. Blue helps reduce appetite. Green is calming. Red heightens emotions. That's why hospitals have a green ambience and restaurants are usually surrounded by orange decor.

Juice fasting is the best way of losing weight, right?

FICTION: Juice fasting is good to clean out, detox, or heal—NOT to lose weight, for several reasons. People who battle weight should not look to juicing as a weight loss diet. They miss the whole point. It's almost more dangerous to "clean out" and then go back to poor eating habits. It is better to learn to eat properly and gradually move into a raw or clean diet. Trying a short juice fast to cleanse the body before your diet is fine. Long-term juicing (or low-calorie diets missing other nutrients) makes the body fat efficient. Juice is the oxidation (breakdown) of a whole, perfect food (fruit or vegetable). The pulp is a natural insulin inhibitor, which is better for weight loss. Juicing is magical for the very ill or exhausted and usually should be supervised when done long term.

Lifting weights creates bulky and stocky women, right?

FICTION: It is physically impossible to build a muscle and gain weight at the same time. When muscle builds, fat burns. Body builders eat massive calories that build bulky tissue. Less weight with more reps can tone a body without making it look bigger.

Everyone needs at least eight hours of sleep, right?

FICTION: The average working adult gets approximately six to seven hours of sleep, which is not enough. A mind that works well needs at least seven and a half to eight hours of sleep a night. A sick or exhausted body needs more, and you can't "make up" your sleep. That means most of us are *enervating* (drawing from nerve energy) ourselves. Rest is the key to all health, mental and physical. However, I have observed that too much sleep is not good for someone. It is a sign of depression or a highly toxic body. A simple twenty-minute nap between the hours of 10:00 AM to 2:00 PM will help remedy this. Resting for one hour (sometimes meditation) is equal to about one half hour of sleep. There's a correlation between obese children and sleep deprivation. The human growth hormone, which is released during sleep, keeps the body in the fat-burning/muscle-building stage. Usually people who are slim and eat small, healthy meals don't need so much sleep. Raw-food dieters only need about four to six hours of sleep a night. Mental activity is far more tiresome on the body than physical exertion.

☞ *Personal Questions: "Dear Barbi"*

Q: When did you realize you had an eating disorder?

A: I think it was when we devoured twenty cases of Girl Scout cookies that we were supposed to sell. Denial obviously takes many forms. When we were young, we knew we had a secret, but then again, we thought everyone did, behind closed doors. We eventually had interventions, which let us know our secret had leaked out. When we went to out mother's AA meetings at a very young age, we could identify with the alcoholic; only our drug of choice was food. This was the problem: We thought the cure was a diet, so we transformed our disease from compulsive overeating to bulimia. We thought, if we could hide our symptoms, then everything would be fine. In the beginning of our career, we felt our lives were unmanageable and that we didn't deserve to be in the limelight while we were sick. Subsequently, we took a sabbatical so we could concentrate on recovering while studying health. Recovery is called a process because you don't wake up one morning and say, "I've got an eating disorder." There are just as many levels to an illness as there are to recovery. It was more important to know what an eating disorder was rather than figure out how it started. As soon as we knew it wasn't about eating or weight appearance (symptom), we *graduated* into healthy thinking.

Q: What made you want to come out of the closet with your bulimia?

A: My sister. She took up took up the whole closet. Actually, we were strongly advised against it but realized that in secrets lie sickness. No one at the time had come out to talk about overeating or barfing. It seemed fashionable to be a drug addict or an alcoholic back then. We surely knew we wouldn't be embraced for being "pigs". Nor did we want to be remembered for bending over a toilet. However, we knew for our recovery, it was important to share just incase we were able to help ONE person. We wanted people to know the HELL behind the glamour facade.

Q: Was "outing" yourselves a good career move?
A: Sure, if we wanted to be the poster girls for *barfing*. Honestly it was the worst career move, even though our career was just seven and a half minutes of fame each. We weren't credible actresses or great singers. We were just a couple of simple models who happen to get a little fame, (or infamy). What man would want to buy our calendar with the mental picture we were describing to our fans? However, we turned a horrible confession into a fulfilling opportunity. Since our "outing," many other celebrities have come out with their eating disorders as well. We were amazed how many people were touched (let alone surprised) by how prevalent this disease is. Women are by far the majority of our fans now, and they are the ones who request photos of us. That's all worth it!

Q: Did Hollywood hurt or help your eating disorder?
A: Which came first: the chicken or the egg? (I don't know. I ate them both.) My sister came first, which means nothing! I believe people are drawn to extreme career choices out of a dysfunctional validation, (getting approval with unhealthy choices). Hollywood was never a dream of ours, unlike most celebrities. We always wanted to be veterinarians, horse trainers, or athletes—NEVER models. We started modeling at the age of seven, so we didn't have much of a choice. Later, we enjoyed the hours and pay that left us free for horses and sports. However, we abused the Hollywood career choice by using it like a carrot on a stick. We thought if we documented ourselves when we were thin (for about five minutes), on a magazine cover, then no one would know about our disease. To force ourselves to starve we used the scare tactic of realizing thousands of people would judge our appearance. That wore off. We were out of control and almost lost our lives because of some of the diet abuse we endured. It was harder to recover in public as well. Everyone watches you if you fall, fail, or slip. It was humiliating but humbling! Now it seems to be a blessing in disguise, as if this suffering was all worth it.

Q: Did having a twin help or hurt your bulimia?
A: Can you spell *codependent?* Having a twin automatically voted us CODEPENDENT! That's one more sickness on top of the eating disorder. If one of us was fat, we were *both* fat. If one of us was well but not the other, we were both sick. If only one of us wasn't ready to work, neither of

us could work. It was enabling having a binge-and-purge buddy. We had to first learn to be independent, because our bottoms were different from each other. We were so used to controlling each other (one of our main character defects). Letting go was the hardest battle we had to endure. I couldn't "give" recovery to my sister any more than she could give it to me. We are grateful, however, that we can share the recovery path together. We make healthier choices together, although they are independently executed. We give each other the freedom of individual choice, which makes a better team.

Q: When exactly were you recovered?

A: I am? No such thing as a cure or instant recovery. It's a process: one day at a time. Every day the recovery is based on the progress (not perfection) of the program the addict works on. It's not about being thin or abstaining from bingeing. That would be like being a dry drunk. A dry drunk still carries the "ism" (intoxicated with the obsession), without having the drug of choice. The alcohol, binge foods, and fat are only a tools or symptoms of a disease. The disease started long before the compulsive overeating. It usually starts out with obsessive-compulsive disorder and progresses into some addiction. We were excessively clean and neat. We were control freaks and had to have everything perfect. If you only work on the symptoms, then the disease can transform, as ours did from compulsive overeating to bulimia. Recovery started long before we could see any weight loss. Mentally, we surrendered the obsession. That was a relief!

Q: How do you know if someone has an eating disorder?

A: A big clue would be a lock on the refrigerator, like I had. But you can't judge a book by its cover. Instead of looking at the obvious, I'd look for the clues of any disorder: control issues, denial, obsession, ritualistic behavior (OCD) dictated by fear, shame-based thinking or grandiosity. They are usually reckless yet they are afraid of taking healthy risks. They also learn live by instinct rather than intuition. These are all characteristics I identify with. Addicts live by magical thinking. They constantly live in the future or the past, yet they indulge (self-absorbed) for one moment only, rather than living *responsibly* in the NOW.

Q: How do you tell someone that you think he or she needs help?

A: Run! No, seriously, you don't for the most part. You can tell people if they ask. Addicts will only be defensive if they are not ready to hear it. What you do have the right to do is to tell them how their behavior (which is not as secret as they think) is affecting you. You do this by discussing YOUR boundaries while offering them help and nonjudgmental support . There's a fine line between helping or pushing them away. The best advice I can give is to get on their level, instead of being condescending, by sharing your experience, strength, and hope. I tell people I want to be surrounded by healthy people or people who are seeking progress. I then share my character defects so they can relate to where I'm coming from. Perhaps I won't have the same drug of choice, but I can connect on some level. Most people have some type of addictive behavior. That's why sharing in group therapy works best.

Q: What is your diet and exercise plan like today and what do you still have a problem with?

A: My only problem now is my sister. Honestly, at one time every type of food was a trigger food for bingeing. Nothing seemed safe. At first our *abstinence* was simply NOT eating compulsively, over exercising or purging . We would plan three healthy but hearty meals with only a few hours of exercise, which was a BIG change for us. We couldn't diet or think of ways to condone eating (like laxatives or marathon sports). Gradually we incorporated better health habits. We noticed that, when we surrendered the obsession to be thin and made HEALTH our goal, it was easier. It wasn't about being "good" or "bad." It was about making healthier choices. Therefore, one day at a time, we progressed without looking for the perfection of a life-changing regimen. The insanity was lifted as soon as we let go of focusing on food and the body. We've evolved slowly into, by and large, a RAW diet. Our diet abuse caused many health problems, and this was our way to remedy them: Our exercise routine is never more than two hours a day. However it is hard to give up exercise to rest, no matter how sick or tired we are, which still is a problem we are working on. Things that are trigger foods we have as allowed/disallowed eating, so we don't blow our abstinence. My treats at this point in my recovery are far healthier than what they were in the beginning of my recovery. Sugar, meat, and junk food is never a problem, because it has become so unfamiliar to my sister and me. We don't relate to them, because they are out of our *systems*, physically and mentally. Food replacements helped that habit in the beginning. When we wanted something junky, we would create a healthy alternative that did the job!

Q: Did you think your image hurt women or exploited women?

A: Although I agree that I exploit my sister, I don't think we exploited women anymore than we exploited twins. Actually, if you think about it, it is men who seem to be exploited by images that are manipulated and packaged by women for money: men's money. Modern-day people have choices. Regardless if some of us make poor choices, as we all have, we are still able to choose what we want to buy or what we want to project. I do think, however, we did a disservice to women with eating disorders. My sister and I were so wrapped up in our own insecurities; we couldn't have imagined that we would impact anyone, much less women. However, when we did realize that our packaged image (through bulimia) affected women negatively, we decided to come out with our eating disorder. Ironically, it is women who now embrace our calendars, posters, and other merchandise, which they say motivates and inspires them. That makes us feel good that something nice came out of this ugly disease. It also gave us a podium for our biggest passion: animal charities!

CHAPTER 14:
PET HEALTH TIPS

Animals need more nutrition than what is found in most commercial pet foods. Most cat and dog foods are low quality and are the waste products of our own food. Worse, if the ingredients state there are byproducts, it could mean the product includes parts of diseased animals that were euthanized. Corn byproducts are bad for people as well as animals. That is why more cats and dogs are sick today with human diseases (like cancer) than several years or decades ago. Whether it's animal medicine or human medicine, big business seems to be the priority rather than a cure. In general, animals thrive on the same nutritionally balanced diet as humans. It also holds true that, if a food is unhealthy for a person (salt, sugar), then it's also unhealthy for your pet. Natural remedies are usually a better solution to combat illness and health problems.

There is controversy as to whether dogs and cats can or should be complete vegetarians. Some claim the cruelty of slaughtering selected animals for the existence of others is hypocritical. Dogs are mostly carnivores. However, I have observed some dogs become less aggressive on a vegetarian diet. Though vegetarian diets seem to make dogs happier and calmer, some veterinarians claim that it can really make your dog sick and weak due to malnutrition. Cats are complete carnivores, so a complete vegetarian diet would be robbing them of nutrition that is vital for their survival. The lack of taurine, which is found primarily in meat, can cause convulsions or seizures, if not complete death, for cats in particular. Cats and dogs that don't have any nutritional foods added to their meals, like vegetables, have the risk of kidney or liver problems, particularly from a rich and acidic diet. Some experts swear that a diet of dry food is sufficient for their pet because it contains a lot of roughage and is great for their teeth. Still, dry food alone can dehydrate your pet. I have found that adding a little bit of ground flaxseed meal, ground sunflowers, and wheatgrass powder is very good for indoor pets and is comparable to expensive vitamins that are sometimes loaded with sugars and unhealthy ingredients.

I have also found that dogs and cats turn to grass or sometimes fruit when they are unhealthy. They also know instinctively when to fast (sick, depressed, etc.). The chlorophyll in grass neutralizes poisons and helps their bodies' pH balance.

Animals can benefit people mentally and physically. I have heard that there is proof that the cat's purr can help osteoporosis and the "hypnotic" vibration is soothing and healing. Unconditional love from your pets helps depression and heart problems, lowers blood pressure, and so much more. Obviously, a dog forces a person to exercise. Giving love to your pet and receiving love from your pet helps both immune systems.

When in doubt, go natural. Example: Horses naturally graze with their heads stretching downward. Instead, horse owners prefer feeding concentrated foods in feed bins that are place in high areas. This restricts their natural neck placement, which disrupts a horse's natural flow of enzymes. This can then promote diseases such as colic.

Purebreds are the subject of many debates. Breeding enhances certain flaws and diseases in the animal. For instance, over-breeding can cause a calcium loss that affects the pet's nervous system. Mutts are the healthiest pets. And of course, one of the cruelest acts to animal kind is declawing a cat or clipping dogs' ears and tails. Aside from being unnatural, the animal lives in constant pain. Cat's defense mechanism is that it can mask extreme pain. Therefore people assume many times that a cat is fine when it is not. Many times the side effect of declawing shows up later in another internal disease like kidney failure.

Most importantly, exercise is necessary for all pets. This means, whatever pet you may have, give it the opportunity to move or exercise. I think it's cruel when I see even the tiniest pet in small living quarters. That is the pet's home, not a decoration for your house or office. Cats should be able to run around. Horses should exercise daily or have room to wander around. Dogs should have room to run around as well, during a daily walk. Dog walking (primarily with a choker) is an exercise that teaches the dog to focus and listen, and is it also good for a neurotic, shy, or aggressive dog because it tires the dog into submission and trust. Walking your dog also improves your relationship with your dog, teaching him that you are in charge. You should walk the dog on your left side, slightly in front of you, to teach them the dog you are the leader of the pack, because dogs are pack animals. A treadmill can be used for dogs, much like the hot-walker is used to walk horses. Dog walking is known to help combat depression, anxiety, and constipation. This is a healthy relationship that your dog will appreciate.

Although everything suggested in this chapter should be checked by your veterinarian, it's best to keep your pet's diet simple, natural, and nutritious.

QUICK HEALTH TIPS FROM A-Z

☞ Arthritis: Sunshine, EFA oils, massages, calcium supplements like bone meal.

☞ Bad breath: Super-greens (spirulina, barely grass, etc.). All greens neutralize poisons.

☞ Coat and skin: EFA oils, brushing, combing, massaging the coat, and sunshine. Too many baths are unnatural and rob the pet's coat of its natural oils.

☞ Constipation: Animals should be regular. The animal's health can be determined by looking at the pet's stools (for worms, parasites, etc.). Fiber and vegetables are great for both cats and dogs. Manx cats have a problem with constipation and diarrhea, therefore, they need high-fiber foods added, like pumpkin. Aloe vera is a gentle laxative that also helps with diarrhea. EFA oils are also excellent. Exercise and drinking lots of water also helps regularity.

☞ Dehydration: Fruit such as watermelon helps prevent dehydration. This is because the sodium in the fruit holds the water and natural sugar in the fruit, supplying the pet with energy. Fresh water is vital but can also be a diuretic.

☞ Depression: Dogs and cats, in particular, should never be left alone. A pet companion is necessary if they are mostly home alone. In addition to a nutritious, balanced diet, sunshine and exercise helps keeps your pet happy.

☞ Exercise: All pets should be exercised daily. Dogs need the walks more than room to run on their own. Exercise helps fight anxiety, depression, aggression, and constipation, and it creates a bond with your dog. Hamsters and other rodents need exercise wheels and plenty of space.

☞ Flea, worms, and parasites: To get rid of these put B vitamins, brewers yeast or garlic in their meals (horses included). Seaweed baths, or tea-tree oil baths are helpful.

☞ Infections, colds, and other diseases: Fresh air, super-greens, vitamin C powder, liquid diets, lots of fresh water, EFA oils, and plenty of rest. Some claim yogurt naturally fights bacteria, but usually dairy is not recommended for pets.

☞ Pregnancy: Several meals throughout the day, vitamin C, super-foods, EFA oils, and sunshine. Kittens and puppies need to eat more frequently than adult pets.

☞ Sleeping quarters: Cats and rodents are nocturnal and sleep many hours. They prefer dark, private places that are warm.

☞ Sunshine: Just like people, most horses, dogs, and cats like to sunbathe. They receive the same benefits that we do from the vitamin D. Sunbathing helps their sleeping patterns as well.

☞ Vitamins: Make your own. With cats and dogs, mix ground flax, sunflower, and wheatgrass together for all around good health; this is better than vitamins loaded with sugar.

☞ Vital dog food ingredient: Amino acid arginine

☞ Vital cat food ingredient: Amino acid taurine

☞ Weight problems: Several mini-meals throughout the day, EFA oils, high-fiber foods, plenty of exercise, and plenty of love to help fill their void.

CHAPTER 15:
FORTY DAYS AND FORTY NIGHTS

Inspirational Stories and Good Charity Options

Attention Readers: We want to take every reader who has suffered as we have down the path of hope. Let my sister and I take your hand and adopt you as our "triplet." We want to share our most embarrassing stories and other people's inspirational stories. If you feel alone and desperate, we know how you feel. We went from trailer trash to decadent divas and back to recycled trash: very humiliating.

Forty Days and Forty Nights was used as this chapter's title because it was the most humiliating of all the attempted diets we've actually admitted to. *Forty Days and Forty Nights* was the time my boyfriend locked my sister and I in our three-story apartment. We were attempting to fast for *forty days and forty nights*. We wanted to take the *vow of hunger!* It seemed easy as long as we had a little help from God (hence the fast days intended). On our tenth day, we ended up using our bed sheets as ropes to escape through our window and made a beeline to the nearest convenience store. We repented all the way. At least we kept to our word…sort of. We binged for forty days and forty nights thereafter.

Nothing is worse than being famous just long enough to have everyone watch you bottom out for a longer period of time than you were famous. There were uncomfortable situations, like being *recognized* or *busted* in the middle of our binges. That wouldn't be so embarrassing, except that it happened to be on the same day that we swore we were "totally recovered," on *national TV!* How could anyone recognize us under all those crumbs?

It's also pretty embarrassing to have someone ask you if you are pregnant when you're not. Worse, I would reply yes because explaining my binge belly would be more embarrassing. Most people assumed culinary arts was our major in school. Our favorite pastime game was "guess what the neighbors are eating." Like narc dogs, we could smell the butter and salt our neighbors sprinkled on their potatoes. Anytime we gave directions to someone, they would always include food landmarks—"two blocks down from the donut shop; make a right at the pancake house; cross the street at the yogurt shop." Yes, we've used every diet trick and remedy for weight loss, which always backfired. Let us share some of our "bottoms" (We've got enough for everyone.) so you don't have to feel alone or ashamed.

251

TWO BIG BOTTOMS: BOTTOMING OUT

Bottomed Out #1: What is it about other people's refrigerators? It's taboo. It appears "free," not necessarily in cost but in calories. I thought my binge weight wouldn't show up on the scale, *if no one knew*. I felt like a CIA agent: undercover, pretending to do dishes or clean the kitchen. My mission: retrieve food without evidence. I'd always come prepared with my backyard detective kit. It included rubber gloves to clear myself of any DNA residue. First I would carefully dismantle the victim's treat in the refrigerator. My tongue was like an artist's spatula. I gloated like a cat burglar. Then I bloated like a pig. After devouring the free calories, I would then remold the treat before I was a fugitive on the run. Usually I'd pray for an earthquake, flood, fire—*anything* to camouflage my "wipe-out" raid. Needless to say, my sis and I are no longer trusted in kitchen areas. Friends actually seal their refrigerators off, like a crime scene.

Bottomed Out #2: Shane cannot sing, dance, or act. Nevertheless, I was *so* jealous because she could puke like a pro. She could actually vomit on command with just one delicate and nimble finger. Shane tried to coach me in her style of fine vomiting techniques. If I could "Rotor Rooter" a plunger down my throat or "blast" dynamite out my butt. I would, but nothing worked! While listening to my sister "abort" billions of calories in the restroom, I seemed to be finding the weight she was losing. Although she resembled the skull on the poison sign,
THIN = BEAUTY! Heart attacks, rotten teeth, etc. were trivial side effects for her.

Bottomed Out #3: The car was our favorite food retreat because it was our quick and private fast-food restaurant on wheels. I could have fed the starving kids in India with all the food crumbs left on my car floor. One time, the police pulled us over, thinking we were drunk when we simply OD'd on sugar. We thought that, by wearing dark sunglasses (at night) and layers of clothes, we were in disguise. Wrong! We looked like drug lords! Another time, an overzealous fan followed our fast-food restaurant on wheels for miles until we threatened to call the police. The good Samaritan was just trying to innocently point out that we had left some of our groceries, on top of the car. We embarrassedly snapped back, "we know" and drove off as if we were in <u>complete </u>control!

Bottom Out #4: My sister and I would rotate playing food cop so one of us would stick to a diet. This way, at least <u>one</u> twin could lose weight. The twin who was allowed to binge had enough *fuel* to hold the other twin hostage on some severe diet. If the starving twin wanted to binge, she had to be clever enough to outsmart her own mind, since we thought alike. There was a God.

One night my sister forgot to lock her binge cupboard. I "creepy crawled" so slowly, knowing every creak and crack would awaken her from her sugar coma. There it was, teasing me in the moonlight glare: her unfinished ninth course, CHOCOLATE CAKE with her folk still attached. I could feel myself melt as my fingers gently squeezed the fork, gracefully dangling like a Christmas ornament. BANG! Bright lights immediately spotlighted me. "Put your hands in the air; *slowly* step away from the cake." I should have known my sis took delight in setting me up!

Bottom Out #5: I wanted extreme methods to make me diet. One time, my friend offered her electrical zapper, which helped her quit smoking. She agreed it would be great for my next diet invention. This little electrical box had simulators that would deliver painful shocks. It worked Pavlovian style. She suggested that I bring my forbidden binge foods over to her place so she could "zap" my cravings away for each food. I suggested bringing the "zapper" to the supermarket. It turned out to be too exhausting. I guess it slipped my mind that I craved EVERYTHING! I almost electrocuted myself. Next, I decided to get my wisdom teeth removed, not because it was necessary but because it was a guaranteed diet plan. All my friends lost weight because their mouths were packed and sore. Unfortunately, this surgery made me discover new ways of eating food without teeth—via powder form. I crushed every goodie I craved and smeared it on my gums, like a cocaine addict.

Bottom Out #6: When I lived in Hawaii, I had to endure the hurricane season. On one occasion a hurricane wiped out most of the island. While most people attended to the disaster's damage, I went looking for my favorite dessert shack. It had been completely wiped out! Suddenly the island felt like a pebble. It was too small to supply any of my cravings. It was also too many miles of ocean to travel, to find anything that resembled my cravings. I placed flowers on the grave site of the beloved little dessert hut that once fed me.

Bottom Out #7: I tried to incorporate spiritual means into my diets. In other words, I would negotiate with God to try to lose weight. I thought that if I fasted for forty days and forty nights, like the Bible mentioned, I would be blessed and weight would drop off. Many times, I wanted to take the "vow of hunger." If certain saints could live solely on a communion wafer, then it wouldn't be farfetched for me to use my own fanatic methods. But I needed the help of God. Then I had the idea that if I worked in my church's kitchen the "devil" (food) couldn't tempt me. This was the place to cast the demons of hunger right out of me. It was like having a video camera on me 24/7. I was unable to sneak any food; God was omnipresent and omniscient. Unfortunately, the food appeared blessed and therefore inviting. My weight gain felt blessed as well.

INSPIRATIONAL STORIES FROM OTHERS

Anonymous Story 1

This woman wrote us on the internet, following a TV special. The TV special had a post-chat one-to-one on the Internet so we could talk with individuals.

"Annie" said she was on the brink of suicide because she was depressed over her extreme weight gain. She never heard anyone in the media talk about compulsive overeating as a disease. And sshe never heard of someone talking about recovery with a disease. People always told her she just needed "willpower and a good diet to stick with." She heard us claim diets make you fatter and compulsive overeating has nothing to do with willpower. She asked us if there was any hope for her. We told her she was half well by just admitting she was a compulsive overeater. Then we suggested that she worked on her shame, not her dieting. We told her she was struggling against chemicals and hormones in her body that created an insatiable "thirst" for food and that it was not in her control. We stressed that her life had become unmanageable and out of control because her focus was on the food and the weight and not what she was eating over. No one becomes "large" from loving food. She took our recommendation to follow up and join twelve-step meetings with other compulsive overeaters. This way she could share and not feel alone. She was so happy there was a nonprofit organization with others who suffered just like her. She was actually excited that there was an alternative path and didn't need to resort to suicide. She wrote us later to tell us she bought our book and shared it with her support group. By the time she wrote us back, she was already sponsoring another newcomer in her support group. She remembered us saying that the best compliment was hearing how we have helped others. She agreed, stating it was nice to be on the other end, helping someone else like we did with her.

Anonymous Story 2

A young girl came up to us following a lecture we had given at a high school. She waited until everyone had left, terrified that people would know what she did behind closed doors.

"Sharon" said that she would go on the Internet to secretly congregate with other wannabe anorexics so they could all share their tricks. Her family and friends were concerned but trusted that she was just "going through a phase." It was hard to keep up the lies, her friendships, school, and the front she was putting on. She was exhausted. The more shame she felt, the more she wanted to disappear into extreme anorexia. When people told her "anorexics die," all she could hear was that she was noticed for being thin. This created a "thirst" to continue, because she wanted to be a "better" anorexic. Her health problems were starting to manifest. She thought there was no turning back. She was in tears when she admitted to my sister and me that she felt alone until she heard our stories about laxative abuse and extreme dieting. The anorexic Internet group omitted the down side to anorexia. She was so inspired that there was life after anorexia she read our book cover to cover. The jargon hit home with her because everyone else told her she would be "well" if she just gained weight. I don't talk about weight with anorexics. Weight is only the symptom. Usually people only focus on weight. Later she wrote us that she joined an outpatient clinic for eating disorders. She made friends with other recovering anorexics and shared recovery stories instead of tricks with them. She thanked us for not only saving her life, but giving her one.

Anonymous Story 3
This gentleman approached us with his story at a book signing.
"Scott" stood in line awhile, hoping that we would have time to hear his story. He was buying the book for his sister, who had seen one of our TV shows. He had known that his sister, a dancer, was bulimic for years. It was something no one talked about. However, her whole personality changed and she was acting like a drug addict. She lost her desire to dance because her bulimia progressed into body dysmorphia. Her obsession with her body image left no time for anything but bingeing and purging. Scott said his sister "Ashley" saw our TV show and decided to come clean about her bulimia. She thought she was the only person to steal food or lie about her addiction. Ashley told Scott that she related to my sister and my story about our extreme ways to get rid of food, which escalated daily. When I was up to 100 laxatives and 10 hours of exercise a day, where could I go from there? That was exactly what she was asking herself. Ashley bargained with Scott and her family. She said she would go to an Overeaters Anonymous meeting, if they went to Al-Anon meeting. She told Scott that she heard us say "it's a family disease; everyone is affected and should work their own programs." This gave her relief because she wanted to choose recovery on her own, without having to *answer to* an overly concerned family. Scott wanted to respect her request but still support her. He thought our book was a sweet, silent support for her.

Anonymous Story 4
We met a young woman at a convention where we spoke about eating disorders.
"Janet" introduced herself as the organizer for all the convention's events. She had a lot of pressure on her and an impeccable record of efficiency. Many of the events at the convention had to do with addiction. She never identified with any of the stories that the addicts told. She always saw herself in total control, as a "perfectionist." Those were the exact terms I used as symptoms of some addictions or eating disorders. She

thought control and the desire to have everything "perfect" was a sign of discipline and professionalism. Part of her discipline was to look the part she was playing as the perfect executive. Janet said that eating made her anxious and it was the easiest thing to control. She just didn't eat. Everyone complimented her and thought she was perfect for the job because she had everything, including her weight, under control. When she heard me say that people mistake ritualistic control for discipline she said she went to the restroom in order to "break down in tears." It especially hit home with her when I was saying that people who carry too much responsibility on the outside disregard their insides. She didn't want anyone at the convention to notice how human she was, because she had put too much energy into her image. Nonetheless, she said, if we could publicly display our disease and all the embarrassing behaviors we've used to feed our addiction, she now felt "safe" enough to be honest about herself. Janet said that she thought her personality was just helping people. Control was just needed for perfection. She told us that our speech taught her that you can't help someone else until you humbly admit your own faults. Janet got more out of that short speech than a lot of people do during years of therapy. You can see the glass as half full or half empty, and she choose to see it three-quarters full.

Anonymous Story 5
This young lady came up to us in a hotel.
"Connie" came up to us with her friend and said she had been waiting for the day to meet us. She said at one school event where we spoke, they would not let her and her friend in because they were "gay." Following the event, she went out and bought our book. She admitted to having an eating disorder but never connected her eating disorder with the pressure of outside judgment. She dealt with the *shame* by turning to food. She later learned that my sister and I were raised by a gay mother and were discriminated against because of it. That compelled Connie even more to meet us. I do not put up with any type of discrimination or bigotry whatsoever. However, I learned that we have no control over others and their cruel or unfair reactions. This doesn't mean that we need to be burdened with shame because of their misguided judgments. My sister and I told Connie that we were flattered that she went out of her way to seek us out. We advised her to go to GAY therapy groups or twelve-step meetings. We stressed that, as long as she thought *she* was the problem instead of having a problem (eating disorder), she was *never* going to win her battle with food. In these gay therapy groups, she could discuss eating disorders and be open about being gay. The relief of letting go of her secret would help lift her obsession with food. We also suggested reporting this intolerance and discrimination to certain organizations. Learning to not react doesn't mean that we need to walk on eggshells or be people pleasers. Connie felt as good as we did that we all connected on several mutual levels. When you open up, it's amazing how many people will be able to relate.

Anonymous Story 6

This young lady was a successful woman in Hollywood. She was beautiful, intelligent, and always looked as if she had it all together.

"Gina" had grown up in the "biz," surrounded by famous celebrities. She married another high-profile person and had a baby while trying to juggle her career. Everyone around her advised drugs, steroids, and plastic surgery to get back to her perfect figure. The new rage for male and female celebrities is to use synthetic HGH to cheat their way beyond normal standards into perfection. HGH causes you to be in the fat-burning/muscle-building process at an accelerated rate. Sure these people look unnaturally good, particularly when they brag they don't work out or eat right. We told Gina there is a price to every shortcut: diets, plastic surgery, drugs, or hormones. I know people who swore by those means. It did the job for them at the time. However, they paid for it eventually. Our laxative abuse, as well, could be considered drug abuse. We also paid dearly for it. Everything, including drugs and hormones, is filtered through the liver. All drugs and hormones deplete your own natural chemicals and hormones and enhance tumor and fibroid growth. Gina took our advice and went the natural way to bounce back by juicing and eating raw. Furthermore, she hand-blended all her baby's "raw" baby food. Plastic surgery, drugs, or synthetic hormones could have NEVER put the sparkle in their eyes or create the glow they manifested, like the raw diet we suggested did. Some people can cheat some of the time, but anyone can change their eating habits all of the time, without any of the adverse effects that drugs and surgery have. Incidentally, Gina's baby never gets ear infections, digestion problems, sleep problems, or any other illnesses like all her friend's toddlers continually have.

Anonymous Story 7

This forty-something woman tried for years to get pregnant and eventually gave up. She really didn't have an eating disorder, except when she had female problems. Her bleeding fibroids left her feeling weak. She developed other related problems because her doctors continued to symptom-chase. Her doctors suggest to eat meat for the iron and to eat sugary carbs for to get more energy. She lived on coffee, ice cream, and hamburgers. Although she was far from fat, her eating habits were obsessive and made her feel ashamed. "Pam" was on the birth control pill for her acne and bleeding problems. Ironically, we told her that her acne was from her poor diet and hormone imbalance. She was scheduling a hysterectomy because she had developed severe endometriosis. This was devastating because it meant that she was never going to be able to have children. Her doctors told her she was sterile and didn't need her female organs, because she was about to go through menopause. We suggested our diet and giving supplements a try before she turned to radical surgery. She had nothing to lose while waiting for her insurance to go through. Most importantly, I had her get off of all *coffee,* meat, and sugar. Then, for her anemia, I had her juice greens for the chlorophyll. We suggested sea greens for energy and salmon instead of meat. She loaded up on all the EFA's in food and supplement form. Then I suggested bioidentical progesterone cream from the health food store. That relieved her painful bleeding and helped her regularity. When she went back to see her doctor, both Pam and her doctor were shocked. She had NO trace of endometriosis. Her fibroids shrank. But the biggest shock was that she was PREGNANT! No one will really know if it was just one thing or all the radical changes I had her make that turned a crisis into a dream for her. Her bonus was she finally had clear skin for the first time in years.

Anonymous Story 8

This gay friend of ours has a profitable job in Hollywood. He has always been in good shape and has never had any symptoms of any eating disorder. "Tom" would find himself really bored when he was home alone at night. He was used to being invited to all the Hollywood parties and premiers, which was a part of his job perks. He never had any addiction to speak of, but he started the habit of eating to put himself to sleep at night. He was in perfect shape, so he didn't worry about putting on weight. He found that he was starting to prefer time alone with his bedtime treats. He asked my sister and me if this ritual was something to worry about. There's nothing wrong with eating treats before bedtime, if it is a once in a while thing and you don't have any weight or eating disorders. Tom's physical activity would prove that weight was never going to be an issue. However, he was starting to cancel important evening events he was invited to. These events were important for his career and usually very exciting. We told Tom that possibly the bedtime treats were hiding another problem he hadn't faced. Perhaps he felt uncomfortable constantly having to be "on" for his work and events and wanted some time off from all the excitement. Perhaps he didn't feel like himself around people who had to project a perfect image continually. Whatever it was wasn't the important thing, it just wasn't fulfilling enough, although everyone envied him. We suggested that he do something that was the opposite of being around packaged people—to surround himself with people who were interested in developing their inner selves. A perfect way to connect and contribute is working with charities. He enjoyed animals and couldn't own one where he lived. We suggested getting involved with an animal adoption center. This way he could get his down time without totally becoming isolated. He could be around animals he could help. Tom ended up being able to bring home little foster animals once in a while. Instead of his bedtime treat ritual, he has a little critter who fills that void. We were glad to make both Tom and his little foster critters happy.

Anonymous Story 9

This little girl was a stepdaughter of a relative. She, too, had grown up in a dysfunctional family. She had alcoholism and eating disorders as her only role models.

"Debbie" was a darling little girl who was very overweight and fighting the constant cruel remarks made to her daily. Her family would tell her that her weight didn't matter and that she was beautiful, regardless of what anyone else said. I personally wanted to spend one weekend with her. Although she was only eight years old, she was an extremely bright little girl. She wanted me to teach her how to diet so she wouldn't be teased. I wanted to teach her how to eat and how to respond with a positive goal as opposed to fear and shame. I knew she was bright enough to understand the simple biology of the body. I told her that certain foods cause an allergic type reaction that makes the body produce fat. I told her it was a healthy reaction for the body to gain weight when certain foods are introduced into it. I never used the word "bad" or "good" but said "healthy" and "unhealthy." Nor did I use denial. The world is a cruel place and avoiding the purple elephant in the middle of the living room doesn't make hurt feelings go away. Debbie was a beautiful little girl, but that was not important. Instead of leaving the obsession on her "outsides", I wanted her to focus on her health. Like a science class, I made simple analogies that created simple solutions so she could connect the dots. So Debbie wouldn't continue to eat over her shame, I gave her simple exercises that made her feel good about herself and taught her to think about her health, not her appearance. It was as if it was a game. I asked her questions like, "If I ate carrots, what could I expect? If I ate chocolate, what could I expect? If my feelings are hurt, what can I do to feel better?" I reminded her that she had a choice in everything she ate and how she responded to others. Just because we don't have control over other people doesn't mean we need to respond to them the way they expect. I also told her to empathize with people who purposefully make hurtful statements, because they are reacting from pain, ignorance, or fear. If Debbie reacted defensively or from pain, that was the response that was expected. However, not responding can completely disarm the culprit, taking away that person's power. Debbie learned that simple biology makes health a sure thing, and the byproduct will be proper fitness for an eight-year-old girl. Most of all, Debbie learned that changing her eating habits was a *process* that didn't need to be perfect. The process had choices. The choices are simple biology that will eventually achieve her goal. She found her own power in being able to not react out of shame but rather empathetically to others who weren't able to be empathetic. Debbie now teaches her other little friends about lifestyle choices, which has really built up her confidence.

Anonymous Story 10

This gentleman was a trainer to the stars. My sister and I used to work out with him because he was so inspiring. He had an impressive clientele.

"Chris" had a fifteen-hour-a-day workout schedule seven days a week. It seemed to grow constantly. Chris had to turn down clients because he was in such high demand. His girlfriend, an athlete as well, could hardly keep up with him. With what little time he had off, he would plan some athletic event like a race. He constantly had to outdo himself and raise the bar. "Jenny," his girlfriend, was bothered by his obsession to be perfect. When they went to the gym, Jenny would notice Chris observing himself in the mirror only to be distraught over what he saw—or what he thought he saw. Jenny said Chris would think he was starting a tire rim around his perfect physic. None of us could see it, let alone tell him he was wrong. He saw what he saw. This created an unending obsession to punish himself for not appearing as a trainer should appear. Chris was so exhausted that at one point he actually considered liposuction. He realized that the time off required for healing was going to throw his whole routine off. Then there would be more to worry about than just a tire rim. Chris would refuse to take his shirt off, fearing that people would see his tire rim rather than the eight-pack he worked so diligently for. At this point, Chris was actually destroying himself trying to achieve something that wasn't' necessary. This is body dysmorphia. My sister and I suggested Jenny attend an Al-Anon meeting. Jenny brought Chris's family, who were also concerned about Chris's strange self-perception. It was becoming alarming. I also gave Jenny our book, which detailed several options, like interventions and the best way to construct an intervention. Subsequently, they found a professional and put together an intervention. The potency of the intervention made it clear to Chris that it wasn't about how he looked or his career. He could see that he was drowning in an obsession over something he perceives in his mind that wasn't accurate. As soon as he saw it as an addiction, which he had always thought was a sign of not having discipline, he wanted to address it immediately. Chris eventually agreed to attend therapy with his girlfriend. He didn't realize that trying to fix his problem was the problem. Chris never lost the perception of his tire rim. However, it was such a relief for him to let it go as an obsession that wasn't important. It wasn't worth killing himself over it or making his family worry about it. Though Chris's perception may never be normal, his obsession went from his body to his priorities. Most of all, Jenny and Chris's family realized everyone is involved with any type of addiction and they couldn't work Chris's program. Therefore, they continued group therapy to work their own program and tried not to control Chris. It is always easier to surrender something when you surround yourself with a support group. Incidentally, Chris and Jenny were also able to work out their other problems in therapy, mostly because Chris now has a lot more available time, compared to the *exhausting* schedule he had previously.

"Compassion, in which all ethics must take root, can only attain its full breadth and depth if it embraces all living creatures and not limit itself to mankind." Albert Schweitzer

FAVORITE CHARITY: ANIMALS!!!

Charity itself is therapy for the soul and recovery from any disease. It teaches you to connect and contribute, reach out, practice gratitude, and live in the NOW. Most of all, it releases you from any self-obsession. When you are focusing on something other than yourself without a motive to profit, you learn true humility. When we are wrapped up in ourselves, our perception is misguided because everything is attached to the ego. A common character defect of addicts is thinking that they are different, that their problems are the worst and no one will understand. When you help others in need or contribute to the world in some way, you suddenly see the big picture and somehow your little problems don't seem so bad or different. Our parents believed in contribution, so they taught my sister and me to involve ourselves in various charities, which helped combat depression. We were involved in every charity from pediatric AIDS to eating disorders. However, I must admit our favorite charity is one that has anything to do with animals. Both my sister and I were always a bit uncomfortable with people because we always thought that we were constantly being judged and weren't good enough (self-absorbed). Animals didn't care if I was fat, skinny, successful, or not. It was my first spiritual epiphany connecting with animals. It was one living creature connecting with another. I saw God's innocent creations and experienced unconditional love when I was with animals. Just because we can use animals doesn't mean we should. I think we have a responsibility to take care of our little pets because they depend on us.

My sister and my first pet was a little turtle: Timothy, the turtle. My sister and I were surrounded by so much turmoil and alcoholism; it was nice to have our little pets to turn to. We learned responsibility at a very young age. The next pet we insisted on was a little hamster we rescued from school. We didn't like students using the little rodent as a pleasure toy, ignoring its fear and needs. Our parents later granted our requests to take in strays that we would befriend. It felt good, no matter how bad our surroundings were, that there was a little warm animal waiting for me to come home. We knew how it felt to be neglected and didn't want to pass on our pain to them. Instead we received unconditional love from these little animals. We noticed that our pets had feelings like we did. They didn't just get hungry or tired. They wanted love, affection, and they were curious or felt sad. Each pet, we noticed, took on its own personality. If we were gone, our pets felt hurt or betrayed. If you did something to irritate them, they would get annoyed. This was amazing to us as kids. Subsequently, when we moved onto a ranch and our father wanted to "raise" our food, it didn't seem natural to eat little critters that had feelings. It wasn't *what* were we having for dinner but *who* were we having for dinner. Uncommon or not, we became vegetarians early in our lives. It was our selfish disease that turned us back into carnivores later on. Ironically, recovery has brought our diet full circle. The way we eat and the way we think are very related. Besides loving animals, live food seemed more natural to eat than dead meat. But that is a personal choice that I'd rather educate people about than push on others. Anyone who practices vegetarianism for the sake of animals is contributing toward animals in some way every day. I like to focus on preventing cruelty toward animals and helping the overwhelming pet population at shelters (adoption, spaying, neutering).

Regardless of whether you are a vegetarian or not, a little service dedicated to animals is very rewarding. There are so many ways of expressing your love for animals or some kind of pet charity. If you can't rescue or adopt a shelter animal, then go volunteer your time. Perhaps you can spare a little love, which goes along way with these animals who feel abandoned, alone, scared, and betrayed.

There are animal lovers who gather and capture strays, neuter or spay them, and then mark them and turn them loose. There are organizations that help without any cost. You don't always need to give monetary donations. Your time is just as precious and very rewarding. I think it is so selfish when people don't even want to hear the sad stories of these poor abandoned pets. They think their lives are better when they don't hear about such sadness. I'll never understand why people want the perfect prototype purebred when little mixes are more fun to watch grow into a surprise. Most people don't even realize that you can find your preferred purebreds at the shelters. Most breeders overlook animal humanity when it comes to costs and only think of the pet as a commodity or expense. The profit not the pet's new home is the usual motive.

Numerous religions revere animals. The Torah doesn't allow any animal to suffer. The Bible states "dominion over beast," which means we have a responsibility toward them. Hindus are vegetarians who revere the cow because of the maternal quality of giving milk, which saves a lot of hungry people. Unfortunately, I have met a lot of animal rescuers who have become atheists because they witnessed so much cruelty toward innocent animals who did nothing wrong. The world can be perceived a cruel and unfair, but we can make a difference, even in a small way.

The rewards you receive are beyond what you give. Owning a pet helps reduce stress, improve cardiovascular health, and lower your cholesterol levels. I've heard about the claim that the vibrations from a cat purring can improve the symptoms of osteoporosis. I've also heard about people who suffer from compromised immune systems or HIV/AIDS have been shown to get worse if their pets are taken away and show marked improvement when the pets are returned. Everyone has heard about the amazing effect that animals have on the elderly as well—so much so that it is becoming common for animals to be brought into retirement homes and to hospice centers for people suffering from chronic diseases like Alzheimer's. It's been shown that dogs can detect cancer before conventional medicine can. It's true your pet can sense when you are not well. There are programs that match handicapped kids with gentle horses no one wanted because they had a few problems. There's a new animal rescue program that pairs abandoned or abused animals with children who were abandoned and abused with very good results. I have learned that this is healing for both and teaches kids to empathize instead of continuing the pattern of abandonment or abuse. Animals are proven to stimulate the release of good brain chemicals, like serotonin, and hormones that help counter depression and fight addiction. We learn responsibility because these little beings depend on us and don't have a voice or choice like we do. We can practice tolerance and acceptance, instead of taking animals that are perfect. It's been known that animal vivisection (live surgery) is not only unnecessary cruelty, but is dangerous to humans. Its purpose is not to help humans; it is more of a political policy that helps fight lawsuits and support insurance. It's a known fact that animals' reactions are sometimes quite the opposite of humans'. If I'm different from my twin sister in many ways, then an animal may have an opposite reaction of a human to a certain drug, chemical, or experiment. A big part of any disease is isolation. Having a pet is a good conversational piece or an excuse to meet someone if you are too shy. There are parks and animal gatherings where people bring their pets and intermingle with other pet owners. This is a good way of connecting with others without obsessing about your own insecurities.

True crime experts note that criminals start torturing animals before they move to humans. Animals can't speak out or defend themselves. I think you can judge a person by the compassion they show to animals. People pleasers or people stuck on their image are only interested in how they appear to other people. My suggestion for a good choice of anonymous charity work is working with animals! Simple compassion and regard for animals tells me a lot about someone who wants to develop their own self-worth and humility.

GOOD CHARITY OPTIONS:

✓ Twelve-step programs: You can volunteer your time at any of the twelve-step programs like Compulsive Overeaters Anonymous.

✓ Reputable nationwide or local community organizations (homeless shelters or local religious foundations): Around the holidays, food is such a battle for my sister and I. When you feed the homeless or volunteer your time with underprivileged kids or abandoned pets, it relieves your compulsion to overindulge.

✓ Children's hospital's and convalescent homes: When you volunteer time with sick children, the elderly, or even people affected with the AIDS virus, you objectively observe individuals who are fighting to live. Addictions are a self-destructive disease, a slow death that we put on ourselves. Helping ill people can inspire addicts to choose recovery rather than a self-destructive path. It's a good wake-up call for someone who takes their life for granted. My sister and I are working with an organization that is trying to place animals with sick or old people. That's a two-way charity.

✓ Local animal shelters and rescue organizations: These organizations can always use any type of volunteer work. Abandoned pets are cage stressed, lonely, and starved for any type of attention. Dogs need to be walked and cats need to stretch out or explore. All baby animals need to be comforted and bottle-fed. All animals need to be groomed so they can find a good home. These animals are so low-maintenance; they are content just to be petted. It is better to donate your time or pet supplies rather than money, so you know your gift goes straight to the animals!

✋ **Warning: I think it is very important to do extensive research for any charity you want to be involved with, like we did. Ask questions, be "hands on" and work with them. Most of all, have other unbiased administrations and research organizations rate and investigate them. Various organizations, such as governmental agencies are able to check up on the charity's background and any possible misconduct. I am very surprised that many celebrities endorse their name to well known animal organizations that have felony animal abuse charges filed against them. Just because an organization or celebrity is famous doesn't mean that they are a good choice.**

☺ *Best Friends (Animal Sanctuary) is our favorite charity organization. North Shore Animal League, The Paw Project, Feral Cat Alliance, Pooch Heaven, New Leash On Life, and Cat Crossing are also excellent.*

THE BARBIS' GLOSSARY

These simple, straightforward definitions are relevant to the context of this book. The glossary contains only limited information but may be helpful in understanding many of the terms used throughout.

Acid – A substance that release hydrogen ions. Acidosis is an increase in hydrogen ions and a major cause of exercise fatigue. Acids can be either organic or inorganic compounds.

Acidophilus – Beneficial, live bacteria essential for healthy intestinal function.

Acidosis – A blood condition in which the bicarbonate concentration is below normal. It is often produced by the fermentation of proteins and carbohydrates because mineral salts are not present in food.

Acute illness – A sickness that comes on quickly and may cause severe symptoms but is of a short duration.

Adrenal glands – Glands situated on top of the kidneys that secrete different types of hormones.

Aerobic – With oxygen. Aerobic exercise utilizes oxygen in the fuel burning process; it encompasses any type of sustained and rhythmic movement. The main fuels for aerobic energy are carbohydrates and fats.

AIDS – Acquired immune deficiency syndrome.

Aloe vera – A juice or gel-like substance derived from the Aloe plant; it prevents scarring from wounds, burns, and abrasions. Aloe juice is sometimes used for digestion and as a natural laxative.

Allergen – A substance that provokes an allergic response.

Allergy – An inappropriate defensive response by the immune system to a normally harmless substance.

Amino acid – The building blocks of proteins; any of twenty-two nitrogen-containing organic acids essential for synthesizing proteins in your body. Fourteen are non-essential, while eight are essential (obtained through diet).

Anaerobic – With little or no oxygen. Anaerobic exercise utilizes a limited amount of oxygen in the fuel burning process, as in stop-and-go activities like weight lifting and wind sprints. In these activities, glycogen is immediately available to the muscles and the liver for short bursts of exercise.

Anemia – A hemoglobin deficiency in blood that affects its ability to carry oxygen to the bodily tissues.

Antacid – A substance that neutralizes acid in the stomach.

Antibody – A protein molecule that neutralizes a specific invading organism in the body.

Antioxidant – A protective substance that inhibits destructive oxidation reactions at the cellular level. Examples include vitamins C and E, the minerals selenium and germanium, some amino acids, etc.

Ascorbic acid – Vitamin C compound found in citrus fruits and green vegetables that helps heal and fight infections. The symptoms of a deficiency are anemia and being prone to bleed and bruise easily.

Astragalus root – Astragalus membranaceus. An herb that helps fight extreme fatigue and aids the immune system.

Autoimmune disorder – A condition in which the body's immune system rejects and attacks the body's own tissues. Examples include multiple sclerosis, rheumatoid arthritis, systemic lupus erythematosus, etc.

Autolysis – A process whereby the bodily tissue is broken down by the action of enzymes contained in the tissue affected; self-digestion. The body literally feeds on itself, breaking down less important tissue to feed vital tissue. Like a potato in water growing roots, this is the same process that occurs when fasting and during ketosis.

Bacteria – Single-celled microorganisms. Harmful bacteria can cause disease; friendly bacteria aid digestion, protect the body, and engage in other vital functions.

Bee pollen – A natural substance collected by bees from male seed flowers, mixed with secretions from the bee and molded into granules. Bee pollen is high in vital nutrients and amino acids; it can be used to combat allergies.

Bee propolis – A product collected by bees from the resin under the bark of certain trees. It is an antibiotic substance that boosts immunity and fights infection.

Benign – Considered harmless or not cancerous.

Bentonite – A natural clay substance used for elimination of the body's toxins and bacteria.

Beta-carotene – The chemical precursor to vitamin A; an antioxidant.

Bile – A compound made in the liver, stored in the gall bladder, and secreted in the small intestine when needed. It readies fats and oils for digestion. Bile is alkaline; it acts to counteract acidity in the stomach.

Bioflavonoids – Plant compounds found in citrus fruit and green leafy vegetables. Known collectively as vitamin P, they exhibit antioxidant properties and are sometimes prescribed for allergies and inflammations, as they act to strengthen cellular membranes by maintaining the resistance of capillary walls to permeation and change of pressure. They are essential for the absorption of vitamin C.

Boron – A trace mineral found in legumes and some fruit; it may help prevent bone loss and arthritis. It is beneficial for bone and muscle building.

Bran – *The outside shell of the grain with the highest form of fiber content; it helps digestion, elimination, and other health functions.*

Brewer's yeast – *A rich source of protein, B vitamins, and amino acids and minerals such as chromium. It helps steady blood sugar and metabolism, reduces serum cholesterol, and raises levels of HDL. It also aids healing by producing large amounts of collagen; it improves skin texture and blemishes. Intake of Brewer's yeast should be avoided during yeast infections.*

Bromelain – *A natural enzyme found in pineapple that aids metabolism and energy, relieves muscle pain and swelling, and promotes wound healing. Found in wine and cheese.*

Broom foods – *High-fiber, wholesome foods including bran, grains, fruits, and vegetables.*

Canola oil – *The oil from the rapeseed plant; high in monounsaturated fat.*

Capillaries – *Tiny blood vessels that allow the exchange of nutrients and wastes between the bloodstream and cells.*

Capsium – *A catalyst that synergistically enhances other herbs. Promotes thermogenesis, aiding weight loss and increasing circulation.*

Carbohydrate – *An organic substance or large group of compounds, including sugar, starch, and cellulose. It is found in living tissue and food, almost always of plant origin, and is broken down for the major source of energy in the diet.*

Carcinogen – *A substance that may cause cancer.*

Carob powder – *Natural, sweet, powdered sugar similar to chocolate, but it contains less fat and no caffeine.*

Carotene – *A yellow to orange pigment that is converted into vitamin A in the body.*

Cell – *A small, complex organic unit consisting of a nucleus, cytoplasm, and a cell membrane. All living tissues are composed of cells.*

Cerebral – *Pertaining to the brain.*

Charcoal – *A safe, nontoxic agent that relieves gas and diarrhea and many digestive disturbances.*

Chelated – *Bound to an amino acid for better absorption. When attached to minerals, it enables better assimilation. Remember, if your minerals are not ionic, they are merely crushed rocks. Every extra help improves assimilation.*

Chiropractic – *A system of healing based on the belief that disorders and imbalances generally result from misalignments of the vertebrae.*

Chitosan – *A marine fiber concentrate that adheres to and binds lipids in the stomach, causing fat and weight reduction.*

Chlorella - *A single-cell algae plant rich with protein, fiber, beta-carotene, and other high-quality nutrients. Boosts energy and the immune system.*

Chlorophyll - *The green color of plant tissues; essential to the production of carbohydrates by photosynthesis. Chlorophyll-rich products can be taken raw as diet supplements.*

Cholesterol - *A sterol that naturally occurs in bodily tissues. A necessary constituent of cell membranes for the transport and absorption of fatty acids. Excess cholesterol is a threat to health. Yet insufficient cholesterol is dangerous as well. Healthy, normal cholesterol levels range between 180 to 200 mg/dl.*

Chromium - *An essential trace mineral found in brewer's yeast, organ meats, whole grains, and cheese. In the body, chromium helps stabilize insulin production, thus causing weight reduction. Chromium also helps even out blood sugar and reduce blood fat content and cholesterol.*

Chromium picolinate - *The combination of chromium and picolinic acid, a natural substance secreted by the liver and kidneys. Chromium helps level the body's insulin. Controversial studies show that it may build muscle, promote growth, and help heal.*

Chronic illness - *A disorder that persists for a long duration, such as hay fever or diabetes.*

Citric acid - *An organic acid found in citrus fruit. Helps pH balance.*

Co-enzyme - *A molecule that works with an enzyme to enable it to perform its specific function. Co-enzymes are necessary in the utilization of vitamins and minerals.*

Co-enzyme Q10 - *A vitamin-like antioxidant compound that helps fight heart disease and high blood pressure, improves athletic performance, and boosts immunity.*

Colic - *A malfunction of the digestive system involving abdominal pain, distension, and a painful intestinal spasm.*

Colloids - *A suspension composed of a continuous medium throughout which small particles are dispersed small particles, 1 to 1000 nm in size, as opposed to crystalloids, particles smaller than colloids that are capable of forming a true solution. Colloids can pass through semi-permeable membranes; crystalloids cannot. The body is able to digest and recognize colloids as opposed to crystalloids which, due to their ability to rush throughout the digestive tract, are not absorbed (unless chelated, etc.). Unless in food, certain supplements such as freeform amino acids, minerals, etc., will usually not be absorbed.*

Complex darbohydrate - *A type of carbohydrate comprised of long-stringed molecules; it is converted into blood glucose slowly. Sources of complex carbohydrates also contain fiber. Good sources of complex carbohydrates include whole grains and wheat cereals.*

Creatine - *An amino acid that is a constituent of the muscles of vertebrates. Naturally occurring in meat; when taken as a supplement, it increases muscular cell water retention, allowing increased energy for muscular contraction, thus facilitating muscle gain.*

Cross-linkage - Refers to the phenomenon of amino acid linking. Sun damage causes cross-linkage in our skin. Overcooking of food causes cross-linkage, thereby reducing assimilation and usability of the food.

Cruciferous - A term used to refer to a group of vegetables including broccoli, Brussels sprouts, cabbage, cauliflower, and turnips, which have cross-shape blossoms. These vegetables may help prevent colon cancer.

Dementia - A permanent acquired impairment of intellectual function.

Dermis - The layer of skin that lies underneath the epidermis.

Detoxification - The act of reducing the buildup of poisonous substances.

DHEA - Dehydroepiandrosterone; a steroidal hormone produced in the adrenal glands (a precursor to testosterone). Its synthetic form is a nutritional supplement used to cause an increase in lean muscle mass. Best if taken when you are over forty years of age.

Diabetes - A disease that occurs when the pancreas fails to produce adequate insulin. Symptoms are mental confusion, coma, blindness, and poor circulation.

Diet - A food plan that restricts calorie consumption, often to 1,000 calories or below, and does not incorporate balanced nutrition principles.

Dimethylglycine - (B15) a tissue oxygenator; used by athletes for top endurance.

DNA - Deoxyribonucleic acid. A substance in the cell nucleus that contains the cell's genetic blueprint and determines the type of life form into which a cell will develop.

Dopamine- A kind of neurotransmitter formed in the brain that is essential for normal function of the nervous system. Lack of this causes Parkinson's disease.

Dulse - A sea vegetable used as a salt substitute or as a diet tea.

Edema - Water retention. A condition that causes the body to bloat from spilled cellular fluids. A common response of the lymphatic system, it is the body's way of searching for protein. It normally occurs during dieting or fasting. Since protein cannot be stored in the body, during fasting, the lymphatic system searches for available protein, robbing bodily tissues. Sometimes, even when not dieting, one can still bloat. It is due to the fact that the body is then searching for extra protein to build antibodies to combat infection. Eating protein produces a dehydrating effect.

EDTA - Ethylenediaminetetraacetic acid. An amino acid that fights free radicals and enhances minerals.

EEG - Electroencephalogram. A graph used to measure brain activity.

EKG - Electrocardiogram. A graph that monitors and measures heart function.

Eicosanoids - A form of fatty acids found primarily in fish oils. These are mini-hormones within our cells that help dictate every action in the body. Good eicosanoids can reduce inflammation, strengthen the immune system, and lower blood fat and cholesterol. Taken in excess, they can reduce the blood-clotting capability. Bad eicosanoids contribute to pain, bleeding, etc. Aspirin is a blocker of bad eicosanoids. Essential fatty acids are the building blocks of eicosanoids. Linoleic acid is the only truly essential fat.

Electrolytes - Vital mineral compounds that maintain the body's fluid balance; they are capable of conducting electrical impulses.

Emulsion - A mix of two liquids that do not mix with each other, such as oil and water. Emulsification is the first step in the digestion of fat.

Endocrine system - The system of glands that secrete hormones. Endocrine glands include the pituitary, thyroid, thymus, and adrenal glands, pancreas, ovaries, and testes.

Endorphins - They are composed of amino acids made by the pituitary gland and act on the nervous system. These types of peptide hormones bind to opiate receptors found mostly in the brain. These feel-good chemicals are released, causing a morphine-type effect (a runner's high). These natural opiates increase pain tolerance and create feelings of well-being.

Enervate - When there is a lack of strength, energy is drawn from nerves.

Enzymes - Protein catalysts that initiate or speed chemical reactions in the body.

Epidermis - The outer layer of skin.

Essential - A necessary nutrient. It is not manufactured by the body and must be supplied in the diet.

Essential fatty acids - Linoleic acid, linolenic acid, and arachidonic acid are major components of all cell membranes. They help energy production and endocrine system function, regulate hormone and metabolic functions, ease PMS and menopause symptoms, and more.

Ester C - A buffered version of vitamin C, from a natural source. This form of vitamin C stays in the body longer since vitamin C is water soluble and Ester C is not.

Estrogen - A female reproductive hormone produced primarily in the ovarian follicles and stored in fat. The more fat you eat, the more estrogen you store. A high-fiber, low-fat diet drops the level of estrogen in the body; a extremely high level is associated with PMS, irregular periods, uterine fibroids, breast and ovarian cancers, and a late (or dangerous) menopause. This hormone is naturally occurring in seeds, vitamin E, wheat germ, dong quai, yams, etc. If you have fibroids, reduce these foods, especially caffeine. Too much vitamin C, citrus, or even carbohydrates can mimic estrogen and destroys your B vitamins, which causes a hormonal imbalance. Tofu and other soybean products contain phytoestrogens (plant estrogen) that help regulate estrogen levels in the body.

Fat- A soft, greasy, solid substance occurring in organic tissue.

Fat-soluble - Capable of dissolving in fat and oils.

Fatty acids - Organic acids from which fat and oils are made.

Fiber - The indigestible portion of plant matter. It is capable of binding to toxins and escorting them out of the body.

Flaxseed oil - High in Omega 3, an excellent source of unsaturated fatty acids.

Fo ti - A flavonoid-rich herb used for energy and circulation.

Free radical - An atom or group of atoms that has at least one unpaired electron. Free radicals can attack cells and cause the body damage.

Fructose - A simple fruit sugar.

Fungus - A class of organisms that includes yeasts, molds, and mushrooms. Some are capable of causing severe disease.

Gamma linoleic acid (GLA) - Naturally occurs in primrose oil, borage oil, or black currant oil. A source of energy that helps regulate hormonal balance and metabolism.

Gamma oryzanol - A substance naturally occurring in rice bran oil that has hormonal and vitamin-like effects on sex organs.

Garcinia cambogia - An Indian fruit used as a curry ingredient. It also contains active ingredients that aid weight reduction.

Garlic - Therapeutic food with antioxidant properties that stimulates the liver to identify toxins and fight disease and infection.

Germanium - A trace mineral excellent for the immune system and energy.

Germinate- (Of a seed or spore) begins to grow and put out shoots after a dormancy period.

Ginger - A spicy herb that aids digestion and alleviates headaches and other conditions.

Ginkgo biloba - A leaf or leaf extract that fights the aging process, improves circulation, increases memory, and has antioxidant properties.

Ginseng - A tonic herb that provides energy, helps stress and fatigue, builds endurance, stimulates brain activity, aids memory, and enhances male reproductive and circulatory systems.

Gland - An organ or tissue that secretes a substance for use elsewhere in the body rather than for its own functioning.

Globulin - Protein found in the blood that contains disease-fighting antibodies.

Gluconeogenesis - Glucose formation in the body from a non-carbohydrate source, like from protein or fats. During fasting, this process starts when the body is finished with ketosis.

Gluconeogenesis usually starts after twenty-one days of fasting. Unlike in ketosis, during gluconeogenesis the body does not directly use fat for energy; it first converts fat or protein into glucose, thus destroying important organic tissue.

Glucose - A simple sugar present in blood as blood sugar. It is the main source of energy for the body's cells.

Gluten - Protein found in many grains.

Glycemic index - The relative potency of carbohydrates and their propensity to raise and stabilize blood sugar. Low glycemic means small rises in blood sugar and insulin release. High glycemic means rising quickly in excess, creating a blood sugar and insulin imbalance.There are advantages to consuming lower glycemic foods like lentils rather than high-glycemic foods like potatoes.

Glycerin - A naturally occurring carbohydrate-like substance found in coconuts. Used in natural cosmetics as a smoothing agent.

Glycogen - A tasteless polysaccharide that serves as the principal carbohydrate used by the body for energy. It is stored in the liver and muscles.

Gotu kola - A caffeine-free stimulant herb. Helps restore energy and aid healing.

Green tea - A tea that has powerful antioxidant and anti-allergenic properties. Used mostly for energy and clear thinking. Rich in flavonoids.

Guarana - A rainforest shrub from South America. Contains natural caffeine and guaranine, which provides long-lasting energy without the highs and lows..

Hemoglobin - A red protein containing iron responsible for transporting oxygen in the blood or vertebrates.

HIV - Human immunodeficiency virus; the virus that causes AIDS.

Homeopathy -A medical methodology based on the belief that a disease can be treated with natural substances in minute amounts that in large quantities would produce symptoms of the disease.

Honey - A sweet viscous fluid produced by bees from the flower nectar and stored in nests or hives. Used as a natural raw sweetener; twice as sweet as sugar. May have antibiotic and antiseptic properties; contains vitamins and minerals.

Hoodia gordonii- A cacti plant native to South Africa that contains a natural appetite suppressant and libido enhancer.

Hormones - Essential substances produced by the endocrine glands that regulate many bodily functions.

Human growth hormone - Somatotropin, a polypeptide hormone secreted by the pituitary gland, that promotes growth before puberty and after puberty and keeps the body in the muscle-

building/fat-burning process. Growth hormone can also increase your bone mass. Inhibitors are insulin and the aging process. Growth hormone release is enhanced by sleep, protein intake, fasting, and anaerobic exercise.

Hydrochloric acid - An inorganic acid produced in the stomach to aid in digestion.

Hydrogenation - The amount of hydrogen atoms involved in chemical processes of fatty acid molecules.

Hypoallergenic - Having low capacity for inducing allergic reactions.

Hypoglycemia - Low blood sugar. Symptoms include fatigue and weakness, headache and irritability, and panic attacks and anger.

Hypotension - Low blood pressure.

Hypothalamus - A portion of the brain that helps regulate metabolic activities, including body temperature and the hunger response.

Immune system - A combination of functions and processes constituted by the interaction of many different organs, cells, hormones, and proteins. Its chief function is to identify and eliminate foreign substances, such as harmful bacteria.

Immunity - The ability to resist disease or infection.

Infection - An invasion of bodily tissues by disease-causing organisms such as viruses, fungi, or bacteria.

Insomnia - The inability to sleep.

Insulin - A hormone secreted by the pancreas that regulates the metabolism or glucose (sugar) in the body. Insulin allows cells to absorb and utilize glucose. It stimulates glucose uptake by the liver and muscles and converts excess glucose into fat storage. Exercise helps lower the amount of insulin needed to function optimally. An over-release of insulin is usually the basis of any weight problem and disease. Therefore, a properly balanced ration of protein/fat/carbs can help insure continuous insulin balance, without causing an over-release.

Intestinal flora - "Friendly" bacteria in the intestines; essential for digestion.

IU - International unit reserved for some vitamins and minerals. A measure of potency based on an accepted international standard.

Kava - A Polynesian shrub, Piper methysticum, of the pepper family. When taken as an herbal supplement, it acts as a relaxant and mood enhancer.

Ketosis - The act of burning fat without burning glucose, which changes the acid/alkaline pH balance of your blood and can ultimately lead to coma and death. It usually occurs in diabetics who lack insulin to metabolize carbs but can also affect strict dieters who consume insufficient and dangerously low levels of carbohydrates. Telltale signs include foul-smelling breath and urine.

Kola nut - A seed from a tropical tree. A natural and rich source of caffeine and theobromine. Has stimulant effects without the highs and lows of coffee, which contains hydrocarbons.

Kosher- Authentically proper and ritually pure.

L-Carnitine - An amino acid that aids fat metabolism.

L-Tryptophan - An amino acid that stimulates serotonin and may ease depression and insomnia.

Lactase - An enzyme that converts lactose into glucose; necessary for the digestion of milk and milk products.

Lactic acid - Acid that results from anaerobic glucose metabolism. This organic acid is found in certain foods, including certain fruits and sour milk. It is also produced in the muscles during strenuous exercise. The buildup of lactic acid in the body causes muscle fatigue. This form of lactic acid (blood and muscles) is a product of the transformation of the carbohydrate (glucose) and glycogen.

Lactose intolerance - Inability to break down and digest milk. Lactose is a substance found in milk and milk products. Inadequate production of lactase (see our enzyme section) in the small intestine results in the body's inability to digest lactose. Lactose intolerance is rare (but dangerous) in children but common in adults. With age, the body's ability to digest lactose (milk sugar) lessens. Drinking milk after infancy results in an improved lactose tolerance.

Lecithin - Fatty acid found in egg yolks and soybean products that protects against heart disease, lowers cholesterol, and boosts memory. Sometimes considered one of the B vitamins.

Lipid - A chemical family name for fats and related compounds including choline, gamma-linolenic acid, inositol, lecithin, and linoleic acid.

Lipoprotein - A protein molecule that incorporates a lipid. Lipoproteins act as agents of lipid transport in the lymph system and blood.

Lymphatic system (and lymph nodes) - A system of vessels and nodes transporting lymph, a clear fluid that can coagulate, resembling blood plasma. It contains white blood cells. The lymphatic system moves nutrients (oxygen, etc) to cells and transports cell waste and cell poisons away from tissues. This process doubles as the body's vital sewer system. Nodes are organs located in the lymphatic vessels that act as filters, removing toxic and foreign material.

Macrobiotics - A diet based on eastern philosophy focused on balancing the yin and yang energies of foods. The macrobiotic diet incorporates whole grain cereals, millet, rice, and vegetables with beans.

Malabsorption - The body's inability to absorb nutrients from the intestinal tract.

Melatonin - A hormone secreted by the pineal gland whose secretion is affected by the amount of light received by the retina. Taken as a supplement, it naturally enhances sleep and eases falling asleep.

Metabolism - Physical and chemical processes necessary to sustain life, including the production of cellular energy and synthesis of biological substances.

Microgram - A measurement of weight equivalent to 1/1,000,000 of a gram.

Milligram - A measurement of weight equivalent to 1/1,000 of a gram.

Minerals - Naturally occurring inorganic substances present in plants and animals. Essential for human life.

Miso - A fermented soybean paste. A therapeutic food that fights free radicals, helps the immune system, and lowers cholesterol. Miso is a base for soups, sauces, dressings, dips, spreads, and cooking stock and is a healthy substitute for salt.

Mitochondrion - A cellular power source, controlling cell metabolism and generating energy from energy sources such as fat.

Molasses - An unsulphured byproduct of sugar refinement with high mineral content. Good for hair growth and natural hair color.

Neurotransmitters - Brain chemicals or chemical substances (such as dopamine) that transmit nerve impulses.

Norepinephrine- A hormone and a neurotransmitter secreted by the adrenals. It affects blood pressure.

Nucleic acids - A class of chemical compounds found in all viruses and plant and animal cells. Examples are RNA and DNA.

Nutrient - A substance that is needed by the body to maintain life and health. There are four basic nutrients: protein, carbohydrates, fat, and water.

Oats and oat brain - Beneficial grain and fiber sources that lower cholesterol and aid digestion and excretion. Oats are excellent as a long-term metabolic stimulant that, in their purest form, have been known to help combat addictions.

Octacosanol - Wheat germ derivative excellent for energy.

Oils (natural, vegetable) - Natural oils that contain vitamins and essential fatty acids.

Omega 3 oils - Essential fatty acids that prevent blood clotting, high cholesterol, and high triglyceride levels. They improve stamina and hasten metabolism.

Organic - Foods that are grown without synthetic chemicals such as pesticides and hormones.

Oxalic acid - A white, water-soluble, poisonous acid found in such foods as spinach, sodas, coffee, cocoa, chocolate, etc. It robs the body of nutrients, especially calcium.

pH - Potential of hydrogen. A scale used to measure the acidity or alkalinity of substances. A pH of 7 is considered neutral; numbers below 7 show increasing acidity; numbers above 7 show increasing alkalinity. Too much alkalinity is from too much carbon dioxide (hyperventilating). The alkaline-acid ratio in the blood is normally 7.4 pH. Since the body cannot tolerate excess acids from the diet, it robs alkali in the body to neutralize excess acidity. Bodily pH is maintained in the kidneys (by the process of throwing off hydrogen ions from acids in the urine). The lungs excrete carbon dioxide (carbonate acid). The skin excretes hydrogen ions through sweating.

Pectin - A colloidal carbohydrate of high molecular weight; occurs in ripe fruit, especially in apples. Pectin helps with constipation.

Peptide- Molecule chain of two or more amino acids.

Pituitary - A gland located at the base of the brain that secretes hormones, regulating growth and metabolism.

Prostaglandin - A class of hormone-like chemicals that are made in the body from essential fatty acids and have important effects on organs. They influence the secretion of hormones and enzymes and regulate inflammatory response, blood pressure, and blood clotting.

Protein - A class of complex, nitrogen-based, organic compounds constituted of different amino acids. Protein is the basic element of all animal and vegetable tissue, and lack of sufficient protein can cause edema, muscle atrophy, and even worse conditions. Excess protein has a dehydrating effect on the body, and it leeches nutrients.

Psyllium husks - Fibrous seed husks from plants; they promote intestinal function and elimination, decrease appetite, and blood sugar suppress swings.

Pycnogenol - A strong bioflavonoid extract containing powerful antioxidant and memory enhancing capabilities.

Pyruvate - A naturally occurring substance that is important for energy metabolism. It is a byproduct of carb and fat metabolism.

RDA - Recommended daily allowance. The amount of a vitamin or other nutrient that should be consumed daily in order to prevent nutritional deficiency of that vitamin/nutrient and promote health. The U.S. Food and Drug Administration determines RDA.

Red blood cell - A blood cell that contains hemoglobin and transports oxygen and carbon dioxide in the bloodstream.

Retinoic acid - Vitamin A acid. A form of retinoic acid is the active ingredient in the medication Retin-A.

Rice syrup - Sweetener that is made of a complex carbohydrate; increases energy.

RNA - Ribonucleic acid. A complex protein found in plant and animal cells that carries coded genetic information from DNA in the cell nucleus to protein-producing cell structures called ribosomes, where these instructions are translated into the form of protein molecules, the basic components of all living tissue.

Royal jelly – A secretion from queen bee's nurse workers that is rich in vitamins, minerals, enzymes, and amino acids; it may be a natural antibiotic.

Salad – A Latin word for salt. Vegetables are excellent natural sources of sodium. Sodium supplementation is not generally needed (Do not eat table salt). The body distinguishes sodium from other salts. Potassium is an excellent salt substitute, as it reacts with hydrochloric acid in the stomach to produce sodium.

SAM-e – (S-adenosylmethionine) a naturally occurring compound in all living things which becomes depleted as we get older or sick. It has many functions but mainly helps joints in the body. It is also a mood stabilizer. It cannot be found in your diet.

Saturated fat – Fat that is solid at room temperature. Saturated fat is of animal origin although some forms of it, like coconut oil and palm oil, come from plants.

Sea vegetables – Dulse, hijiki, kelp, and others. Rich sources of protein, minerals, and vitamins.

Serotonin – Both a neurotransmitter and hormone. An organic compound formed from tryptophan that is in animal and human tissue, especially the brain and blood serum. It is responsible for the transmission of impulses between nerve cells. Serotonin is in the intestines and the brain. It is essential for relaxation, sleep, concentration, complacency, and satiety.

Simple carbohydrate – A type of carbohydrate that is rapidly digested and absorbed into the bloodstream. Glucose, lactose, and fructose are examples of simple carbohydrates.

SOD (superoxid dismutase) – An antioxidant enzyme that helps neutralize free radicals.

Sorbic acid – An organic acid used as a food preservative.

Spirulina – High-protein algae rich in B vitamins and beta-carotene. Its high chlorophyll content helps digestion.

Sprouts – Sprouted seeds of alfalfa, red clover, mung bean, radish, sunflower, etc. It is a highly nutritious food and a good source of protein; chlorophyll; vitamins A, C, B, and E; minerals; and trace minerals.

Sublingual – Placed under the tongue.

Suma – An herb used for energy since ancient times. Promotes hormonal balance.

Thermogenesis – The body's ability to produce heat by burning calories. Stimulants such as caffeine increase thermogenesis. Normal body temperature is about 98.4 degrees, or anywhere from 96 degrees to 99 degrees Fahrenheit. Starving reduces body temperature. A temperature below 94 degrees or above 110 degrees may cause death.

Tofu – A cholesterol-free soybean food that contains complete protein (all essential amino acids).

Toxicity – The quality of being poisonous.

Toxin - A poison that impairs the health of the body.

Triglyceride - A compound consisting of three fatty acids plus glycerol. Triglycerides are the form in which fat is stored in the body; the primary type of lipid in the diet.

Triticale - A grain hybrid formed by crossing wheat and rye.

Unsaturated fat - Dietary fat that is liquid at room temperature. Unsaturated fat comes from vegetable sources and is a good source of essential fatty acids. Examples are flaxseed oil, sunflower oil, safflower oil, and primrose oil.

Valerian Root - A powerful sedative herb used to treat stress, gas, and cramps and to provide general pain relief.

Vegan- A diet with only plant products. Some vegans don't use animals products for anything.

Vinegar - A diluted and impure form of acetic acid . Varieties are brown rice, balsamic, apple, cider, herb and other sources. Food preserver that also helps digestion.

Virus - A minute disease-causing organism composed of a protein coat and a core of DNA and/or RNA. Because viruses are incapable of reproducing on their own, they must reproduce inside the cells of an infected host. Unlike bacteria, antibiotics do not affect viruses.

Vitamins - One type of approximately fifteen types of organic substances that are essential in small quantities for life and health. Need to be supplied in the diet.

Water- One of the four basic nutrients (protein, carbohydrates, fat, and water). Our bodies are made up of approximately 70 percent water. The body can live without food for approximately five weeks; the body cannot survive without water for more than 5 days.

Water-soluble - Capable of dissolving in water.

Wheat germ and wheat germ oil - An embryo of the wheat berry rich in B vitamins, protein, vitamin E, and iron.

Wheatgrass - A storehouse of vitamins, minerals, amino acids, and enzymes used in diet supplementation. This powerful super-food cleanses and balances the body.

White blood cells - Blood cells that fight infection and repair wounds.

Yeast - A type of a single-celled fungus. Certain types of yeast cause infection.

Yerba mate - An herb used for energy and cleansing.

Yohimbe - An herb that purportedly aids in bodybuilding; some claim it has testosterone-stimulating capabilities.

ABOUT THE AUTHORS

Shane and Sia, known as the Barbi Twins, shot to fame with their own comic book, record-breaking *Playboy* covers, merchandise, and top-selling calendars, worldwide. The Barbi Twins became international celebrity models and household names with their highly-rated *E! True Hollywood Story, 48 Hours,* and other cover stories.

These 5'9" blonde twins started modeling at the age of seven. These native Californians initially wanted to be veterinarians. Struggling with the life-and-death epidemic of eating disorders, the Barbi Twins instead used this top-rated subject to help other women. Armed with degrees in nutrition, biochemistry, and kinesiology, the Barbi Twins are currently sought out as eating-disorder spokeswomen for universities nationwide. As health authors, their initial book, *Dying to Be Healthy,* received great reviews and major coverage in the media.

The Barbi Twins have a new health show that will coincide with their new product line. This will include their own health magazine, vitamins, and other health-related products, which will be distributed in retail stores nationwide.

All proceeds will be donated to **ANIMAL CHARITIES** to make a better and healthier world for animals.

www.ingramcontent.com/pod-product-compliance
Lightning Source LLC
Chambersburg PA
CBHW061338280526
45784CB00001B/57